Procter & Gamble Pharmacist's Handbook

Second Edition

Procter & Gamble
Pharmacist's Handbook

Second Edition

Edited by
Dennis B. Worthen, Ph.D.

Contributing Authors
Walter Stanaszek, Ph.D., R.Ph.
Mary Stanaszek, R.R.A.
Robert Holt, M.A., R.Ph.
Bruce Carlstedt, Ph.D., R.Ph.
Steven Strauss, Ph.D., R.Ph.

CRC PRESS

Boca Raton   London   New York   Washington, D.C.

Library of Congress Cataloging-in-Publication Data

Main entry under title:
Procter & Gamble Pharmacist's Handbook, Second Edition

Full Catalog record is available from the Library of Congress.

© 2001 by CRC Press LLC
Originally Published by Technomic Publishing
First CRC Reprint 2002

No claim to original U.S. Government works
International Standard Book Number 1-58716-123-0
Library of Congress Card Number 2001092386
Printed in the United States of America 1 2 3 4 5 6 7 8 9 0
Printed on acid-free paper

Contents

SECTION FIVE

SECTION SIX

SECTION SEVEN

Letter to Students

Procter&Gamble

Dear Pharmacy Student:

Procter & Gamble is pleased to provide you with a personal copy of *The Pharmacist's Handbook.* We believe you will find this a useful reference in college and throughout your professional career.

Pharmacy is an essential part of the health care delivery system and pharmacists are critical in helping their patients achieve optimal outcomes from their medication therapy. Patients view the pharmacist as a highly credible and trusted source of health care advice. Communication with patients or caregivers and with other health care professionals is fundamental to the pharmacist's role as a drug therapy expert. Several sections within this text covering abbreviations, definitions, terminology, etc. should be useful in your college coursework and in future communication needs critical to your practice.

As a future pharmacist, you must also ensure your personal professional development. You may have already identified individuals as professional mentors and professional societies that can contribute to your professional growth. As a practicing pharmacist, you will also begin a journey of life-long learning and development to maintain your expertise in drug therapy and stay abreast of issues impacting the profession. Sections on professional associations and the Pharmacist Code of Ethics have been included in this text to support your professional development and growth.

Please accept our best wishes from Procter & Gamble for every success during pharmacy school and in your future as a pharmacist.

Sincerely,

Janelle Sobotka

Janelle Sobotka, Pharm.D.
Pharmacy Relations Manager

Dedicated to Pharmacy Students and Practicing Pharmacists and their work to ensure positive medication outcomes in the patients they serve.

Preface

An important skill in the pharmacist's professional life is the ability to communicate accurately and comprehensibly. This skill is especially critical when one considers the audiences that the pharmacist communicates with.

The pharmacist is in a unique position, and has a real responsibility, to understand the language of both the professional and lay audiences. It is through this understanding that the pharmacist can help patients to realize the best possible benefits from their therapies.

The *Pharmacist's Handbook*, Second Edition, is designed as a tool to help the pharmacist in the role of a communication facilitator. The different sections are designed to help foster communication and understanding with both the professional and lay audiences. For example, the Inverted Medical Dictionary Section provides a beginning point to convert lay terminology into more technical vocabulary. This is the point where one may use a regular medical dictionary for a full definition if that is needed. Other sections provide technical terminology, such as eponyms and abbreviations that will provide a reference for your own understanding and conversion to language that your patients will be able to understand. Also, there is information included in sections to help you and provide a one stop reference for items such as normal laboratory values, conversion factors, and weights and measures. This edition also includes information on herbal nomenclature as well as a glossary of managed care terms that will be helpful in understanding the language of the payer and insurance community.

Each of these sections provides a reference to information that is important for the pharmacist to understand and use as part of providing pharmaceutical care.

We hope that you will find the *Handbook* a useful tool. We wish you every success in providing the best possible pharmaceutical care for your patients.

DENNIS B. WORTHEN, PHD
Executive Director
The Lloyd Library and Museum
Cincinnati, OH

UNDERSTANDING MEDICAL TERMINOLOGY

The study of medical terminology is integral to any study of the health care system. Like any other field, health care has its own special language, and an understanding of that language is necessary for an understanding of the discipline.

Since medical terms do not vary in meaning from one generation to another or from one community to another, they are extremely precise in their definitions and allow those in the health care community to converse with each other with exactitude. This exactitude, however, is lost to those who do not understand the language. Therefore, it is important for the pharmacist to be well versed in medical terminology, especially in the role of the provider of pharmaceutical care.

In the community practice setting, pharmacists frequently provide the initial access to the health care system. They are often asked by patients to make sense of the technical language and help them achieve the full benefit from their therapeutic regimen. In the hospital and clinic, pharmacists often counsel patients either during the hospital stay or as part of the discharge planning. Here also, the ability to influence the patient to receive the full potential of the medical therapy is dependent on the pharmacist's ability to understand and communicate with both health care professionals and patients.

Fundamentals of Medical Terms

INTRODUCTION

Like every other specialized discipline, the practice of medicine has evolved its own language over the years, using terminology not found in the general vocabulary. An understanding of medical terminology requires two basic elements: (1) some knowledge of the body structure and functions and (2) familiarity with meanings of the prefixes, suffixes, and roots comprising medical terms.

Most medical terms are composed of roots or stems derived from Greek or Latin and used in combination with prefixes and suffixes. These language sources are used interchangeably, such as in the term *appendicitis* containing the Latin *appendix* and the Greek suffix *-itis*. Terms derived from Greek and Latin have the advantage of being precise and unchanging. They have the same meaning in all countries; therefore, medical terminology is a universal language.

The fundamental method for building a medical vocabulary consists of analyzing a word by identifying its root, suffix, and prefix. Most medical terms are derivative; that is, they consist of a combination of two or more roots or word elements rather than a single Greek or Latin word. The identification of a term through structural analysis involves determining the meaning of each of its components that will either reveal the exact definition of the word or convey its applied meaning.

> Example: *myopathy* = *myo* (root meaning "muscle")
> + *pathy* (suffix meaning "disease")

Some words are comprised of more than one root, each of which retains its basic meaning. Such words, referred to as compounds, are very commonly found in medical terminology.

> Example: *osteoarthritis* = inflammation of the bone joints
> *osteo*, = meaning bone (root)
> *arthro*, = meaning joint (root)
> *itis*, = meaning inflammation (suffix)

For some medical terms, both the Greek and Latin spellings have been adopted as acceptable forms, so the spelling of a root can vary from one term to another. It is imperative, therefore, that a medical dictionary be consulted to determine the correct spelling of unfamiliar words. Because an incorrect spelling can convey an inaccurate impression, diagnosis, condition, or procedure, phonetic spelling has no place in the medical field.

As spelling of a root can vary, so too can pronunciation. Pronunciation of medical terms can be difficult initially, since no rigid rules can be followed. In addition, some words may be acceptably pronounced in more than one way. Common usage prevails; discrepancies in pronouncing medical terms will be found even in the same location.

> Example: *ab do″ men*   or   *ab″ do men*
> *lab″ o ra tory*   or   *la bor″ a tory*
> *du″ o de′ num*   or   *du od′ e num*
> *bar bit″ u rate*   or   *bar″ bi tu′ rate*

Those pronunciations of which the reader is unsure should be determined from a medical dictionary. Repeated spoken use of the terms is the most helpful tool in acquiring mastery of expression.

The point of studying suffixes, roots, and prefixes is to refine the ability to analyze unknown words and derive an accurate meaning. How to go about that may initially seem backwards, but the definition of a term or its applied meaning can usually best be determined by beginning the analysis with the suffix and proceeding to the root and then the prefix. The reason is that the suffix often gives the general context, part of speech, or activity involved; the root then may determine the part of the body, the basic action, or other specific application or meaning. The prefix usually provides restriction or modification of the understanding derived from the suffixes and roots.

SUFFIXES

True suffixes consist of one or more syllables added to root words to modify the meaning and/or to indicate the part of speech—that the completed word is either a preposition or an adverb. Many endings, however, are nouns or adjectives added to a root to form a compound word. Such nouns and adjectives are not true suffixes; they are combinations of true suffixes and roots and may be referred to as combining forms or pseudosuffixes.

> Example: *-gloss*   (tongue)   Root
> *-al*   (related to)   True suffix
> *-glossal*   (related to the tongue)   Pseudosuffix

These compound endings may then be added to other prefixes or roots, as in the word *hypoglossal*. Because words are built of prefixes, roots, and suffixes, reasons arise to include multiple restrictions or modifications on the root, so a single word may contain more than one suffix at a time.

Table 1.1 includes some commonly used word endings, along with their meanings and examples of their use in medical terms. Tables 1.2 and 1.3 list suffix endings denoting physiology, symptoms, and procedures. A study of true suffixes apart from their association with specific use—as,

Table 1.1 Suffixes: Commonly Used Word Endings.

Suffix	Meaning	Example
-able	ability	palat*able*
-ible		flex*ible*
-ile		frag*ile*
-ac	related to,	cardi*ac*
-al	concerning,	abdomin*al*
-an	pertaining to	ovari*an*
-ar		ocul*ar*
-ary		papill*ary*
-ic		pyogen*ic*
-ical		pract*ical*
-ory		sens*ory*
-tic		orthodon*tic*
-ate	action	puls*ate*
-esis		enur*esis*
-ure		meas*ure*
-form	resemblance,	veri*form*
-oid	like	fibr*oid*
-e	agent	lactago*gue*
-er		inhal*er*
-ician		phys*ician*
-ist		urolog*ist*
-or		levat*or*
-eal	of that kind,	poplit*eal*
-eous	pertaining to	calcan*eous*
-ose		adip*ose*
-ous		mucin*ous*
-esis	condition,	par*esis*
-ia	state	dysplas*ia*
-iasis		cholelith*iasis*
-id		flacc*id*
-ism		catabol*ism*
-ity		hyperacid*ity*
-osis		diverticul*osis*

continued

Table 1.1 (continued).

Suffix	Meaning	Example
-tia	condition, state	prociden*tia*
-tion		malabsorp*tion*
-y		gout*y*
-cle	small	corpus*cle*
-cule		mole*cule*
-culun		tuber*culum*
-culus		duct*ulus*
-et		pip*et*
-ium		endocard*ium*
-ole		arterio*le*
-olum		hordeo*lum*
-olus		bo*lus*
-ious	capable of, causing	infect*ious*

Table 1.2 Suffixes: Symptomatic and Miscellaneous.

Suffix	Meaning	Example
-agogue	producer, leader	sila*lagogue*
-agra	attack, seizure	pod*agra*
-algia	pain	neur*algia*
-aphia	touch	ambly*aphia*
-ase	enzyme	lip*ase*
-atresia	abnormal closure	proct*atresia*
-cele	hernia, swelling	hydro*cele*
-chesia	discharge of	uro*chesia*
-chezia	foreign substance	hemato*chezia*
-cide	destroy, kill	germi*cide*
-cleisis	closure	entero*cleisis*
-didymus	cojoined, twin	atlo*didymus*
-dymus		triopo*dymus*
-dynia	pain	pleuro*dynia*
-ectasis	expansion, dilatation	angi*ectasis*
-ema	swelling, distention	emphys*ema*
-emia	blood	septic*emia*
-ferent	bear, carry	ef*ferent*
-ferous	to bear, produce	ossi*ferous*
-fuge	expel, drive away	centri*fuge*
-genic	producing, origination	broncho*genic*
-iasis	presence/formation of	nephrolith*iasis*
-id	secondary lesion	tubercul*id*
-ide	a binary compound	chlor*ide*
-ine	a nitrogenous compound	morph*ine*

Table 1.2 (continued).

Suffix	Meaning	Example
-ite	division	metabol*ite*
-itis	inflammation	arthr*itis*
-lemma	sheath, envelope	neuri*lemma*
-logy	science/study of	cardio*logy*
-lysis	dissolving, reduction	hemo*lysis*
-mentia	mind	de*mentia*
-metry	measure/instrument	opto*metry*
-meter		cranio*meter*
-nomy	law	taxo*nomy*
-ol	alcohol, phenol	ethan*ol*
-oma	tumor	carcin*oma*
-opia	slight defect	ambly*opia*
-opsia	condition of vision	xanth*opsia*
-ose	sugar	gluc*ose*
-osis	abnormal condition	dermat*osis*
-pagus	to fasten together	diplo*pagus*
-pathy	disease	myelo*pathy*
-penia	lack, deficiency	leuko*penia*
-phagia	to eat, swallow	dys*phagia*
-phasia	speech	dys*phasia*
-philia	to love, to crave	hemo*philia*
-phobia	to fear	photo*phobia*
-plasia	development	hyper*plasia*
-plegia	paralysis	hemi*plegia*
-pnea	breathing	dys*pnea*
-poiesis	make, produce	hemo*poiesis*
-ptosis	to fall	blepharo*ptosis*
-rrhagia	excessive discharge	meno*rrhagia*
-rrhea	flow	leuko*rrhea*
-rrhexis	rupture	cardio*rrhexis*
-scope	instrument for viewing	broncho*scope*
-spasm	involuntary contraction	entero*spasm*
-stalsis	constriction	peri*stalsis*
-stasis	at a standstill	hemo*stasis*
-staxis	hemorrhage	epi*staxis*
-taxis	involuntary response to stimuli	rheo*taxis*
-thyma	condition of mind	cyclo*thymic*
-tome	cutting instrument	osteo*tome*
-tonia	stretching, causing tension	hyper*tonia*
-ule	small	tub*ule*
-uria	condition of the urine	glycos*uria*
-vert	turn	di*vert*
-vorous	to eat	herbi*vorous*

Table 1.3 Suffixes: Surgical/Diagnostic Procedures.

Suffix	Meaning	Example
-centesis	puncture, aspiration	thoracentesis
-clasis	fracture	osteoclasis
-desis	fusion	arthrodesis
-ectomy	excision	gastrectomy
-lysis	freeing	enterolysis
-ography	process	roentgenography
-oscopy	look within	cystoscopy
-ostomy	form an opening	colostomy
-otomy	incision into	laparotomy
-pexy	fixation, suspension	hysteropexy
-plasty	repair	blepharoplasty
-rrhaphy	suture	herniorrhaphy
-tripsy	crushing, friction	lithotripsy

for example, those dealing with diagnostic terms—is difficult and necessitates repetition. For this reason, all of the true suffixes are introduced in this chapter and then presented again in specific areas to reinforce their common usage. Their sheer number makes learning these suffixes a daunting task, but careful review and repetition of these suffixes in a large number of terms simplifies the problem. In addition, the tables are useful for reference long after their original study.

ROOTS

The word *root* or *stem* is the fundamental or elementary part of the word that conveys its primary notion or significance. Modification of the basic meaning is then made by the addition of prefixes, suffixes, or other roots. The root should not be confused with a prefix or suffix, regardless of the position of the root within a word. Prefixes come at the beginning and suffixes at the end of a word, but a root can appear anywhere, including before or after another root. The roots (since there may be more than one) give the word its primary meaning; prefixes or suffixes, however, serve to modify that meaning. Those roots used in medical terminology generally indicate an organ or part of the body.

The term *combining forms* is often encountered in the study of medical terminology. A combining form of a root is created by the addition of a vowel, usually *o*, to the word root. This is done primarily for ease in pronunciation. These are, therefore, convenience forms and do not influence the meaning of a word root.

Example:	(Combining Form)	*gastro-*
	(Root)	*gastr-*
	(Medical Terms)	*gastr(o)*dynia
		*gastr*algia
		*gastr*itis

Some roots end in vowels, so frequently there is no need to add a vowel to these roots to create a combining form. Further, the addition of a vowel would place two vowels in succession. Thus, a vowel is usually not added if the word root ends in a vowel and two vowels would be in sequence.

Example:	*celio-*	(Root meaning abdomen)
	-oma	(Suffix meaning tumor)
	celioma	(tumor of the abdomen)

A medical dictionary should be consulted whenever correct spelling is in question.

The list in Table 1.4 contains many commonly used roots or combining forms that do not readily fall into the body system classifications or that apply to more than one. Since the meaning of a word can be determined by knowledge of its basic parts, these examples should illustrate the value of learning root words as a basis for understanding medical terminology.

PREFIXES

Prefixes are the most frequently used elements in the formation of medical terms. Most prefixes are commonly used in everyday language and are not unique to medical terminology, so those wanting to learn or improve their mastery of medical terminology have a sound basis on which to build.

Prefixes may be adjectives, adverbs, or prepositions that are used to indicate various relationships or conditions of the root word. Most prefixes have a final vowel that is deleted if the following root or stem begins with a vowel.

Since prefixes originate from both Latin and Greek, two different prefixes may have the same meaning. For example, the prefixes *poster-* and *retro-* both indicate "behind," as in the terms *posterior* and *retrograde*. Conversely, multiple meanings may be associated with a single prefix because of multiple sources for the prefix; *meta-*, for example, can mean both "over" and "after change."

True prefixes are distinguished from roots in that they serve only to modify the meaning of the root and have no significance alone. Roots that are used at the beginning of words are not considered to be true prefixes.

	Example:	Prefixes	Roots
		*hyper*trophy	*hepato*megaly
		*brady*cardia	*osteo*myelitis

The prefixes listed in Tables 1.5 through 1.8 have been grouped according to the type of relationship or conditions that they identify. The examples serve to illustrate how prefixes are joined to root words.

Table 1.4 Roots: Combining Forms, Miscellaneous.

Root	Meaning	Example
abdomin-	abdomen	*abdomin*al
actino-	ray, radiated structure	*actino*genic
adipo-	fat	*adipo*se
aer-	air, gas	*aero*gram
alge-	pain	*algo*spasm
alveo-	hollow	*alveo*lus
ambulo-	walk about	*ambul*atory
aneurysmo	widening	*aneurysmo*rrhaphy
ankyl-	crooked, attached	*ankyl*osis
astro-	star	*astro*cyte
auto-	self	*auto*clasis
blast-	bud, germ	*blast*ocyte
blenno-	mucus	*blenno*rrhea
bucc-	cheek	*bucc*inator
calori-	heat	*calori*genic
celio-	abdomen	*celio*ma
coeli-		*coeli*oma
cervico-	neck	*cervico*brachial
chir-	hand	*chiro*megaly
chron-	time	*chrono*graph
clas-	smash, break	osteo*clasis*
clin-	bedside	*clin*ical
coleo-	sheath	*coleo*cele
crymo-	cold	*crymo*philic
cryo-		*cryo*extraction
crypt-	hidden	*crypt*ogenic
cycl-	round, recurring	*cyclo*tropia
cyt-	cell	*cyt*ology
desm-	fibrous connection	*desmo*dynia
ergo-	work	*ergo*phobia
eury-	broad	*eury*cephalic
febri-	fever	*febri*le

Table 1.4 (continued).

Root	Meaning	Example
gero-	aged	*gero*ntology
glio-	glue	*glio*ma
glyco-	sugar, sweet	*glyco*suria
gony-	knee	*gony*ocele
gust-	taste	*gust*ation
helio-	sun	*helio*therapy
hidro-	sweat	*hidro*sis
histo-	tissue	*histo*logy
hydro-	water	*hydro*cele
hypno-	sleep	*hypno*tic
iatro-	medicine, physician	*iatro*genic
ictero-	jaundice	*ictero*genic
iso-	equal	*iso*tonic
kinesio-	movement	*kinesio*logy
lapar-	loin, flank	*lapar*otomy
lepto-	slender, thin	*lepto*dermic
lip-	fat	*lip*oma
litho-	stone	*litho*genesis
lyso-	dissolving	*lyso*genic
macro-	large, long	*macro*nychia
mal-	ill, bad, poor	*mal*absorption
megalo-	large	*megalo*cyte
mero-	part	*mero*tomy
micro-	small	*micro*gram
mio-	less, smaller	*mio*sis
morpho-	form	a*morpho*us
muco-	mucus	*muco*purulent
myco-	fungi	*myco*logy
myx-	mucus	*myx*edema
necro-	death	*necro*sis
nocto-	night	*nocto*uria
nycto-		*nycto*philia
noso-	disease	*noso*poietic
not-	the back	*not*algia
oligo-	few, little	*oligo*uria
omo-	shoulder	*omo*dynia
omphalo-	umbilicus	*omphalo*tomy
oneir-	dream	*oneir*ism
oxy-	sharp, keen	*oxy*cephalic
pachy-	thick	*pachy*onchia
paleo-	old	*paleo*genetic
pan-	all	*pan*arthritis
papillo-	pustule	*papill*oma
papulo-		*papulo*squamous
patho-	disease	*patho*logy

continued

Table 1.4 (continued).

Root	Meaning	Example
pedia-	child	*pedia*trics
pedo-	foot	*pedo*graph
pero-	deformed	*pero*brachius
phago-	devour, eat	*phago*cyte
phanero-	appear, visible	*phanero*sis
photo-	light	*photo*phobia
phren-	mind, diaphragm	*phren*ic
phthisio-	wasting, atrophy	*phthisio*logy
phyco-	seaweed	*phyco*bilins
physio-	nature	*physio*logy
phyt-	plant	hemato*phyte*
platy-	flat, broad	*platy*podia
pod-	foot	*pod*iatrist
pros-	forward, anterior	*pros*ademic
prosop-	face	*prosop*oneuralgia
psychr-	cold	*psychr*algia
puri-	pus	*puri*lent
pyo-		*pyo*genic
pyro-	fever, heat	*pyro*genic
radio-	ray	*radio*therapy
schisto-	split, divide	*schisto*celia
scirrh-	hard	*scirrh*osity
scler-		*scler*oderma
sit-	food	*sit*ophobia
somni-	sleep	in*somnia*
sphygmo-	pulse	*sphygmo*manometer
splanchn-	viscera	*splanchn*ic
staphylo-	grapelike cluster	*staphylo*toxin
stear-	fat	*stear*rhea
steat-		*steat*olysis
steno-	narrow, contracted	*steno*sis
stereo-	solid, three dimensional	*stereo*scope
stetho-	chest	*stetho*scope
sthen-	strength	mya*sthen*ia
strepto-	twisted, curved	*strepto*bacillus
thanat-	death	*thanat*ology
theco-	sheath	*theco*dont
thermo-	heat	*thermo*meter
thrombo-	clot	*thrombo*cyte
tome-	cutting instrument	micro*tome*
top-	place, topical	*top*ectomy
topo-		*topo*graphy
trachelo-	neck	*trachelo*dynia
ul-	scar, gingiva	*ul*orrhagia

Table 1.4 (continued).

Suffix	Meaning	Example
vermi-	worm	*vermi*fuge
viscer-	organ	*viscera*
vita-	life	*vita*min
xeno-	strange, foreign	*xeno*phthalmia
zoo-	animal	*zoo*logy

Table 1.5 Prefixes: Location, Direction, Tendency.

Prefix	Meaning	Example
a- an-	without, not	*a*phasia *an*emia
ab- apo- de-	away from	*ab*ductor *apo*physis *de*capitate
ad-	to, toward, near	*ad*nexia
ambi- amphi- ampho-	both	*ambi*dextrous *amphi*bious *ampho*terism
ana-	up, apart, across, back again, excessive	*ana*catharsis *ana*stasis
ante- fore- pre- pro-	before, forward	*ante*partum *fore*head *pre*natal *pro*cidentia
anter-	in front of	*anter*ograde
anti- contra- counter- ob-	against, opposite	*anti*toxin *contra*ceptive *counter*irritant *ob*dormition
cata- kata- circum- peri-	down, according to around, about	*cata*tonic *kata*thermometer *circum*flex *peri*carditis
co- com- con- sym- syn-	together, with	*co*arctation *com*missure *con*ductor *sym*physis *syn*arthrosis
dextro-	to the right	*dextro*version
di- dis-	apart from	*di*astemia *dis*sect

continued

Table 1.5 (continued).

Prefix	Meaning	Example
dia- per- trans-	through, across	*dia*phragm *per*forate *trans*ection
dorsi- dorso-	back	*dorsi*flexion *dorso*lateral
e- ec- ex-	out from	*e*nucleate *ec*toblast *ex*acerbation
ecto- exo- extra- extro-	outside	*ecto*derm *exo*genous *extra*cellular *extro*vert
em- en- im- in-	in	*em*pyema *en*arthrosis *im*paction *in*flammation
endo- ento- intra-	within	*endo*cardium *ento*cele *intra*ocular
epi-	upon, over	*epi*gastric
eso-	inward	*eso*tropia
extra- hyper- per- pleo- super-	more, excessive	*extra*ocular *hyper*trophy *per*tussis *pleo*morphic *super*numerary
gen-	producing, coming to be	*gen*etics
homo-	same	*homo*geneous
hyper-	above, over	*hyper*trophy
hypo- infra- sub-	below, under, beneath, less, deficient	*hypo*tension *infra*orbital *sub*cutaneous
im- in- ir- non- un-	not	*im*miscible *in*articulate *ir*reducible *non*toxic *un*conscious
inter-	between	*inter*costal
intro-	into	*intro*version

Table 1.5 (continued).

Prefix	Meaning	Example
ipsi- iso-	same, equal	*ipsi*lateral *iso*metric
juxta-	near	*juxta*position
latero-	to the side	*latero*flexion
levo- sinistro-	to the left	*levo*version *sinistro*cardia
medi- mes- mid-	in the middle	*medi*al *meso*cephalic *mid*brain
meta-	over, after, change	*meta*stasis
opistho- poster-	behind, backward	*opistho*tic *postero*median
para-	beside, near	*para*centesis
post-	after, behind	*post*partum
primi- prot-	first	*primi*para *proto*derm
re-	again	*re*habilitation
retro-	backward, behind	*retro*grade
super- supra- ultra-	above, excessive	*super*natant *supra*renal *ultra*sonic
tel- tele- telo-	end, distance	*tel*ediastolic *tele*opsia *telo*phase
trans-	across, through	*trans*plant
ventro-	anterior	*ventro*fixation

Table 1.6 Prefixes: Size, Condition, State.

Prefix	Meaning	Example
allo-	not normal	*allo*tropic
ambly-	dim, dull	*ambly*opia
aniso-	unequal, dissimilar	*aniso*cyosis
atel-	imperfect	*atel*ectasis
atreto-	lack of opening	*atreto*cystia
bio-	relation to, life	*bio*logy
brachy-	short	*brachy*cephalic
brevi-		*brevi*collis

continued

Table 1.6 (continued).

Prefix	Meaning	Example
brady-	slow	*brady*cardia
caco-	bad, ill	*caco*genic
cry-	cold	*cry*osurgery
dolicho-	long	*dolicho*sigmoid
dys-	difficult, painful	*dys*pnea
eu-	well, easily, good	*eu*phoria
haplo-	single, simple	*haplo*id
heter-	different, other	*heter*ochylia
holo-	entire	*holo*graphy
homeo-	like, similar	*homeo*stasis
homo-		*homo*geneous
ischio-	suppress, restrain	*isch*uria
leio-	smooth	*leio*myoma
malaco-	soft	*mala*cia
medulo-	marrow	*medullo*blastoma
mis-	bad, wrong, improper	*mis*carriage
mogi-	painful, difficult	*mogi*phonia
myel-	marrow	*myel*oma
neutro-	neither	*neutro*phil
poikilo-	varied	*poikilo*derma
poly-	many, much	*poly*uria
presby-	old	*presby*opia
proto-	first, original	*proto*vertebra
pseudo-	false	*pseudo*pregnancy
sclero-	hard	*sclero*sis
scoli-	cruved, crooked	*scoli*osis
tachy-	fast	*tachy*cardia
torsi-	twist	*torsi*on
trachy-	rough	*trachy*phonia
varico-	twisted, swollen	*veric*ose
xero-	dry	*xero*cheilia

Table 1.7 Prefixes: Number, Measurement.

Prefix	Meaning	Example
mono-	one	*mono*cyte
uni-		*uni*lateral
bi-	two, twice	*bi*furcation
bin-		*bin*aural
di-		*di*cephalus
diplo-		*diplo*coccus
dis-		*dis*mutase

Table 1.7 (continued).

Prefix	Meaning	Example
ter- tri-	three, third	*ter*tiary *tri*ceps
quad- tetra-	four	*quad*ruplet *tetra*plegia
penta- quinqu- quinti-	five	*penta*valent *quinqu*evalent *quinti*para
hex- sex-	six	*hex*asaccharide *sex*tuplet
hept- sept-	seven	*hept*achromic *sept*ipara
octa-	eight	*octa*gonal
nona-	nine	*nona*n
deca-	ten	*deca*meter
micro-	one one-millionth	*micro*gram
milli-	one one-thousandth	*milli*liter
centi-	one one-hundredth	*centi*meter
deci-	one tenth	*deci*gram
hecto-	hundred	*hecto*liter
kilo-	thousand	*kilo*gram
demi- hemi- semi-	half	*demi*lune *hemi*cardia *semi*conscious
ambi- amphi- ampho-	both	*ambi*dextrous *amphi*bious *ampho*teric
multi- poly-	many	*multi*para *poly*chromatic

Table 1.8 Prefixes: Color.

Prefix	Meaning	Example
chroma-	color	*chroma*tography
alb- albumin- leuk-	white	*alb*inuria *albumin*uretic *leuk*emia
amaur-	dark	*amaur*osis

continued

Table 1.8 (continued).

Prefix	Meaning	Example
chlor- verdin-	green	*chlor*anemia *verdo*hemoglobin
ciner- glauc- polio-	gray	*ciner*itious *glauc*oma *polio*myelitis
cirrh- flav- lute- xanth-	yellow	*cirrh*osis *flavo*protein *lute*in *xanth*oma
cyano-	blue	*cyano*mycosis
erythr- rube-	red	*erythr*ocyte *rube*lla
melan- nigro-	black	*melan*oma *nigro*sine
purpur-	purple	*purpur*a

BODY AS A WHOLE

Medical terms describing position or direction relative to the body are expressed in terms of the "anatomical position": the human body standing erect, arms at the sides and the palms of the hands turned forward. This reflects the **anterior** (*anter/o*) or front side, also called the ventral or belly side. The combining form for **posterior** is *poster/o*, meaning "back"; **dorsal** (*dors/o*) also refers to the back side of an organism. The combining form for the side is *later/o*. **Unilateral** (*uni* = one) would denote one side, while **bilateral** (*bi* = two) means two or both sides. **Medial** pertains to the middle. Other combining forms referring to locations on the body include *super-*, meaning superior (e.g., superficial); *dist-*, meaning far or distant (e.g., distal); *proxim-*, meaning near (e.g., proximal); *caudo-*, meaning tail or lower part (e.g., caudal); and *cephal-*, meaning head (e.g., cephalad).

The abdomen is divided into nine anatomic regions. The right and left **hypochondriac** regions are those lying beneath (hypo-) the ribs, although the term also describes a person who is overly concerned with health and may imagine illness (named for the region of the body that was thought to be the seat of the disease). Between the hypochondria is the **epigastric** (*epi* = upon, *gastr* = stomach) region. The right and left **lumbar** regions are separated by the **umbilical** (naval) region. Below are the **hypogastric** and left and right **inguinal** or iliac regions. Areas in the abdominal cavity are also divided by quadrants, designated as right upper quadrant (**RUQ**), left upper quadrant (**LUQ**), right lower quadrant (**RLQ**), and left lower quadrant (**LLQ**).

The body has two principal body cavities designated as the **ventral** (front) and **dorsal** (back). The smaller dorsal cavity contains the cranial and spinal cavities. The ventral cavity contains the thoracic (chest) cavity, separated from the abdominal cavity by the **diaphragm**. Lowest is the pelvic cavity. The serous membrane lining these two (abdominopelvic) cavities is called the **peritoneum**. Organs within the cavities are sometimes referred to as **viscera**.

INVERTED MEDICAL DICTIONARY

Unlike a normal dictionary, an inverted medical dictionary does not provide definitions. Instead, it starts with a common term (or the definition) and then supplies the correct technical term. This tool is especially valuable when one is trying to determine what the correct technical term might be for a non-technical or lay term.

EPONYMS

The eponym is a specialized form of technical terminology. An eponym is a shorthand to describe a specific disease, condition, or syndrome by using the proper name of the person who first described it or the patient. For example, Paget's disease is a shorthand description for osteitis deformans, a generalized skeletal disorder characterized by thickening and softening of bone, and is named after James Paget, a London surgeon who first described the condition. Amyotrophic lateral sclerosis was named Gehrig's (or Lou Gehrig's) disease after the New York Yankee baseball star, who was diagnosed and later died from the disease.

ABBREVIATIONS

Abbreviations are used as shortened forms of disease names, diagnostic procedures, anatomical terms, quantities, routes of administration and practically anything else that appears in clinical use. The sheer number of abbreviations in common use precludes simplicity; instead, they often add to the confusion. It is important to be sure that an unfamiliar abbreviation is verified if there is any doubt about its true meaning.

TERMS USED IN PRESCRIPTION WRITING

Latin and abbreviations still form much of the prescription vocabulary. This list of terms provides the English equivalent for both the prescription term and its common abbreviation.

Inverted Medical Dictionary

A

abdomen, upper part
midriff

abdominal cavity distension
celiectasia

abdominal fluid
ascites

abdominal fissure
hologastroschisis
a narrow opening or crack of considerable length and depth

abdominal gas
tympanism
swelling of the abdominal area due to intestinal gas

abdominal incision
celiotomy
a cut into the abdominal cavity
laparotomy
through the loin or flank

abdominal pain
formen
severe griping or colicky pain

abdominal wall suture
celiorrhaphy
laparorrhaphy

abnormal blood pressure
dysarteriotony

abnormal development
teratogenesis

abnormal formation
cacogenesia
cacogenesis

abnormal sensation
paresthesia
as of burning, prickling, or tingling

abnormal sense of taste
dysgeusia

abnormal size of head
macrocephalia
macrocephaly

abnormal sweating
diaphoresis

abnormal thirst
anadipsia
dipsosis

abnormal tissue development
dysplasia

abortion
embryotocia

absence of anatomical parts
agenesis
organ or part

(development)
agnathia
lower jaw
amastia
mammary glands
amelia
limbs
amyelia
spinal cord
anandria
male characteristics
anephrogenesis
kidney tissue

23

absence of anatomical parts (development) (cont.)
anorchism
    testes
apneumia
    lungs
apodia
    feet
aprosopia
    face
arhinia
    nose
asternia
    sternum
atrichosis
    hair

absence of life
abiosis

absence of menstruation
amenorrhea

absence of pleasure
anhedonia
    from acts that would otherwise be pleasurable

absorbent
desiccant
exsiccant

acetone bodies in blood
acetonemia

Achilles tendon pain
achillodynia

Achilles tendon suture
achillorrhaphy

acid, excessive
acidosis
    in body fluids
supersalt
    in salt

acid measurer
acidimeter

acidity deficiency
hypoacidity

activity deficiency
hypopraxia

"Adam's apple"
prominentia laryngea
    prominent area in front of the neck

adenoids inflammation
adenoiditis

adenoids knife
adenomatome
    surgical instrument for cutting adenoids
adenotome
    surgical instrument for cutting a gland or adenoids

adenoids excision
adenoidectomy

after intercourse
postcoital

after surgery
postoperative

after vaccination
postvaccinal

air bacteria collector
aerobioscope
    device to determine bacterial content in the air

air-breathed measurer
aeroplethysmograph
    instrument to measure the amount of air breathed out (exhaled)

air dust measurer
aeroscope
    instrument used in determining the purity of the air
konometer
    instrument for counting the number of dust particles in the air

air/gas anywhere in body
pneumatosis
    in any abnormal location

air/gas in brain ventricles
pneumocranium
pneumocephalus

air/gas in heart chambers
pneumatocardia

air/gas in intestines
aerenterectasia
meteorism
tympanites
    also in abdomen

air/gas in joints
pneumarthrosis

air/gas in peritoneal cavity
aeroperitoneum
aeroperitonia

air/gas in pleural cavity
pneumothorax

air/gas in skull
epidural aerocele
usually caused by fracture

air/gas in spinal canal
pneumorrhachis

air/gas under the skin
pneumoderma
subcutaneous emphysema

air/gas in urine
pneumaturia

air/gas vaginal distention
aerocolpos

air in heart
aerendocardia

air-inspired measurer
inspirometer
instrument to measure the force, frequency, or volume of inhaled air

air in mediastinal tissues
pneumomediastinum

air in pericardial sac
pneumohydropericardium

air/saliva swallowing
aerosialophagy
sialoaerophagy
entry of of air and saliva into the stomach

air swallowing
aerophagia
aerophagy

air/water treatment
aerohydropathy
aerohydrotherapy

albumin measurer
albuminometer
instrument to measure albumin contents, especially in the urine

albumin in urine
albuminuria
noctalbuminuria
excess albumin in urine passed at night

alcohol in urine
alcoholuria

alertness of mind
eunoia

alimentary canal
enteron

alimentary canal lacking
agastric .

alkalinity in blood
alkalemia

alkalinity in urine
alkalinuria

allergic disease
allergosis
any disease resulting from allergy

allergic reaction
atopy
specifically with strong familial tendencies

allergic skin disorder
allergodermia

altered hematin in urine
urohematin
urofuscohematin
red pigment in urine

altitude sickness
Acousta's disease

ambisexual
hermaphroditism
hermaphrodism
condition of having both ovarian & testicular tissue

amebas in urine
ameburia

amines in urine
aminuria

amino acids in blood
aminoacidemia
presence of the enzyme in excessive amounts

amino acids in urine
acidaminuria
aminoaciduria

ammonia compounds in blood
ammoniemia

ammonia in urine
ammoniuria

amnion inflammation
amnionitis

amnion lacking
anamnionic
anamniotic
without the membrane normally surrounding the fetus

amnion ruptured
amniorrhexis

amnion fluid escaped
amniorrhea

amount desired
ad lib (ad libitum)
as desired

anatomy study
morphology
study of the structure and forms of organisms

anesthesia below waist
para-anesthesia
affecting only the lower half of the body

anesthesia by cold
cryanesthesia
refrigeration anesthesia

anesthesia by electricity
electroanalgesia
electronarcosis
insensitivity to pain by use of electrical current

anesthetic measurer
anesthesimeter

aneurysm repair
aneurysmoplasty
arterioplasty

aneurysm suture
aneurysmorrhaphy

aneurysm of vein/artery
phlebangioma
phlebarteriectasia

angel dust
phencyclidine (PCP)
"street drug" subject to abuse

angle measurer
goniometer

animal anatomy
zootomy

animal breeding
zoogony

animals, collectively
fauna

antibody producer
antigen
anything that produces antibodies

antimony poisoning
stibialism

antrum (sinus) operation
antrostomy
antrotomy
opening of the antrum for drainage purposes
antrectomy
excision of the antrum

anus aperture lacking
aproctia

anus artificial
colostomy
creation of an artificial anus in the abdominal wall by surgical means

anus inflammation
periproctitis
perirectitis
inflammation of the connecting tissues around the rectum or anus
proctitis
rectitis
inflammation of the rectum or anus
sphincteritis
inflammation of the anal sphincter muscle

anus pain
proctagra
proctalgia
proctodynia
proctalgia fugax
sphincteralgia

anus proximity
perianal
surrounding the anus

anus specialist
proctologist
physician who specializes in treating anal conditions

anus stricture
proctostenosis

anus viewer
anoscope
instrument to examine anus and rectum

aorta inflammation
aortitis
mesaortitis
inflammation of the middle layer of the aorta
periaortitis
inflammation of the tissues surrounding the aorta

aorta membrane
endaortitis

apathy
ameleia
indifference

apex inflammation
apicitis
of a tooth root or a lung

aponeurosis inflammation
aponeurositis

aponeurotic operation
aponeurotomy

aponeurotic suture
aponeurorrhaphy

appendages
adnexa
anatomical parts that are cojoined

appendages of the eye
adnexa oculi
the lacrimal glands

appendages of the uterus
adnexa uteri
oviducts and ovaries

appendix inflammation
appendicitis

appendix operation
appendectomy

appetite in excess
bulimia

appetite lacking
anorexia

appetite unnatural
allotriophagy
pica
appetite for unusual or harmful substances
chthonophagia
chthonophagy
geophagy
desire to eat earth, clay, chalk, etc

application
epithem
anything placed on a wound or sore spot

arachnoid membrane inflamed
arachnitis

arm amputation
brachiotomy

arm lacking
monobrachius
congenital deformity

arm largeness
macrobrachia

arm pain
brachialgia

arm smallness
microbrachia

armless/headless
acephalobrachia
born without head and arms

armpit
axilla

aromatic urine
uraroma

arrow poison
curare
ukambin

arsenic treatment
arsenotherapy
use of arsenic agents to treat disease

arson compulsion
pyromania

arterial pressure low
hypopiesia

artery calcification
arteriostosis

artery calculus
arteriolith

artery constriction
arteriarctia
arteriostenosis

artery crusher
angiotribe
instrument for crushing an artery embedded in the tissue

artery degeneration
arteriasis
arteronecrosis

artery dilatation
arteriectasis
arteriomotor

artery disease
arteripathy

artery hardening
arteriosclerosis

artery inflammation
arteritis
exarteritis
of the outer layer
mesarteritis
of the middle layer
panarteritis
of all the arteries
periangitis
of outside tissues around an artery
periarteritis
of the outer layer and tissues surrounding an artery
polyangitis
perivasculitis
involving multiple blood vessels
stetharteritis
of the arteries of the thorax

artery narrowing
arteriostenosis
constriction or compression inhibiting the flow of blood

artery operation
arteriectomy
arteriotomy
arterioplasty

artery pressure measurer
hemadynamometer
instrument to measure the blood pressure within the arteries

artery rupture
arteriorrhexis

artery small
arteriole

artery spasm
arteriospasm

artery suture
arteriorrhaphy

artery twisting
arteriostrepsis
to stop a hemorrhage

artery/vein communicating
anastomosis

artery x-ray
arteriography

articulation difficulty
dyslalia

articulation inflamed
osteoarthritis
degenerative disease of a joint

artificial anus
enteroproctia

artificial intelligence
computer reasoning

artificial substitution
prosthesis
artificial parts to the body
prosthetist
specialist in artificial substitution
prosthodontics
branch of dentistry devoted to the restoration of teeth

asbestos inhaled
asbestosis

asexual reproduction
agamogenesis
agamogenetic
agamogony

astigmatism measurer
astigmatometer
astigmometer
instrument to measure the extent of blurred and imperfect image due to imperfect refraction

athlete's foot
dermatophytosis
tinea pedis

atmospheric humidity measurer
hygrometer
instrument to measure moisture in the air

atmospheric study
meteorology

atomizer
nebulizer

atrophy diffuse
panatrophy
   of several parts

atrophy of skin
atrophoderma
   decrease in size or wasting away
atrophodermatosis
   of the cutis

attachment
bonding
   to object or person

attic operation
atticotomy
   opening of the tympanic attic

attraction
tropism
   involuntary attraction of an animal or
   vegetable organism toward a more desirable spot

attraction to corpses
necromania
   also desire for death

attraction/rejection of sun
heliotaxis
heliotropism
   phenomenon where plants or plant organs have a tendency to lean toward
   or away from the sun

autopsy
necropsy

aversion to food
anorexia nervosa
apocleisis
apositia

aviator's disease
aeroneurosis
   a nervous disorder

axes equal
homoaxial
homaxonial

B

bacilli in blood
bacillemia

presence of a type of rod-shaped bacteria in the blood

bacilli in urine
bacilluria

back
dorsalis
   posterior

backing-up
regurgitation

backward bent
retroflexion

backward displacement
retroposition

bacteria in blood
bacteremia
endotoxemia

bacteria collector
aerobioscope

bacteria largeness
macrobacterium
megabacterium
   bacteria of unusually large size

bacteria study
bacteriology

bacteria in urine
bacteriuria

bad breath
halitosis
ozostomia
stomatodysodia
*bromopnea**
   *obsolete term

bad taste sensation
cacogeusia

bag of waters
amniotic sac

baldness (see hair loss)

ball-and-socket
enarthrosis
   such as knee joint

barber's itch
mentagra
sycosis

base of skull
basicranial

beaded hair
moniliform hair
congenital disease of scalp

beast transformation
lycanthropy
individual believes to be a wild beast

bedclothes plucking
carphology
floccillation

bedsore
decubitus ulcer

bedwetting
enuresis

before birth
antenatal
antepartum
prenatal
the period of time preceeding birth

before death
ante mortem

behind the ear
postaurical

behind the eye
postocular

belching
eructation

belief of smaller body
micromania

belief of one's divinity
theomania

belief that one is a dog
cryanthropy

bend
geniculum
the bend in an organ

beryllium disease
berylliosis
lung disorder caused by exposure to
fumes or dust particles of beryllium

between attacks
interictal
intercritical

between cartilages
intercartilaginous
interchondral

between cell divisions
interphase

between cells
intercellular

between eyelids
interpalpebral

between lobes
interlobar
between the projecting parts of an
organ or other structure

between muscles
intermuscular

between nostrils
internarial

between nuclear layers
internuclear
of the retina

between parietal bones
interparietal
also between the walls of any cavity

between ribs
intercostal

between similar structures
interspace

between teeth
interdentium
interdental
interocclusal

between thighs
interfemoral

between two adjoining surfaces
interproximal

bile duct dilation
cholangiectasis

bile duct inflammation
angiocholitis
cholangiolitiis
cholangitis
periangiocholitis
pericholangitis
inflammation of the tissues surrounding
the bile ducts
pericholecystitis
inflammation around the gallbladder

bile duct operation
cholangiostomy
cholangiotomy

bile excessive formation
hypercholia

bile flow excessive
cholerrhagia
cholerrhagic
cholorrhea
hepatorrhea
polycholia

bile pigments
bilirubin
orange-red
biliverdin
green

bile secretion
choleresis
by liver

bile secretion lacking
acholia

bile in spinal fluid
bilirachia

bile in urine
biliuria
choluria

bilirubin in blood
bilirubinemia
hyperbilirubinemia
excessive amounts in the blood

bilirubin in urine
bilirubinuria

birth control
contraception
contraceptive
prevention of contraception or impregnation by sperm

birth to males
androgenous

birth to one
monotocous

birthmark
nevus

biting self
autophagia
autophagy

black-and-blue marks
livedo
discolored patch on the skin

black-haired
melanotrichous

black sickness
kala-azar
a fatal infectious disease endemic in the tropics

black spot vision
scotodinia
dizziness with blurring of vision and headache

black tongue
melanoglossia

black urine
melanuria

black vomit
vomitus nigar

blackhead
comedo

blackness in organs
melanism
presence of black pigment in tissues, organs, and skin

bladder calculus
cystolithiasis

bladder/cervix
cervicovesical

bladder dilatation
cystectasia
cystectasy

bladder discharge
cystorrhea
mucous discharge from the bladder

bladder examination
cystoscopy
visual examination of the interior of the urinary bladder

bladder fissure
exstrophy
schistocystis

bladder hernia
cystocele
enterocystocele

bladder inflammation
cystitis
cystopyelitis
   inflammation of bladder and pelvis of
   the kidneys
paracystitis
pericystitis
epicystitis
   inflammation of connecting tissues
   around the bladder
pyelocystitis
   inflammation of the bladder and pelvis
   of a kidney
trigonitis
   inflammation of the trigone
cystoureteritis
   inflammmation of bladder and ureters

bladder lacking
acystia
   born without urinary bladder

bladder operation
cystectomy
cystotomy
epicystotomy
vesicotomy
cystolithectomy
cystolithotomy
   removal of calculi from urinary bladder
cystopexy
   fixation of bladder
cystoplasty
cystollytroplasty
cystoproctostomy
cystostomy
neocystostomy
proctocystoplasty
vesicostomy
   repair to the bladder
ureteroileoneocystostomy
   a segment of the ileum is made part of
   the ureter

bladder pain
cystalgia

bladder paralysis
acystinervia
cystoplegia

bladder prolapse
cystoptosis
   the slipping of the urinary bladder from
   its normal position

bladder proximity
paracystic
paravesical

bladder tool
bilabe
   used in removing foreign matters
   through the urethra

cystometer
   instrument to study pressure and capacity of the bladder

cystourethroscope
   instrument to examine posterior urethra
   & bladder

bladder x-ray
cystography
cystourethrography

bleeding after delivery
postpartum hemorrhage

bleeding arrester
hemostat
   an agent/instrument that stops bleeding

blind spot
scotoma
   within the visual field

blindness
amaurosis
amaurotic
typhylosis
amaruosis fugax
   temporary blindness
amblyopia
   dimness of vision
hemeralopia
   day blindness
hemianopsia
   blindness in half of visual field
meropia
   partial blindness
quadrantanopia
quadrantanopsia
   loss of vision in one fourth of visual field

blister causing
epispastic
vesicant

blister groups
herpetiform

blistering disease
pemphigus
various types of skin diseases

bloodw/acetone
acetonemia
in relatively large amounts

blood albumin low
hypoalbuminemia
hypoalbuminosis

blood alkalinity increased
alkalemia

blood alkali measurer
hemoalkalimeter

blood w/ammonia compounds
ammoniemia

blood analysis
hemanalysis
examination of the blood, especially by chemical methods

blood w/bacilli
bacillemia

blood w/bacteria
bacteremia

blood bilirubin excess
bilirubinemia
hyperbilirubinemia
excessive amounts in the blood

blood in bone
hematosteon

blood calcium excess
calcemia
hypercalcemia

blood calcium low
hypocalcemia

blood carbon dioxide excess
hypercapnia
hypercarbia
also increased arterial carbon dioxide tension

blood carotene excess
carotenemia

blood cell
hematocyte
hemocyte

blood cell disintegration
erythrocytolysis
hemocatheresis
hematocytolysis
hemocytolysis
hemocytotripsis
hemolysis
the alteration, dissolution or destruction of red blood cells, caused by a specific agent, toxicity or change in temperature.

blood cell formation
hematogenesis
hematopoiesis
hematosis
hemogenesis
hemopoiesis

blood cell measurer
erythrocytometer
hemocytometer

blood chloride low
hypochloremia

blood w/chyle
chylemia
presence of chyle in the circulating blood

blood/chyle in urine
hematochyluria

blood clot
embolus
hematoma
thrombus

blood clot destruction
thromboclasis
thrombolysis

blood clot operation
embolectomy
thrombectomy
surgical removal

blood clotting agent
prothrombin

blood coagulation disorder
coagulopathy
any disorder
consumptive coagulopathy
disseminated intravascular coagulation

blood w/cystine
cystinemia

blood deficiency
hyphemia
ischemia
oligemia

blood w/diacetic acid
diacetemia

blood disease
dyscrasia
hemopathy

blood disease study
hematopathology

blood drinking
hematophagia

blood elements low
hypocythemia
deficiency of red blood cells

blood w/epinephrine
adrenalinemia
adrenemia

blood w/fat excess
hyperlipemia
hyperlipidemia
hyperlipoidemia
lipemia
lipidemia
lipoidemia
presence of an abnormally large
amount of lipids in the blood

blood w/fibrin
fibremia
fibrinemia

blood filtration
hemofiltration
removal of waste products by passing
the blood through a filter

blood flow
hemokinesis
hemorrhage

blood flow arrest
electrohemostasis
hemostasia
hemostasis
arrest of circulation in a body part or
stagnation of blood

blood flow measurer
flowmeter
hemadrometer

hemadromometer
hemodromometer
hemotachometer
rotameter

blood fluid deficiency
anhydremia
hemoconcentration

blood fluid increase
hemodilution

blood formation
hematopoiesis

blood w/foreign matter
embolemia
usually blood clots

blood formation defective
anhematopoietic
anhematosis

blood freezing point
hemocryoscopy
process of determining the freezing
point of blood

blood gas measurer
aerotonometer

blood w/glucose
euglycemia
glycemia
hyperglycemia
excessive amounts

blood w/gonococci
gonococcemia

blood hemorrhage
hematorrhea

blood w/heparin
heparinemia

blood w/inositol
inosemia

blood w/insulin
insulinemia
excessive amounts

blood iron low
hypoferremia

blood in joint
hemarthrosis

blood w/ketone bodies
ketonemia

blood lacking alkali
acidosis
decrease of alkali in proportion to the acid

blood lacking hemoglobin
oligochromemia

blood lacking lymphocytes
alymphocytosis
lymphopenia

blood w/lactic acid excess
lactacidemia

blood leukocytes deficient
leukopenia

blood measurement
hematometry
used to determine the number and types of cells, formed elements or hemoglobin present

blood w/melanin
melanemia

blood w/methemoglobin
methemoglobinemia

blood w/nitrogen
azotemia
hyperazotemia
uremia
excessive amounts

blood oxalates in excess
oxalemia

blood oxygen low
hypoxemia

blood phosphates high
hyperphosphatemia

blood phosphates low
hypophosphatemia

blood plasma low
apoplasmia

blood platelets low
thrombocytopenia
thrombopenia

blood w/pneumococci
pneumococcemia

blood w/poikilocytes
poikilocythemia
poikilocytosis

blood poisoning
toxemia
toxicemia
poisoning in general
radiotoxemia
poisoning induced by overexposure to radioactive substances
scatemia
poisoning through the intestine

blood w/polypeptides
polypeptidemia

blood potassium elevated
hyperkalemia
hyperpotassemia

blood potassium low
hypokalemia
hypopotassemia

blood pressure
arteriotomy

blood pressure elevated
hypertension

blood pressure estimator
hemomanometer

blood pressure low
hypotension

blood pressure measurer
sphygmotonometer
sphygmo-oscillometer
sphygmomanometer
instrument to measure arterial blood pressure
ochrometer
measures capillary pressure

blood protein high
hyperproteinemia
proteinemia

blood protein low
hypoproteinemia

blood prothrombin low
hypoprothrombinemia
prothrombinopenia

blood recycling
hemodialysis
by diffusion through a semipermeable membrane

blood relationship
consanguinity

blood in semen
hematospermatocele

blood sodium elevated
hypernatremia

blood sodium low
hyponatremia

blood speed measurer
rheometer
instrument to measure the velocity of blood current
stromuhr
instrument to measure the speed of blood flow within blood vessels

blood in spinal cord
hematomyelia

blood w/sodium
natremia
natriemia

blood specialist
hematologist

blood spitting
hemoptysis

blood stone
hemolith

blood in stool
hematochezia
passage of bloody stools

blood study
hematology
hematopathology
hemodiagnosis
hemodynamics
hemorrheology

blood substitute
periston

blood w/sugar
glycemia
hyperglycemia
excessive amounts

blood sugar lacking
aglycemia

blood transfusion
autotransfusion
transfusion of one's own blood

blood in tympanic cavity
hematotympanum
hemotympanum

blood w/uric acid
uratemia
uricacidemia
uricemia
hyperuricemia
excessive amounts

blood in urine
hematocyturia
natriemia

blood w/urobilin
urobilinemia

blood in uterus
hematometra
hematosalpinx
in uterine tube

blood in vagina
hematocolpos

blood vessel calculi
angiolith

blood vessel constriction
vasoconstriction

blood vessel development
angiogenesis

blood vessel dilatation
angiotelectasia
angiotelectasis
hemangiectasia
hemangiectasis
phlebarteriectasia
vasodilation

blood vessel enlargement
angiomegaly
increase in size of blood vessels or lymphatics

blood vessel formation
angiopoiesis

blood vessel hardening
angiosclerosis

blood vessel inflammed
angiotitis
endangitis
endangeitis
endarteritis
inflammation of the blood vessels of the ear

endovasculitis
endophlebitis
   generally inflammation of the intima of
   a blood vessel
endaortitis
endoartitis
   inflammation of the aorta

blood vessel narrowing
angiostenosis

blood vessel nutritional disorder
angiodystrophia
angiodystrophy

blood vessel oozing
angiostaxis

blood vessel operation
angioneurectomy
angioplasty
angiorrhaphy
angiostomy
angiotomy

blood vessel paralysis
angioparalysis
angioparesis

blood vessel rupture
angiorrhexis
rhexis
   rupture of a blood vessel or lymphatic

blood vessel spasm
angiospasm
angiospastic

blood vessel tumor
angioma
hemangioma
   swelling from proliferation of the vessel

blood w/virus
viremia

blood volume high
hypervolemia

blood volume low
hypovolemia

blood vomiting
hematemesis

blood without sugar
aglycemia
aglycemic

blower
insufflator

   instrument used to blow air, gas, water,
   etc. into a body cavity

blue blood
cyanemia

blue hands/feet
acrocyanosis

blue skin
cyanochroic
cyanochrous
cyanoderma
cyanosis

blue sweat
cyanephidrosis
cyanhidrosis
   excretion of sweat with a bluish tint

boat-shaped
scaphoid

boat-shaped head
cymbocephaly
scaphocephaly

body curve measurer
cyrtometer

body deformity correction
orthopraxis

body dryness
xerotes

body in excess
polysomia
polysomus
   developmental anomaly with doubling or
   tripling of the body size

body largeness
gigantism
macrosomia

body measurer
anthropometer
   instrument used for measurements
   of the body
anthropometrist
   operator of the instrument
anthropometry
   art of measuring the body

body odor
bromhidrosis
bromidrosis
bromohyperhidrosis

body pain
pantalgia

body smallness
dwarfism
microsomia
nanism
nanosomia
meromicrosomia
smallness of some body parts

body temperature low
hypothermia
hypothermy

body type
somatotype
constitutional or body type of an individual

boil
furuncle
an abscess

bone
os
ossa

bone cell
osteoblast

bone cutter
osteotome
osteotribe
rongeur

bone death/decay
osteolysis
osteonecrosis
decay in general
osteoradionecrosis
caused by radiation

bone development
osteogenesis

bone development defective
anostosis
osteodystrophy

bone disease
osteochrondrosis
osteopathia
osteopathology
osteopathy
osteopoikilosis

bone enlargement
hyperostosis

bone formation
osteosis

bone formation defective
dysostosis
osteochondrodystrophia
disorder of bone and cartilage formation

bone hemorrhage
osteorrhagia

bone hardening
osteosclerosis

bone inflammation
osteitis
osteoarthritis
bone and joint
osteochrondritis
bone and cartilage
osteomyelitis
bone marrow
osteosynovitis
bone and synovial membrane
osteophlebitis
veins of a bone
osteoperiostitis
bone and periosteum
panosteitis
entire bone
periostitis
petrositis
fibrous membrane covering part of the temperol bone

bone knife
osteotome

bone marrow inflammation
medulitis
medullitis
myelitis
osteomyelitis

bone marrow tumor
myeloma
composed of cells derived from hemopoietic tissues of the bone marrow

bone measurement
osteometry

bone/membrane adhesion
meningosis
as in the skull of the newborn

bone nutrition
osteotrophy

bone operation
ostearthrotomy
ostectomy

osteoarthrotomy
osteoclasis
osteoplasty
osteorrhaphy
osteostixis
osteotomy

bone pain
ostalgia
ostealgia
osteocope
osteodynia
osteoneuralgia

bone regeneration
osteanagenesis
osteanaphysis
reproduction of bone

bone in skin
osteodermia

bone softening
halisteresis
osteomalacia
osteoporosis

bone specialist
orthopedist
physician specializing in diagnosis and
treatment of the skeletal system

bone study
orthopedics
osteology

bone suppuration
ostempyesis
pus in the bone

bone suture
osteorrhaphy
osteosuture

bone tumor
osteocarcinoma
osteochondrofibroma
osteochondroma
osteochondrophyte
osteoclastoma
osteocystoma
osteofibroma
osteoma
osteonucus
osteophyma
osteosarcoma
osteospongioma

border
limbus

both sides
ambilateral

bowels uncontrollable
scatacratia
scoracratia
incontinence of feces

brain
encephalic
encephalon

brain abscess
encephalopyosis

brain atrophy
encephalatrophy

brain calculus
encephalolith

brain disease
encephalosis
organic disease
encephalomeningopathy
disease of brain and meninges

brain extract
sphingomyelin

brain gray matter
cinerea

brain hardness
cerebrosclerosis
encephalosclerosis

brain/head lacking
deranencephalia
born with neck, but no head or brain

brain hemorrhage
cerebral hemorrhage
encephalorrhagia

brain hernia
cephalocele
encephalocele
encephameningocele

brain imperfect
ateloencephalia

brain inflammation
cerebritis
encephalitis
ependymitis
the ependyma
ventriculitis
cerebral meningitis
cerebrospinal meningitis
myeloencephalitis

brain inflammation (cont.)
meningitis
meningocephalitis
meningoencephalitis
  brain and spinal cord
meningocerebritis
  brain and meninges
meningoencephalomyelitis
  meninges, brain and spinal cord
mesencephalitis
  midbrain
periencephalitis
poliencephalitis
  surface of the brain
polioencephalitis
  gray matter of the brain
polioencephalomeningomyelitis
  gray matter of the brain and spinal cord
  meninges
polioencephalomyelitis
poliomyelitis
  gray matter of the brain and spinal cord

brain knife
encephalotome
  instrument used in brain surgery

brain lacking
anencephaly
pantanencephalia
pantanencephaly

brain largeness
macrencephaly
macrencephalous

brain operation
encephalotomy
leukotomy
lobotomy
topectomy
ventriculostomy
ventriculotomy

brain puncture
encephalopuncture
ventriculopuncture
  puncture of the brain substance

brain pus
encephalopyrosis
pyencephalus

brain smallness
micrencephalia
micrencephaly
micrencephalous

microencephaly
  abnormal smallness in size of the brain

brain softness
cerebromalacia
encephalodialysis
encephalomalacia

brain/spinal cord disease
encephalomyelopathy
encephalomyeloradiculopathy

brain/spinal cord inflammation
arachnoiditis
encephalomyelitis

brain/spinal cord lacking
amyelencephalia
amyelencephalus
amyelencephalous
amyelencephalic
amyelia
amyelic
amyelous
amyelus
  congenital absence

brain stone
encephalolith
  a calculus (stone) in the brain or one of
  its ventricles

brain tissue hardening
sclerencephalia
sclerencephaly

brain tumor
encephaloma
glioma
meningioma

brain x-ray
encephalogram

breast atrophy
mastatrophy
mastatrophagia

breast disease
mastopathy
  any abnormal condition of the breast

breast excess number
pleomastia
pleomazia
pleomaziax
polymazia

breast hemorrhage
mastorrhagia

breast inflammation
mastitis
paramastitis
perimastitis
tissues around the breast

breast largeness
macromastia
macromazia
mammose
mastauxe

breast operation
mammectomy
mammoplasty
mastectomy
mastopexy
mastoplasty
mastotomy

breast pain
mammalgia
mastalgia
mastodynia
mazodynia

breast smallness
micromazia
rudimentary presence only

breast tumor
mastoderma
mastochondroma

breath odor
halitosis
ozostomia
ozostomiax
bromopnea*
*obsolete term

breathing absence
apnea

breathing difficulty
atelectasis
dyspnea

breathing fast
tachypnea

breathing machine
respirator

breathing slowness
bradypnea

breathing sound
rale

rhonchus
diagnosed during examination

bronchi inflammation
bronchadenitis
bronchial lymph nodes
bronchiolitis
bronchioles
bronchitis
bronchial tubes
bronchopneumonia
bronchopneumonitis
bronchi and lungs
peribronchitis
peribronchiolitis
tissues surrounding thebronchi/
bronchioles

bronchial calculus
broncholith
the calculus (stone)
broncholithiasis
the medical condition

bronchial dilation
bronchocele

bronchial fistulization
bronchostomy
through the chest wall

bronchial suture
bronchorrhaphy

bronchial viewer
bronchoscope

bruise
contusion

bunion
hallux valgus
deviation of main axis of the great toe

bunion operation
bunionectomy

burning pain
causalgia
persistent severe burning sensation of
the skin

bursa inflammation
bursitis

bursa operation
bursectomy

buttocks pain
pygalgia

buttocks pertaining
gluteal

buttocks too fat
steatopygia

bypass
shunt

C

---

calcified fetus
lithokelyphopedion
lithokelyphopedium
lithopedion
lithopedium
osteopedion*
  *obsolete term

calcium antagonist
calcium channel blocker
slow channel blocker

calcium in bile
calcibilia

calcium in blood
calcemia
hypercalcemia
  excessive amount
hypocalcemia
  abnormally low levels

calcium lacking in diet
calciprivia

calcium regulation
calmodulin
  protein present in all nucleated cells

calcium in tissues
calcinosis

calcium in urine
calciuria
hypercalcinuria
hypercalciuria
hypercalcuria

calculi destroying
electrolithotrity
  disintegration of calculi (stones) in the
  urinary bladder

calculi formation
calciphylaxis
calculosis
lithiasis
lithogenesis

calculi smallness
microlithiasis
microlith

calf-bone
fibula

callosity
heloma durum
  hard corn
helome molle
  soft corn

callus
tyloma

callus formation
tylosis

camphor poisoning
camphorism

cancer
carcinoma
sarcoma
  (see also tumor under specific site)

cancer dissemination
carcinolytic
carcinomatosis
carcinosis
metastasis

cancer formation
carcinogenic
carcinogenesis
  causing cancer

cancer specialist
cancerologist
oncologist

cancer study
cancerology
oncology
cynodont
  a tooth having one cusp or point

capillary dilation
capillarectasia
telangiectasia
trichangiectasia
  obsolete term

capillary disease
capillaropathy
telangiectasia

capillary inflammation
capillaritis

capsule inflammation
capsulitis

capsule instrument
capsulotome
cystotome
surgical instrument for incising the capsule of a lens with cataract

capsule operation
capsulectomy
capsulotomy
capsuloplasty

capsule suture
capsulorrhaphy

carbohydrates in urine
carbohydraturia

carbolic acid in urine
carboluria

carbon compounds in urine
carbonuria

carbon dioxide in blood
hypercapnia
hypercarbia
excessive amounts
hypocapnia
hypocarbia
abnormally low tension of carbion dioxide

carbon dioxide measurer
carbonometer
obsolete device

carbon dust disease
anthracosis

carotene in blood
carotenemia
excessive amounts

carpal bone operation
carpectomy

cartilage cell
chondrocyte

cartilage disease
chondropathy

cartilage formation
chondrogenesis
chondroplasia
chondroplasia

cartilage hardening
chondrocalcinosis

cartilage inflammaiton
chondritis
general term
meniscitis
inflammation of the semilunar cartilage of the knee joint
perichondritis
inflammation of the perichondrium

cartilage knife
arthrotome
chondrome

cartilage operation
chondrectomy
chondroplasty
chondrotomy
meniscectomy
on the semilunar cartilage
thyrochondrotomy
thyrotomy
on the thyroid cartilage

cartilage pain
chondralgia
chondrodynia
chondrodynia
xyphodynia

cartilage softening
chondromalacia
softening of any cartilage

cartilage tumor
chondroadenoma
chondroangioma
chondroblastoma
chondrofibroma
chondrolipoma
chondroma
chondromyoma
chondromyxoma
chondromyxosarcoma
chondrosarcoma
chondrosteoma

casts in urine
cylindruria
presence of renal cylinders or casts in the urine

cataract
phacomalacia
phacosclerosis
sclerocataract
obsolete term

cataract operation
phacocystectomy
phacoerysis

cat's whiskers
vibrissa
applies to hair in the nose

cecum calculi
typhlolithiasis

cecum dilatation/distention
typhlectasis

cecum enlargement
typhlomegaly

cecum hernia
cecocele
typhlocele*
*obsolete term

cecum inflammation
cecitis
typhlenteritis
typhlitis
typhlodicliditis
inflammation of the iliocecal valve

cecum operation
cecectomy
cecotomy
cecostomy
typhlectomy
typhlostomy

cecum suture
cecorrhaphy

cell counter
cytometer
glass slide or chamber used in counting
and measuring

cell deficiency
cytopenia

cell death
necrocytosis

cell destroyer
cytocele
cytoclasis
cytotoxic

cell development
cytogenesis

cell dissolution
cytolysis

cell division
mitosis

cell fusion
plasmatogamy
plasmogamy
plastogamy
union of two or more cells with preserva-
tion of the individual nuclei

cell granulation
emiocytosis
exocytosis
release of secretory granules or droplets
from a cell

cell largeness
macrocyte

cell membrane
plasmalemma

cell-produced poison
endotoxin

cell repair
cytothesis
repair of injury to cells

cell rupture
erythrocytorrhexis
plasmorrhexis

cell size equal
isocellular

cell smallness
microcyte

cell stimulus
cytropism
tendency of cells to move toward or
away from stimuli

cell study
cytogenetics
cytology

cerebellum lacking
notanencephalia
born without cerebellum

cerebral convolutions lack
agyria
born without cerebral convolutions

cerebral hemispheres fused
cyclencephalia
cyclencephaly

cyclocephalia
cyclocephaly

cerebrospinal
encephalorrhachidian

cerebrospinal sugar
glycorrhachia
in the fluid
hyperglycorrhachia
excessive amounts

cerebrum/cerebellum lacking
anencephalia
anencephaly

cerum excess
ceruminosis

cervix/bladder
cervicovesical

cervix inflammation
cervicitis
trachelitis
cervicocolpitis
cervix and vagina

cervix operation
cervicectomy
trachelectomy
trachelopexy
tracheloplasty
trachelotomy
trachelorrhaphy

Cesarean birth
partus caesarius

change
metamorphosis
in form, structure or function

change of life
climacteric
menopause

cheek
bucca
mala

cheek cleft
meloschisis
congenital condition

cheek inflammation
melitis
general term
gnathitis
also of the jaw

cheek pertaining
malar
cheek or zygoma
buccogingival
cheek and gums
buccolabial
cheek and lip
buccolingual
cheek and tongue
buccopharyngeal
cheek and pharynx

cheekbone
os zygomaticum

cheeselike
tyroid

chemical attraction
chemotaxis
property of cells to be attracted to or re-
pelled by chemical stimuli

chemical breakdown
catabolism
often accompanied by the liberation of
energy

chemical change
metabolism

chest
pectus
thorax
especially the anterior wall

chest deformity
thoracococyllosis
thoracocyrtosis
thoracogastroschisis
thoracomelus
thoracoschisis

chest disease
thoracopathy

chest examination
stethoscopy
by means of listening to the cardiac and
respiratory sounds

chest measurement
stethogoniometer
stethometer
thoracometer

chest narrowness
stenothorax
thoracostenosis

chest pain
stethalgia
thoracalgia
thoracodynia
thoracomyodynia

chest operation
thoracectomy
thoracentesis
thoracolysis
thoracoplasty
thoracopneumoplasty
thoracostomy
thoracotomy

chest spasm
stethospasm

chewing
mastication

chewing incomplete
psomophagia
psomophagy

chewing force measurer
phagodynamometer
instrument to measure the force
exerted

chicken breast
pectus carinatum
prominence of the sternum

chickenpox
varicella

childbearing
texis

childbirth
tocus
tokus
oxytocia
oxytocic

childbirth dry
xerotocia

childbirth normal
eutocia

childbirth psychosis
tocomania
postpartum psychosis

childbirth study
obstetrics
tocology

children perversion
pedophilia
sexual perversion

children physician
pediatrician
pediatrist

children study
pediatrics

chill of death
algor mortis

chin/lip
labiomental

chin operation
genioplasty

chin smallness
microgenia

chlorides in blood
hyperchloremia
high levels
hypochloremia
low levels

chlorides in urine
chloriduria
chloruresis
hyperchloruria
high levels
hypochloruria
low levels

cholesterol in blood
cholesteremia
cholesterolemia
hypercholesterolemia
excessive amounts
hypocholesteremia
low levels

cholesterol in tissues
cholesterosis
cholesterolosis

cholesterol in urine
cholesteroluria

choroid inflammation
choroiditis
general term
choroidocyclitis
choroid and ciliary processes
chorioretinitis
choroid and retina

chronaxie measurer
chronaximeter

chyle in blood
chylemia

chyle deficiency
achymia
hypochylia
oligochylia

chyle in excess
hyperchylia
polychylia

chyle forming
chylifacient
chyliferous

chyle lacking
achylia
achylous
absence of normal intestinal fluid produced during digestion

chyle in pericardium
chylopericardium

chyle in peritoneum
chyloperitoneum

chyle/lymph in urine
chyluria

ciliary body destruction
cyclodiathermy

ciliary body inflamed
cyclitis
general term
cyclochoroiditis
ciliary body and choroid

ciliary body knife
cyclotome

ciliary body operation
cyclectomy
cyclodialysis
cyclotomy

ciliary muscle paralysis
cycloplegia
cycloplegic
pertaining to muscles surrounding the eyeball

ciliary operation
ciliarotomy
zonulotomy

cirrhosis of liver
hepatocirrhosis

clap
gonorrhea

clavicle operation
clavicotomy

clavicle/sternum angle
sternoclavical angle

cleft extremity
schistomelus
individual with one or more cleft limbs

cleft face
schistoprosopus

cleft palate
palatoschisis
palatum fissum

cleft tongue
schistoglossia
congenital fissure of the tongue

clitoris enlargement
clitoromegaly

clitoris inflamed
clitoriditis
clitoritis

clitoris operation
clitoridectomy
clitoridotomy
clitoroplasty

clotting
coagulation
changing from liquid to solid or solid to gel
electrocoagulation
using an electric current

cloudiness measurer
turbidimeter
instrument for determining the extent of cloudiness in a liquid

clubfoot
talipes equinovarus

clubhand
talipomanus

clumsy with either hand
ambilevous
ambisinister

clustered
agminate
agminated

clusterlike
botryoid
racemose

coccyx operation
coccygectomy

coccyx pain
coccyalgia
coccygodynia

coexistence
mutualism
symbiosis
living together of organisms of different
species for common advantage

coin-shaped
mummiform
mummular

coitus climax unreached
anorgasmy

coitus interrupted
coitus interruptus
onanism

coke
cocaine

cold
algid

cold anesthesia
cryanesthesia

cold pain
cryalgesia
psychralgia
pain produced by application of cold

cold sensitiveness
cryesthesia
hypercryalgesia
hypercryesthesia

cold sore
herpes simplex

cold/warm sensation
psychroesthesia
feeling of cold in warm parts of the body
and of warmth in cold parts

colon disease
enteromycosis

colon disease (*continued*)
enteropathogenesis
enteropathy

colon distention
pneumocolon

colon inflammation
colitis
general term
mucocolitis
mucous membranes
paracolitis
outer tissues of the colon
enterocolitis
enteritis
small intestine and colon
perisigmoiditis
sigmoiditis
sigmoid fold of the colon
coloproctitis
colorectitis
proctocolitis
rectum and colon
proctosigmoiditis
rectum and sigmoid colon
rectocolitis
rectum membrane & colon

colon largeness
megacolon
macrosigmoid
megasigmoid
sigmoid colon

colon operation
colectomy
colotomy
enterocentesis
enterocolectomy
enterocolostomy
enteroenterostomy
enterolysis
enteropexy
enteroplasty
hemicolectomy
lumbocolostomy
lumbocolotomy
pancolectomy
rectosigmoidectomy
sigmoidectomy
sigmoidotomy
sigmoidopexy
sigmoidoproctostomy
sigmoidorectostomy
sigmoidosigmoidostomy
typhlostomy

typhlotomy
ureterocolostomy
ureteroenterostomy
ureterosigmoidostomy

colon smallness
microcolon
often arising from a decreased functional state

colon suture
colorrhaphy

color blindness
achromate
the individual
achromatopsia
general term
daltonism
red-green
color amblyopia
partial
cyanopia
cyanopsia
all objects appear blue
deuteranopia
red
dyschromatope
difficulty distinguishing colors
monoblepsia
monochromasy
monochromatism
monochromatic
only one color perceived
protanomaly
protanopia
defective red vision
xanthocyanopsia
yellow and blue visible, not red

color blindness detector
anomaloscope
leukoscope

color intensity measurer
chromatometer
colorimeter

color normal
normochromic

colored cell
chromocyte

colored sweat
chromhidrosis

colorless cell
achroacyte

column of liquid curve
meniscus
the curved surface of a column of liquid

compression
tamponade

compulsive touching
phaneromania

concave skull
clinocephaly
condition where the top of the head is saddle-shaped

concentration lacking
aprosexia

conduct study
praxiology

condyle operation
condylectomy
condylotomy

conflicting mental forces
ambivalence

conjunctiva dryness
xerophthalmia

conjunctiva inflammation
conjunctivitis
blepharoconjunctivitis
conjunctiva & eyelids

conjunctiva mucous flow
ophthalmoblenorrhea

conjunctiva operation
conjunctivoplasty
logadectomy
peritectomy
peritomy

conjunctiva patch
pinguecula
a whitish spot on the conjunctiva

conjunctiva tumor
conjunctivoma

conjunctiva varicosity
varicula
swelling of the veins of the conjunctiva

convulsion
paroxysm

coordination defective
hyposynergia
chalcosis

cord operation
 chordotomy
 cordectomy
 cordotomy
  surgical procedure on the spinal cord

corn
 clavus
 heloma

corn surgery
 helotomy

cornea curve measurement
 keratometry

cornea disease
 keratopathy

cornea with fat
 corneal steatosis
 lipoidosis corneae

cornea growth
 keratoma
 keratosis

cornea inflammation
 keratitis
  general term
 keratoconjunctivitis
  cornea and conjunctiva
 keratoiritis
  cornea and iris
 keratoscleritis
 sclerokeratitis
  cornea and sclera
 sclerokeratoiritis
  cornea, sclera, and iris

cornea inspection
 keratoscopy

cornea knife
 keratome
 keratotome
  surgical instrument used to cut into the
  cornea

cornea largeness
 macrocornia
 megalocornea

cornea opaque ring
 arcus cornealis
 arcus juvenilis
 arcus lipoides
 arcus senilis

cornea operation
 keratectomy
 keratoleptynsis
 keratophakia
 keratoplasty
 keratotomy
 kerectomy

cornea outer layer
 ectocornea

cornea protrusion
 keratectasia
 keratoconus
 keratoglobus

cornea puncture
 keratocentesis
 keratonyxis

cornea rupture
 keratorrhexis
  due to trauma or perforating ulcer

cornea/sclera bulging
 staphyloma
 staphylomatous

cornea smallness
 microcoria
 microcornea

cornea softness
 keratomalacia
  due to disease or Vitamin A deficiency

cornea spot
 albugo
 leukoma
 walleye

cornea ulcer
 keratohelcosis
 ulcus serpens

cornea viewer
 keratoscope

corpulence
 adiposis
 obesity

cotton-mill fever
 byssinosis

cough
 tussis

counting inability
 anarithmia

crack
cocaine

cranial gas/air
erpidural aerocele
accumulation of gas or air in the skull, usually after a fracture

cranial hernia
hydrencephalocele
hydrencephalomeningocele
notencephalocele
notencephalus

cranial knife
craniotome
instrument used to perforate the fetal skull

cranial operation
cephalocentesis
craniotomy

cranial pressure measurer
cephalohemometer

craving
parepithymia
abnormal longing

crib death
sudden infant death syndrome

critical stage
acme

crosslike
cruciform

croup
laryngitis

crystals in urine
crystalluria

cup-shaped
scyphiform
schyphoid

curvature of spine
kyphosis
hunch back
lordosis
leaning backward
scoliosis
lateral curvature

cut
laceration

D

daily recurrence
quotidian

dandruff
dermatitis seborrheica
furfur
pityriasis capitus

"dandruff of the gods"
cocaine

dark vision
scieropia
defective vision with objects appearing dark

darkness measurer
biophotometer
instrument for measuring adaptation to darkness

darnel poisoning
loliism

day blindness
hemeralopia

deafness
anacusis
anakusis

death apparent
anabiosis
anabiotic
involves resuscitation; also used to denote an agent utilized in restoring life

death chill
algor mortis

death by electrocution
electrothanasia

death without pain
euthanasia

decline of disease/fever
catabasis
paracme

decomposition by light
photolysis

deep stained cell
chromatophil
chromophil

deep voice
baryphonia

deer fly fever
tularemia

defecation painful
dyschezia

defective fusion
araphia
dypraphia
dysraphism
holorachiochisis
spina bifida of the spinal column

deficiency of amniotic fluid
oligohydramnios

deficiency of bile
oligocholia

deficiency of blood
oligemia
oligocythemia
oligoplasmia

deficiency of chyle
oligochylia
lack of sufficient digestive fluid

deficiency of hair
hypotrichosis
oligotrichia

deficiency of hemoglobin
oligochromemia
in the blood

deficiency of menstruation
oligomenorrhea
reduction in frequency

deficiency of milk secretion
oligogalactia

deficiency of nutrition
oligotrophia
oligotrophy

deficiency of oxygen
hypoxemia
in the blood

deficiency of phosphates
oligophosphaturia
in the urine

deficiency of saliva
oligoptyalism
oligosialia

deficiency of sodium
hyponatremia
in the blood

deficiency of sperm
oligospermia
oligozoospermia

deficiency of teeth
oligodontia

deficiency of thirst
oligodipsia
abnormal absence of thirst

deficiency of urine
oliguria

deformity generalized
pantamorphia

deformity straightening
orthosis
orthotic

degeneration
retroplasia
decreased cell activity associated with
injury or death

delusion of greatness
megalomania
megalomanic

dental enamel formation
amelification

dentistry
gerodontics
for the elderly
odontology
orthodontics
dental orthopedics
pedodontics
for children

dentition painful
dysodontiasis

depilatory
epilation

depression
melancholia

descent
matrilineal
through the female side

patrilineal
through the male side

designer drugs
street drugs
substance abuse

desire for confinement
claustrophilia

desire for music
melomania

desire to steal
kleptomania

desquamation
ecdysis
casting off of the outer skin

deterioration mental
dementia
due to organic or psychological factor

determining by touch
topesthesia

development of disease
pathogenesis

development incomplete
agenesia
agenetic
agenesis
aplasia

dextrose in urine
dextrosuria*
glycosuria
*obsolete term

diacetic acid in blood
diacetemia

diacetic acid in urine
diacetonuria
diaceturia

diaphragm inflammation
diaphragmitis

diarrhea astringent
albumin tannate

diarrhea of food
lientery
undigested food is evacuated

diastole lacking
adiastole

dietary fiber
cellulose
roughage

dietary treatment
alimentotherapy
dietotherapy
sitotherapy

dietetics
sitiology
sitology

difference in color
heterochromia
heterochromous
between two structures or parts that are normally similar

difference in origin
heterogeneous

differs from normal form
heteromorphous

difficulty in articulation
dysarthria
dyslalia

difficulty in coordination
dyspraxia
dystaxia
dyssynergia

difficulty in defecation
dyschezia

difficulty in speech
dyslogia
dysphasia
dysphonia
dysphrasia
resulting from cortical damage

difficulty in standing
dystasia

difficulty in swallowing
dysphagia
odynophagia

difficulty in teething
dysodontiasis

difficulty in urination
dysuria

difficulty in walking
dysbasia

digitalin-like
apocynein
a glycoside from dogbane with the effect of digitalin

digits fused/lacking
ectrosyndactyl

dilatation of artery
aneurysm

dilatation of heart
cardiectasis

dilator
speculum
instrument to create an opening

dirt/clay eating
geophagia
geophagy
geophagism
geophagist
individual who eats

discharge suppression
ischesis
retention of discharge or secretion

discomfort
dysphonia
feeling of unpleasantness or discomfort

disease of .....
see under specific location

disease classification study
nosology
nosotaxy

disk inflammation
discitis
diskitis

displacement forward
anteversion
anteverted

dog-head shaped
cynocephalus

dosage determination
dosimetry

dosage study
posology
the science of dosage

double chin
buccula

double clitoris/penis
diphallus

double eyelashes
distichiasis

double hearing
diplacusis

double joint
diarthric
relating to two joints

double lip
dicheilia
dichilia

double pupil
dicoria
diplocoria
discoria
presence of a double pupil in the eye

double uterus
didelphia
dimetria

double vision
amphodiplopia
diplopia
monodiplopia

dream analysis
oneiroscopy

drinkable
potable

drop
gutta
abbreviated as ggt and refers to drop of medication (i.e., eye drops)

dropsy of abdomen
ascites

dropsy of the brain
hydrocephalus
retention of fluid

drug action
pharmacodynamics
pharmacology

drug-disease study
pharmacotherapeutics

drug fondness
pharmacomania

drug holiday
drug withdrawal
for brief period during treatment

drug study
biopharmaceutics
pharmacodynamics
pharmacoepidemiology

pharmacology
pharmacognosy

drug treatment
chemotherapy
pharmacotherapy
treatment of disease by means of chemical substances or drugs

drug use multiple
polypharmacy
use of many products simultaneously

drunkard nose
rhinophyma

dry
siccus

dryness
xerotes

dry childbirth
xerotocia
dry labor

dry mouth
xerostomia

dry nasal passages
xeromycteria
extreme dryness of mucous membrane

dry skin
xeroderma
xeronosus
xerosis

drying agent
desiccant

drying out
exsiccation

ductus deferens operation
vasectomy
vasoepididymostomy
vasoligation
vaso-orchidostomy
vasostomy
vasotomy
vasovasostomy
vasovesiculectomy

dullness of intellect
asynesia
asynesis
hebetude
lack of easy comprehension and practical intelligence

dumping syndrome
gastric emptying

duodenum inflammation
duodenitis
periduodenitis
tissues around the duodenum

duodenum operation
duodenectomy
duodenotomy
duodenocholecystostomy
duodenocystostomy
duodenocholedochotomy
duodenoenterostomy
duodenojejunostomy
pancreatoduodenectomy
duodenostomy

duodenum suture
duodenorrhaphy

duodenum x-ray
duodenogram

dura mater
pachymeninx
outer membrane of the brain

dura mater disease
pachymeningopathy

dura mater inflammation
pachymeningitis
perimeningitis
peripachymeningitis

dura mater operation
duraplasty

dwarf
nanus
nanous

dwarfism
nanism

E

ear damaging
ototoxic
having a toxic action upon the ear

ear deformity
otocephaly

ear disease
otopathy
otosclerosis
tympanosclerosis

ears excessive
polyotia
born with more than two ears

ear hairs
tragal

ear hemorrhage
othemorrhagia
otorrhagia

ear implant
auditory prosthesis
cochleal prosthesis

ear inflammation
barotitis
otitis
otoantritis
otomycosis
otopyosis
panotitis
perilabyrinthitis
inner ear
pyolabyrinthitis
labyrinth with pus
tympanitis
eardrum
tympanomastoiditis
eardrum and mastoid cells

ear largeness
macrotia

ear mucous discharge
otopyorrhea
otopyosis
otorrhea

ear murmuring
syrigmus

ear-nose-throat specialist
otorhinolaryngologist

ear-throat study
otolaryngology

ear operation
myringotomy
ossiculectomy
ossiculotomy
otoplasty

ototomy
stapedectomy
stapediotenotomy
tympanectomy
tympanoplasty
tympanotomy
vestibulotomy

ear-originated
otogenic
otogenous

ear external lacking
anotia

ear polyp
otopolypus

ear purulent drainage
otopyorrhea

ear smallness
microtia

ear study
otology
otolaryngology
ears and throat
otoneurology
includes nerves
otorhinolaryngology
ears, nose, and throat
otorhinology
ears and nose

ear thickness
pachyotia

ear tube
cochlea
organ of hearing in the central ear

ear viewer
otoscope

eararache
otalgia
otodynia
otoneuralgia

eardrum
tympanic membrane

eardrum infection
mycomyringitis
myringomycosis

earth eating
geophagia
geophagism
geophagy

geophagist
 individual involved

earthworm
lumbricus

earthworm-like
lumbricoid

eating animal food
carnivorous
zoophagous

eating aversion
apocleisis

eating in excess
polyphagia
bulimia
hyperphagia
 binge eating caused by mental disorder

eating fast
tachyphagia

eating one food
monophagism
 habit of subsisting on one type of food

eggwhite-like
glairy

eighth day fever
octan fever

elbow
cubitus

elbow disease/deformity
cubitus valgus
cubitus varus
olecranarthropathy

elbow inflammation
olecranarthritis
olecranarthrocace

elevation
torulus

embryo development
embryogenesis
embryogeny
 period of about the third to ninth week of pregnancy

embryo disorder
embryopathy

embryo nutrition
embryotrophy

embryo operation
embryectomy

embryotomy
embryoctony

embryo study
embryology

EMG syndrome
exomphalos, macroglossia, and gigantism
 also known as Beckwith-Wiedemann syndrome

endocardium inflamed
endocarditis

enlargement of ...
 see under specific organ

entrance
introitus

epididymis inflamed
epididymitis
epididymo-orchitis
 epididymis and testis

epididymis operation
epididymectomy
epididymotomy
epididymovasostomy

epigastric hernia
epigastrocele
 hernia in the epigastric region

epigastrium pain
epigastralgia

epiglottis inflamed
epiglottis
 area at the root of the tongue

epiglottis operation
epiglottidectomy

epinephrine in blood
adrenalinemia

epinephrine in urine
adrenalinuria

epiploon/omentum lacking
anepiploic

equal axes
homaxial

equal form
homeomorphous

equilibrium
homeostasis
 state of balance in the body functions

erection persistent
priapism

erector muscle
arrector
a muscle that raises

erotic ecstasy
nympholepsy

erythrocytes color variation
anisochromasia

erythrocyte deficiency
oligocythemia

erythrocytes unequal
anisocytosis

esophagus dilatation
esophagectasia
esophagectasis
megaesophagus

esophagus distention
esophagocele
protrusion of the membrane through a
tear in the muscular coat

esophagus examination
esophagoscopy

esophagus inflamed
esophagitis

esophagus operation
esophagectomy
esophagocoloplasty
esophagomyotomy
esophagoplasty
esophagotomy
esophagoenterostomy
esophagojejunostomy
esophagoesophagostomy
esophagogastrectomy
esophagogastroplasty
esophagogastrostomy
esophagostomy
esophagotomy

esophagus pain
esophagalgia
esophagodynia

esophagus prolapse
esophagoptosia
esophagoptosis

esophagus spasm
esophagism
causing difficulty in swallowing

esophagus stricture
esophagostenosis

esophagus/stomach viewer
esophagoscope

etiology unknown
agnogenic
cryptogenic

evacuation involuntary
scatacratia
scoracratia
incontinence of feces

evacuation opening abnormal
allochezia
allochetia

evil spirit possession
cacodemonomania
belief of possession

excessive acid
acidosis
in blood or urine

excessive activity
hyperanakinesia

excessive hunger
sitomania

exciting heart action
cardiokinetic

exhale/inhale measurer
spirometer
instrument used to measure respiratory
gases

expansion
rarefaction
process of becoming light or less dense

expectorating pus
pyoptysis

external ear
auris externa

extrauterine gestation
metacyesis
ectopic pregnancy

extremity cleft
schistomelus

extremity cold
acrohypothermy

extremity clubbing
acropathy

extremity lacking
acolous
amelia
amelus

extremity pain
melagra

extremity pertaining
acral

extremity senseless
acroanesthesia
lack of feeling

eye
oculus
ophthalmus

eye acuteness equal
isopia

eye adhesion
syncanthus

eye angle study
gonioscopy
examination of the angle of the anterior
chamber of the eye

eye appendages
adnexa oculi

eye choroid hernia
choriocele

eye crossed
convergent strabismus
esotropia

eye discharge
ophthalmorrhea

eye disease
ophthalmopathy
any pathologic condition

eye fluid
aqueous humor

eye fusion
cyclopia
cyclops
synophthalmus

eye hemorrhage
ophthalmorrhagia

eye images equal
isoiconia

eye inflammation
canthitis
canthus of the eye
choroiditis
choroid layer
conjunctivitis
conjunctiva
ophthalmia
ophthalmitis
general term
ophthalmomyitis
eye muscles
ophthalmoneuritis
ophthalmic nerve
panophthalmia
panophthalmitis
entire structure
papilloretinitis
optic disk and retina
parophthalmia
near the eye
scleritis
sclerotitis
sclera
sclerochoroiditis
scleroticochoroiditis
choroid and sclera
scleroiritis
sclera and iris
sclerokeratitis
sclera and cornea
sclerokeratoiritis
sclera, cornea, and iris
xenophthalmia
conjunctiva

eye lacking
anophthalmia
anophthalmos
anophthalmus

eye largeness
buphthalmos
megalophthalmus
megophthalmus

eye layers
choroid
middle, vascular layer
retina
inner layer
sclera
outer layer

eye malformation
cryptophthalmia
cryptophthalmos
cryptophthalmus
congenital deformity

eye mechanical
ophthalmotrope

eye muscle balance
orthophoria
  normal condition

eye muscle measurer
optomyometer

eye nerve paralysis
ophthalmoplegia
  paralysis of the motor nerves of the eye

eye ointment
oculentum

eye operation
canthectomy
canthoplasty
canthotomy
canthorrhaphy
ophthalmomyotomy
ophthalmoplasty
ophthalmostasis
ophthalmotomy
orbitotomy
rhinommectomy
sclerectoirdectomy
sclerectomy
scleroplasty
sclerostomy
scleronyxis
sclerotomy
blepharoplasty
tarsectomy
tarsoplasty
tarsorrhaphy
tarsotomy

eye pain
ophthalmagra
ophthalmalgia
ophthalmodynia

eye pupil contracting
miosis

eye refraction measurer
refractometer
  instrument used to measure the deflec-
  tion of light rays

eye refraction unequal
anisometropia
heterometropia

eye shiny particles
synchysis scintillans
  in the vitreous humor

eye softness
ophthalmomalacia
scleromalacia
synchysis
  abnormal softening of the eyeball

eye specialist
oculist
ophthalmologist

eye steel detector
sideroscope
  instrument used in detecting fragments
  of metal

eye tension measurer
tonometer

eye torsion measurer
clinoscope

eye turned left
levoversion
levoduction

eye turned right
dextroversion

eye turned upward
anaphoria
anatropia
  habit or tendency

eye twitching
blepharospasm
blephaospasmus

eye viewer
auto-ophthalmoscope
ophthalmoscope

eyeball covering
conjunctiva
  also coating inside the eyelid

eyeball dryness preventer
antixerophthalmic
antixerotic

eyeball enlargement
buphthalmia
buphthalmos
buphthalmus

eyeball inflammation
endophthalmitis
  inner tissues
panophthalmitis
  all tissues

trichiasis
trichoma
  caused by misplaced eyelashes

eyeball measurer
exophthalmometer
exophthalmometry
proptometer

eyeball movement
oculogyration

eyeball protrusion
exophthalmos
exophthalmus
ophthalmocele

eyeball recession
enophthalmia
enophthalmos
  recession of the eyeball within the orbit

eyeball rupture
ophthalmorrhexis

eyeball smallness
microphthalmia
microphthalmus
nanophthalmia
nanophthalmos
nanophthalmus

eyebrow loss
madarosis

eyebrows meeting
synophrys

eyebrow wrinkling
ophryosis
  caused by spasmodic twitching of the
  nearby muscles

eyelash loss
madarosis
milphosis

eyelash excess
polystichia
  more than one row

eyelid
blepharon
palpebra

eyelid adhesion
ankyloblepharon
blepharosynechia
symblepharon

eyelid aperature small
blepharophimosis

eyelid contraction
blepharospasm
blepharospasmus

eyelid/cornea adhesion
corneoblepharon

eyelid drooping
blepharoptosis

eyelid edema
blepharedema
  causing a baggy appearance

eyelid growth
xanthelasma

eyelid holder
blepharostat
  speculum for diagnostic or treatment
  use

eyelid inflammation
blepharitis
palpebritis
blepharadenitis
  tarsal glands
blepharitis ciliari
blepharitis marginalis
blepharoconjunctivitis
  fatty glands on the edge of the eyelids

eyelid inversion
entrophe
entropion

eyelid largeness
macroblepharia

eyelid not closing
blepharodiastasis
  abnormal separation or inability to close

eyelid operation
blepharectomy
blepharoplasty
blepharotomy
sphincterectomy

eyelid smallness
microblepharia
microblepharism
microblepharon

eyelid spasm
blepharoclonus

eyelid wink
nictate
nictation

eyelid suture
blepharorrhaphy
tarsorrhaphy

eyelid sweat
blepharochromhidrosis

eyelid softness
tarsomalacia
of the cartilage

eyelid thickness
blepharopachynsis
pachyblepharon

eyelid tumor
blepharoadenoma
blepharoncus
blepharophyma

eyelid varicosity
varicoblepharon

eyelid wart
pladaroma
pladarosis
a soft wartlike growth on the eyelid

eyestrain
copiopia

F

face cleft
schistoprosopus

face defective
prosoposchisis
congenital fissure

face enlargement
pseudoacromegaly

face lacking
aprosopia
congenital defect

face largeness
macroprosopia
megaprosopia
prosopectasia
macroprosopous
the individual

face lift
rhytidoplasty

face narrowness
leptoprosopia

face/neck
cervicofacial

face pain
prosoponeuralgia

face shortness
brachyfacial
brachyprosopic

face smallness
microprosopus

face spasm
prosopospasm
risus sardonicus
facial tic

facial neuralgia
prosopalgia
prosoponeuralgia
tic douloureux

facial paralysis
prosopoplegia
diplegia facial
prosopodiplegia

falling organ
prolapse
ptosis
blepharoptosis
drooping of upper eyelid
gastroptosis
falling of stomach
hysteroptosis
falling of uterus

falling sickness
epilepsy

Fallopian tube calculus
salpingolithiasis

Fallopian tube hernia
salpingocele
salpingo-oophorocele

Fallopian tube inflamed
salpingitis
salpingo-oophoritis
tubes and ovaries
salpingoperitonitis
tubes and peritoneum

Fallopian tube operation
  salpingectomy
  salpingo-oophorectomy
  salpingoovariectomy
  salpingopexy
  salpingoplasty
  salpingolysis
  salpingostomatomy
  salpingostomy
  salpingotomy

Fallopian tube suture
  salpingorrhaphy

Fallopian tube x-ray
  salpingography

false anemia
  pseudoanemia
    pallor of skin without signs of anemia

false joint
  neoarthrosis
  pseudarthrosis

false neuritis
  pseudoneuritis

false pregnancy
  phantom pregnancy
  pseudocyesis

false ribs
  costae spuriae

false smell
  pseudosmia
    sensation of an odor that is not present

false taste perception
  pseudogeusia

false tetanus
  pseudotetanus

false vision
  pseudoblepsia
  pseudopsia
    visual hallucinations

farsightedness
  hypermetropia
  hyperopipresbyopia
  presbyope

fascia inflammation
  fascitis

fascia operation
  fasiectomy

fascioplasty
fasciotomy
fasciodesis

fascia suture
  aponeurorrhaphy
  fasciorrhaphy

fast eating
  tachyphagia

fast talking
  agitolalia
  agitophasia
  tachylogia
  tachyphasia
  tachyphemia
  tachyphrasia

fat
  adipose
  obese
  pimelosis

fat absorption
  lipometabolism
  lipophagy
    ingestion of fat by a fat-absorbing cell

fat in blood
  hyperlipemia
  hyperlipidemia
  lipemia
  lipidemia
  lipoidemia

fat cell
  lipocyte

fat in cornea
  lipoidosis corneae

fat decomposition
  lipolysis
    chemical decomposition

fat decreasing
  lipotropic

fat deficiency
  lipopenia

fat deposits
  adiposis
  lipoidosis
  lipomatosis
  liposis
  steatopygia
    in the cells

fat in feces
pimelorrhea
steatorrhea

fat formation/increase
lipogenesis
lipogenic
lipogenetic
lipogenous
lipotrophy

fat inflammation
pimelitis
inflammation of adipose tissue

fat ingesting
ipophage

fat necrosis
steatonecrosis

fat particle
chylomicron
microscopic particle occurring in chyle
or blood

fat pertaining
aliphatic
sebaceous

fat resembling
lipoid

fat soluble
lipid
liposoluble

fat storing
adipopexis
adipopeptic

fat tumor
lipoma
lipomyoma
lipomyxoma
liposarcoma
pimeloma
steatoma

fat in urine
adiposuria
lipiduria
lipoiduria
lipuria
excretion of lipid in the urine

fat of wool
lanolin

Father of Medicine
Hippocrates
Greek physician 460-377 B.C.

fatty degeneration
steatosis

fatty tumors
adiposis tuberosa simplex
Anders' disease
nodular type, often on the abdomen

fauna and flora
biota

fear of air current
aerophobia

fear of alcoholic beverages
alcoholophobia

fear of angina pectoris
anginophobia

fear of animals
zoophobia

fear of bees
apiphobia
melissophobia

fear of being afraid
phobophobia

fear of being alone
monophobia
morbid dread of solitude

fear of being beaten
rhabdophobia

fear of blushing
ereuthophobia

fear of books
bibliophobia
morbid dread or hatred of books

fear to be bound
merinthophobia

fear of bridge crossing
gephyrophobia

fear to be buried alive
taphophobia

fear of cancer
cancerophobia
carcinophobia

fear of cats
ailurophobia

fear of certain places
topophobia

fear of change
neophobia

morbid aversion to novelty or the unknown

fear of childbirth
maieusiophobia
tocophobia

fear of children
pedophobia

fear of choking
pnigophobia

fear of climbing
climacophobia

fear of closed places
claustrophobia

fear of cold
psychrophobia

fear of colors
chromatophobia
chromophobia

fear of confinement
claustrophobia

fear of contamination
mysophobia
fear of dirt or defilement from touching familiar objects

fear of crowds
ochlophobia

fear of dampness
hygrophobia

fear of darkness
nyctophobia
scotophobia
morbid fear of night or the dark

fear of dawn
eosophobia

fear of daylight
phengophobia

fear of death
necrophobia
thanatophobia

fear of deformity
taratophobia
in others
dysmorphophobia
in self

fear of depths
bathophobia

fear of deserted places
eremophobia
or of solitude

fear of dirt
mysophobia
rhypophobia

fear of disease
hypochondria
hypochondriasis
nosophobia
pathophobia

fear of dogs
cynophobia

fear of dolls
pediophobia
morbid fear aroused by the sight of a child or a doll

fear of draft/wind
aerophobia
anemophobia

fear of drugs
pharmacophobia

fear of dust
amathophobia

fear of eating
phagophobia
sitophobia

fear of electricity
electrophobia

fear of errors/sins
hamartophobia

fear of everything
panphobia

fear of fatigue
kopophobia
ponophobia

fear of feces
coprophobia

fear of fever
pyrexeophobia

fear of filth
rhypophobia
rupophobia

fear of fire
pyrophobia

fear of fish
ichthyophobia

fear of flashing light
selaphobia

fear of food
cibophobia
sitophobia
morbid fear of eating food

fear of forests
hylephobia

fear of fresh air
aerophobia
also of drafts

fear of frogs
batrachophobia

fear of fur
doraphobia
touching fur or skin

fear of germs
microphobia

fear of ghosts
phasmophobia

fear of glass
crystallophobia
hyalophobia

fear of God
heophobia

fear of hair
trichophobia
morbid disgust over loose hair
trichopathophobia
anxiety about one's hair

fear of hearing certain names
onomatophobia

fear of heart disease
cardiophobia

fear of heat
thermophobia

fear of heights
acrophobia

fear of hell
hadephobia
stygiophobia

fear to be home
ecophobia
oikophobia
fear of one's home surroundings

fear of humans
anthropophobia
phobanthropy

fear of ideas
ideophobia

fear of infection
molysmophobia

fear of injury
traumatophobia

fear of insanity
maniaphobia

fear of insects
entomophobia

fear of itching
acarophobia
also fear of parasites or of small particles

fear of jealousy
zelophobia

fear of left side
levophobia

fear of lice
pediculophobia

fear of light
photodysphoria
photophobia

fear of lightening/thunder
astrapophobia
keraunophobia

fear of loneliness
eremiophobia
eremophobia

fear of love
erotophobia
aversion to the thought of sexual love and expression

fear of machinery
mechanophobia

fear of many things
polyphobia

fear of marriage
gamophobia

fear of medicines
pharmacophobia

fear of men
androphobia
the male sex as a whole
anthropophobia
any man or men

fear of metal
metallophobia

fear of meteors
meteorophobia

fear of mirrors
spectrophobia

fear of missles
ballistophobia

fear of moisture/dampness
hygrophobia

fear of motion
kinesophobia

fear of naked persons
gymnophobia

fear of names
nomatophobia
onomatophobia

fear of needles
belonephobia
also of pins and other sharp pointed objects

fear of neglect
paralipophobia

fear of newness
neophobia

fear of night
nyctophobias
scotophobia

fear of nothing
pantaphobia
fearless

fear of novelties
neophobia

fear of odors
bromidosiphobia
osmophobia
osphresiophobia

fear of old age
gerontophobia

fear of open spaces
agoraphobia

cenophobia
kenophobia
also fear of leaving familiar surroundings

fear of own voice
phonophobia
or of any sound

fear of pain
algophobia

fear of parasites
acarophobia
parasitophobia
phthiriophobia

fear of people
anthropophobia

fear of personal uncleanliness
automysophobia

fear of personal odor
bromhidrosiphobia

fear of physical contact
aphephobia
haphephobia

fear of pins
belonephobia
or of any sharp pointed object

fear of places
topophobia

fear of pleasure
hedonophobia

fear of pointed objects
aichmophobia
fear of being touched by the object

fear of poison
iophobia
toxicophobia
toxiphobia

fear of poverty
peniaphobia

fear of prepices
cremnophobia

fear of pregnancy
maieusiophobia
extreme dread of childbirth

fear of projectiles/missiles
ballistophobia

fear of rabies
lyssophobia

fear of railways
siderodromophobia

fear of rain
ombrophobia

fear of rectal disease
proctophobia
rectophobia

fear of red
erythrophobia

fear of religious/sacred objects
hierophobia

fear of responsibility
hypengyophobia

fear of returning home
nostophobia

fear of right side
dextrophobia
   fear of objects to the right

fear of rivers
potamophobia

fear of robbers
harpaxophobia

fear of seas
thalassophobia

fear to be seen
scopophobia
   a dread of being looked at

fear of self
autophobia

fear of sermons
homilophobia

fear of sexual intercourse
coitophobia
cypridophobia

fear of sexual love
erotophobia

fear of sharp objects
aichmophobia
belonephobia
   as needles, pins, or any sharp object

fear of sins
hamartophobia
peccatiphobia

fear of sitting down
kathisophobia

fear of skin of animals
doraphobia

fear of skin diseases
dermatophobia

fear of sleep
hypnophobia

fear of small objects
microphobia
   also fear of parasites or bacteria

fear of snakes
ophidiophobia

fear of society
anthropophobia
phobanthropy

fear of solitude
autophobia
eremophobia
monophobia

fear of sounds
acousticophobia
phonophobia

fear of speaking
laliophobia
   morbid fear of speaking or stuttering

fear of spiders
arachnephobia

fear of stairs
climacophobia

fear of standing
stasiphobia
stasibasiphobia

fear of stealing
kleptophobia

fear of strangers
xenophobia

fear of streets
agyiophobia
   a type of agarophobia

fear of stuttering
laliophobia

fear of sun rays
heliophobia

fear of syphilis
syphilophobia

fear of teeth
odontophobia

fear of thirteen
triakaidekaphobia
triskaidekaphobia
superstitious dread of the number thirteen

fear of thunder
astrapophobia
brontophobia
keraunophobia
tonitrophobia

fear of time
chronophobia

fear to be touched
aphephobia
haphephobia

fear of trains
siderodromophobia

fear of trauma
traumatophobia

fear of travel
hodophobia

fear of trembling
remophobia

fear of trichina
trichinophobia
fear of contracting disease from uncooked meat

fear of tuberculosis
phthisiophobia
tuberculophobia

fear of uncleanliness
automysophobia
fear of personal uncleanliness

fear of vaccination
vaccinophobia

fear of vehicles
amaxophobia
hamaxophobia
fear of meeting or of riding in any sort of vehicle

fear of venereal diseases
cypridophobia
venereophobia

fear of vomiting
emetophobia

fear of walking
basiphobia

fear of water
aquaphobia
potamophobia

fear of wind/draft
anemophobia

fear of women
gynephobia

fear of work
ergasiophobia
ponophobia
aversion to work of any kind

fear of worms
helminthophobia

fear of writing
graphophobia

febrifuge
antipyretic

febrile
pyrectic
pyretic

feces bag
colostomy bag
also ileostomy bag

feces calcified
coprolith
fecalith

feces eating
coprophagy
scatophagy

feces with fat
pimelorrhea
steatorrhea
fatty diarrhea
excessive amounts

feces with pus
pyochezia

feces uncontrolled
incontinence

feeblemindedness
amentia
cretinism

feeding on carrion
necrophagous
refers to decayed or decaying flesh

feeding on food of all kinds
omnivorous

feeding on one food
monophagism

feeding unnatural way
enteral feeding/nutrition
hyperalimentation
parenteral alimentation
rectal alimentation
forms of therapeutic nutritional intake

feeling of discomfort
dysphoria

feeling of superiority
egomania

feeling of well-being
euphoria

feet in excess
polypodia

feet gigantic
acrodolichmelia
large size and disproportionate growth of the hands and feet

feet lacking
apodia
apodial
apodous
ectropody
apody
apus
individual involved

feet largeness
macropodia
megalopodia
pes gigas

feet malformed
peropus

feet shortness
brachypodous

feet sweat increased
acrohyperhidrosis
also applicable to the hands

fertilization
gametogenesis

fetal operation
amniotomy
cephalotomy

fetal surgical tool
cephalotome
cephalotribe

fetal thyroid tumor
microfollicular adenoma

fetus calcified
lithokelyphopedion
lithokelyphopedium
lithopedion
lithopedium
*osteopedion**
*obsolete term

fetus deformity
abrachiocephaly
acephalobrachius
without head and arms
acephalocardius
without head and heart
acephalocheirus
acephalochirus
without head and hands
acephalogaster
twin with pelvis and legs only
acephalopodius
without head and feet
acephalorrhachia
without head or vertebra
acephalostomia
without head
acephalothorus
without head and thorax
acephalus
without head
acheilia
achilia
without lips
acheira
achiria
without hands
acorea
without pupils
acormus
without trunk
acrania
without skull
acystia
without urinary bladder
adactyl
without fingers or toes
agenosomia
agenosomus
without genitalia
aglossia
without tongue
aglossostomia
without tongue or mouth opening

agnathia
 undeveloped or missing jaws
agyria
 without cerebral convolutions
amelia
amelus
 without extremities
ametria
 without uterus
amyelencephalia
amyelencephalus
 without brain and spinal cord
amyelia
amyelic
amyelous
amyelus
 without spinal cord
anadidymus duplicatos
 pelvis and lower extremities united
aniridia
irideremia
 iris lacking
anophthalmia
anophthalmos
anophthalmus
 without eyes
anorchia
 without testes
apleuria
 without ribs
apneumia
 without lungs
apodia
apus
 without feet
aposthia
 without prepuce
aproctia
 without anus opening
aprosopia
 without face
arrhinia
arhinia
 without nose
asternia
 without sternum
astomia
 without mouth
atelencephalia
ateloencephalia
 with imperfect brain
athelia
 without nipple

atrachelocephalus
 head and neck missing or undeveloped
atresia
 imperforation of normal opening
atretocystia
 urinary bladder imperforate
atretogastria
 cardiac/pyloric orifice imperforate
brachycephalia
brachycephaly
 short head
brachychilia
 short lips
brachydactylia
brachydactlic
brachydactyly
 short fingers
brachyglossia
brachyglossal
 short tongue
brachygnathia
brachygnathous
 short lower jaw
brachykerkic
 forearm disproportionate
brachymetapody
 shortness of metatarsals or metacarpals
brachyphalangia
 shortness of phalanges
brachypodous
 short legs
brachyrhinia
 shortness of nose
brachyrhynchus
 shortness of maxilla and nose
brachyskelic
 short legs
abdominal fissure
celosomia
celosomus
schistocelia
schistocoelia
 open body with eventration
cryptophthalmos
 eyelids stuck together
cyclencephaly
cyclocephalia
cyclocephaly
 poor development of the two cerebral
 hemispheres
cyclopia
cyclops
 both eyes fused into one
deranencephalia

fetus deformity (cont.)

deranencephaly
  neck without head
didactylism
  only two fingers or toes
diglossia
  split tongue
dignathus
  two lower jaws
diphallus
  double penis
diplocoria
  double pupil
ectrodactylia
ectrodactyly
ectrodactylism
  fingers or toes missing
ectromelia
  limb missing or defective
ectropody
  without feet
ectrosyndactyly
  fingers/toes fused/lacking
hyperdactylia
hyperdactylism
hyperdactyly
polydactyly
  excessive fingers or toes
hypophalangism
  phalanges missing
hypospadias
  urethral opening abnormal
irideremia
aniridia
  iris lacking
lipostomy
  mouth missing
lithopedion
lithopedium
lithokelyphopedion
lithokelyphopedium
  calcified fetus
lusus naturae
  a monstrosity
melomelus
  rudimentary limb
melotia
  displacement of the ear
meroacrania
  parts of the skull missing
miopus
  additional rudimentary face
monobrachius
  having only one arm
monodactylism

monodactyly
  having only one finger or toe
monophthalmos
  having only one eye
monopidia
monopus
  having only one foot
monorchidism
monorchism
  having only one testis
omacephalus
  parasitic twin with imperfect head and
  no upper extremities
opocephalus
  without mouth and nose
ostembryon
  archaic term for lithopedion
otocephalus
  lower jaw missing
pantamorphia
  general deformity
pantanencephalia
pananencephaly
  without brain
paracephalus
  parasitic twin with defective head,
  trunks, and limbs
paragnathus
  parasitic fetus attached laterally to the
  jaw
peracephalus
  parasitic twin with only legs and pelvis
perobrachius
  forearms and hands malformed
perochirus
  hand absent or underdeveloped
perocormus
perosomus
  defective trunk
perodactylia
perodactyly
  fingers or toes defective
peromelia
peromelus
  malformation of limbs
peropus
  feet defective
perosomus
  body malformed
perosplanchnica
  viscera malformed
phocomelia
polymelus
  excessive number of limbs

polymeria
   additional body parts
polydentia
polyodontia
   excessive number of teeth
polyorchisism
polyorchism
polyorchis
   excessive number of testes
polyotia
   more than one ear
polyphalangia
polyphalangism
   additional phalanx in finger or toe
polypodia
   more than two feet
polythelia
   additional nipples
porencephalic
porencephalous
porencephaly
   insufficient development of the cerebral
   cortex and gray matter
proencephalus
   part of frontal skull missing
prognathism
   projecting jaws
pseudotruncus arteriosus
   defective heart and usually without pulmonary artery
ilioxiphopagus
   having two heads and two chests
schistocormus
   open thorax
schistoglossia
   cleft tongue
schistomelus
   cleft extremity
schistoprosopus
   fissue of the face
schistorrhachis
   open spinal cord
schistosomus
   lateral or middle eventration and defective lower extremities
schistosternia
   sternal fissure
schistothorax
   fissure of the thorax
schistotrachelus
tracheloschisis
   cervical fissure
schizogyria
   partial separation of the cerebral gyri

macropodia
   feet size excessive
symelus
symellus
sympus
   both legs fused together
sirenomelia
sirenomelus
sympus apus
uromelus
   fused legs and no feet
strophocephalus
strophocephaly
   deformity of lower face
sympus monopus
   fusion of legs with foot missing
cyclopia
synophthalmia
synophthalmus
   fusion of eyes and orbits
synorchidism
synorchism
   fusion of testes in the abdomen or scrotum
synotia
synotus
   union or near union of the ears in the
   neck region
tetrabrachius
   double fetus with four arms
tetradactyl
   four digits on each limb
tetramastia
   four breasts
tetrapus
tetrascelus
   four feet
tetramelus
   four legs or four arms
tetrastichiasis
   four rows of eyelashes
tetrotus
   four ears
thoracoceloschisis
   fissure of thorax and abdomen
thoracoschisis
   fissure of thorax
tribrachius
   three arms
tricephalus
   three heads
triencephalus
triocephalus
   no organs of sight, hearing or smell

fetus deformity (cont.)

triophthalmos
combined twins with three eyes
riopodymus
three faces with only one head
triorchidism
triorchis
three testes
triotus
three ears
hyperphalangism
triphalangia
triphalangism
three phalanges in the thumb or big toe
triprosopus
three faces fused into one

fetus first feces
meconium

fetus lacking
afetal

fetus monitor
cardiotography
monitoring of fetal heart rate

fetus nutrition
cyotrophy
embryotrophy

fetus ossified
lithopedion
*ostembryon**
*obsolete term

fever blister
herpes simplex
herpes virus

fever causing
febrifacient
pyrogen

fever induced
hyperthermia

fever lacking
afebrile
apyrexia
apyrexial
apyretic

fever reducer
antipyretic

fibrin in blood
fibremia
fibrinemia

inosemia
presence in the blood, causing clotting

fibrocartilage inflamed
fibrochondritis
inochondritis

fibrous tumor
fibroma
neurofibroma
neuroma

filth eating
rhypophagy
scatophagy
eating of excrement

fingers abnormally long
arachnodactyly
dolichostenomelia

fingers/toes adhesion
ankylodactylia

finger communication
cheirology
chirology
dactylology

finger contracton
dactylospasm

fingers/toes defective
perodactylia
perodactyly
perodactylus
individual involved

fingers of equal length
isodactylism

fingers in excess
hyperdactylia
hyperdactylism
hyperdactyly
polydactylism
polydactyly
congenital development of supernumerary digits

fingers fused
syndactylia
syndactyly
syndactylous
zygodactyly

fingers inflamed
dactylitis

finger/toe lacking
adactyly
ectrodactylia

ectrodactylism
ectrodactyly
monodactylism
monodactyly
oligodactylia
oligodactyly
    congenital absence of one or more dig-
    its

finger largeness
dactylomegaly
macrodactylia
macrodactyly
macrodactylism
megadactyly
megalodactyly
    enlargement of one or more digits

finger shortness
brachydactylia
brachydactyly

finger slenderness
leptodactylous

finger/toe smallness
microdactylia
microdactylous
microdactyly
    smallness or shortness of the fingers or
    toes

finger thickness
pachydactylia
pachydactylous
pachydactyly

fingers unequal
anisodactylous
anisodactyly

fingerprint study
dactylography
dactyloscopy

first milk
colostrum
protogala
    first milk secreted at the termination of
    pregnancy

fish oils
eicosapentaenoic acids
omega-3 fatty acids

fish poisoning
ichthyismus
ichthyism

fish study
ichthyology

fishskin disease
ichthyosis
    thick, scaly skin

fission reproduction
schizogenesis

fissure in abdomen
celoschisis
celosomia
celosomus
kelosomus
    individual involved

fissure of sternum
sternoschisis

fistula operation
fistulectomy
fistuloenterostomy
fistulotomy

five children
quintipara
    woman who has given birth
quintuplet
    one of the children born

five day recurring
quintan
    refers to symptom or disease

five fingered/toed
pentadactyl
pentadactyle

flame imagination
pyroptothymia
    belief of engulfment in flames

flask shaped
lageniform

flat celled
planocellular

flat skull
platycephalic
platycephalous
platycephaly
platycrania
tapinocephalic
tapinocephaly
    having a low, flat shape to the head

flatfootedness
pes planus

flatulence reliever
carminative agent

flea killer
  pulicide

fleeing urge
  poriomania

flesh eater
  anthropophagy

flesh forming
  sarcotic

fleshy tumor
  sarcoma
    malignant tumor of the connective tissue

floating kidney
  nephroptosis

floating ribs
  costae fluctuantes
  costae fluitantes

flora and fauna
  biota
    collectively of a given region

flow of watery fluid
  hydrorrhea

fluid accumulation
  anasarca
    in subcutaneous connective tissue
  ascites
    in abdomen
  dropsy
    old term for edema
  edema
    in tissues
  hydrops
    in any body tissues or cavities
  hydrops fetalis
    in the newborn

fluid in cranial vault
  hydrocephalis
    accompanied by enlargement of the
    head and atrophy of the brain

fluid gravity measurer
  pyknometer

fluid in joints
  hydrarthrosis

fluid, watery
  serum

fluidless
  aneroid
  anhydrous

fly killer
  muscicide

food
  aliment
  nutriment

food aversion
  anorexia nervosa
  sitophobia

food craving
  bulemia
  cissa
  citta
  cittosis
  phagomania
  pica
  sitiomania
  sitomania
    abnormal appetite and/or for abnormal
    substances

food inadequate
  hypoalimentation

food stagnation
  ischochymia
    in stomach

foot burning
  erythromelalgia

foot care
  pedicure

foot doctor
  chiropodist
  podiatrist
  podologist

foot gout
  podagra

foot-joint inflammation
  podarthritis

foot lacking
  sympus monopus
    congenital defect

foot largeness
  macropodia
  pes gigas

foot odor
  podobromhidrosis

foot operation
  tarsectomy
  tarsotomy

foot pain
  podalgia

pododynia
tarsalgia

foot smallness
micropodia
micropus
  individual involved

foot sole
planta pedis

foot sole application
suppedania
suppedanum ·

foot thickness
pachypodous

foot treatment
chiropody

footless
apodia
apody
monopus
sirenomelia
sirenomelus
  congenital absence

footless/headless
acephalopodia
acephalopodius

footprint
ichnogram

forearm
antebrachial
antebrachium

forearm inner bone
ulna

forearm shortness
brachykerkic

foreign body extractor
protractor

foreign substance in blood
embolemia

foreign substance use
ergogenic

foremilk
colostrum

foreskin
prepuce
  free fold of skin that covers the glans
  penis

foreskin lacking
aposthia

foreskin tightness
phimosis
  narrowness of the opening of the prepuce

form equal
homeomorphous

formation of gas
aerogenesis
aerogenic
aerogenous
  production and/or formation of gas

foul breath
halitosis
ozostomia

four arms
tetrabrachius

four breasts
tetramastia

four children
quadripara
  woman who has given birth
quadruplet
  one of the children born

four digits
tetradactyl

four ears
tetrotus

four extremity paralysis
quadriplegia

four eyelash rows
tetrastichiasis

four feet
tetrapus
  congenital deformity

four-footed animal
quadruped

four hands
tetrachirus

four legs/arms
tetramelus
tetrascelus

fracture intentional
diaclasia
diclasis
osteoclasis

freak of nature
lusus naturae
  extensive fetal malformation

freckle
ephelis
ephelides

freezing point finder
cryoscope

frenum operation
frenectomy
frenoplasty
frenotomy

frequent urination
micturitition
nocturia
nycturia
abnormally frequent urge to urinate

front and below
anteroinferior

front and side
anterolateral

front to back
anteroposterior

frontal headache
metopodynia

frost itch
pruritus hiemalis

fructose in blood
fructosemia
levulosemia

fructose in urine
fructosuria
levulosuria
excretion of fruit sugar in the urine

fruit sugar
levulose

function in excess
hyperfunction

function reduced
hypofunction

fundus viewer
funduscope
instrument to view the fundus of the eye

fungus suppressor
antimycotic

fungus disease
actinomycosis
mycosis
tinea
of the hair, skin or nails

fungus study
mycology

funnel chest
pectus excavatum

funnel-shaped
infundibular

fused ears
cyclotus
synotia
synotus

fuzz
pappus
first downy growth of beard

G

gait acceleration
festination
as seen in nervous disorders

gallbladder dilatation/distention
cholecystectasia

gallbladder inflammation
cholecystitis
pericholangitis
tissues around the bile duct
periangiocholitis
pericholecystitis
tissues around the gallbladder

gallbladder pain
cholecystalgia

gallbladder/intestine suture
cholecystenterorrhaphy

gallbladder operation
cholecystectomy
cholecystotomy
cholecystopexy
cholecystorrhaphy
cholecystenterostomy
cholecystocolostomy
cholecystoduodenostomy
cholecystostomy
cholecystogastrostomy
cholecystojejunostomy

choledochectomy
choledochostomy
choledochoplasty
choledochorrhaphy

gallbladder stones
cholecystolithiasis
cholelith
cholelithiasis
presence or formation of gallstones

gallbladder x-ray
cholecystogram
cholecystography

gallstone crushing
choledocholithotripsy
cholelithotripsy

ganglion inflammation
ganglionitis
periganglitis

gas/air in chest
pneumothorax
air or gas with fluid in the chest cavity

gas/air in intestines
aerenterectasia
meteorism
tympanites

gas/air in mediastinum
pneumomediastinum

gas/air in peritoneal cavity
aeroperitonia
aeroperitoneum
pneumoperitoneum

gas/air vaginal distention
aerocolpos

gas/fluid removal
aspiration
suction to remove accumulation from a body cavity

gas in body tissues
aerosis

gas density measurer
aerometer

gas formation
aerogenesis
aerogenic
aerogenous

gas/liquid in tissues
hydropneumatosis

gas pain

tympanism
tympanites
distention due to air or gas in the intestine or peritoneal cavity

gas pressure measurer
manometer

gas in urine
pneumaturia

gas volume gauge
eudiometer
instrument to measure volume

gastric juice hormone
gastrin

gastric secretion lacking
achylia

genetic engineering
biotechnology
recombinant DNA

genital plastic operation
gynoplastics
reconstructive surgery of the female reproductive organs

genitals defective
agenosomia

geographic tongue
erythema migrans linguas
tongue with bare patches and thickened outer covering

germ absorbing
fomes
fomite
inanimate object that may retain infectious germs

germ cell
gonocyte

germ free
gnotobiota
gnotobiote
organisms without any contam-inating microorganisms

German measles
rubella

gestures/signs lacking
animia
loss of ability to communicate by means of gestures or signs
ataxic animia
inability to gesture due to paralysis or physical disorder

ghost hallucination
  phantasmoscopia
  phantasmoscopy

gigantism
  somatomegaly

girdle pain
  zonesthesia
    sensation of tightness in lower abdominal area

gland/adenoids knife
  adenotome
    instrument to incise a gland or to remove adenoids

gland deficiency
  adenasthenia

gland development
  adenogenesis

gland disease
  adenosis

gland enlargement
  adenia

gland fibroid degeneration
  adenofibrosis

gland hardening
  adenosclerosis

gland hyperplasia
  adenomatous

gland inflammation
  adenitis
    gland or lymph node
  adenophlegmon
    gland and connecting tissue
  bartholinitis
    major vestibular glands
  myxadenitis
    mucous gland
  paradenitis
  periadenitis
    tissues surrounding a gland
  perithyroiditis
    thyroid gland capsules
  thyroadenitis
  thyroiditis
    thyroid gland
  strumitis
    goiterous thyroid gland

sialadenitis
sialoadenitis
    salivary gland
skeneitis
skenitis
    glands near the urethra
sublinguitis
    gland under the tongue
submaxillaritis
    submaxillary gland
tarsadenitis
    tarsal gland and plate

gland operation
  adenectomy
  adenotomy
  parathyroidectomy
  parotidectomy
  pinealectomy
  prostatectomy
  prostatotomy
  prostatolithotomy
  sialoadenectomy
  sialoadenotomy
  sialolithotomy
  sialodochoplasty
  suprarenalectomy
  thyroidectomy
  thyroidotomy

gland/organ cells
  parenchyma
    distinguishing cells of a gland or organ

gland pain
  adenalgia

gland softness
  adenomalacia

gland stone
  sebolith
    in a sebaceous gland

gland tissue growth
  adenomatosis

gland tumor
  adenocarcinoma
  adenocystoma
  adenoepithelioma
  adenolipoma
  adenolymphoma
  adenoma
  adenosarcoma

gland in wrong place
  adenectopia
    malposition or displacement of a gland

glandlike
adeniform
adenoid
adenose
adenous

glass tube
buret
burette
pipet
pipette
graduated tube used to deliver a measured amount of liquid or gas

glasslike
hyaline
hyaloid
vitreous

glaucoma operation
sclerostomy

globular tumor
spheroma

globulin in urine
globulinuria

glucose in blood
glycemia

god of medicine
Aesculapius
Asklepios
Greek god of medicine

goiter
thyrocele
chronic enlargement of the thyroid gland

goiter inflammation
strumitis

goiter operation
strumectomy

gold therapy
chrysotherapy
treatment of disease by the administration of gold salts

gonococci in blood
gonococcemia

gout in foot
podagra
especially of the great toe

gout in knee joint
gonagra

gout in neck
trachelagra

gout reliever
antarthritic
antiarthritic
uricosuric

gouty deposit in joint
arthrolith
tophus
chalkstone*
*obsolete term

grafting
heteroosteoplasty
heteroplasty
grafting a bone taken from an animal
heterotransplantation
grafting any part taken from a different species
homograft
homoplasty
homotransplantation
grafting taken from same species

gravel in urine
uropsammus

gray matter inflammation
poliomyelitis
of the spinal cord

grayness of hair
canities
poliosis

greasy
oleaginous

greatness delusion
megalomania
megalomaniac

green sickness
chlorosis
chlorotic
anemic disease in young females

green vision
chloropsia

groin area
inguinal

groin pain
inguinodynia

groove between nates
gluteal furrow
sulcus gluteus

groove on brain
sulcus
a depression on the brain surface separating the folds

growth
accretion

gum
gingiva
pertaining to area of the mouth

gum abscess
gumboil
parulis

gum bleeding
ulorrhagia

gum inflammation
gingivitis
gingivoglossitis
gums and tongue
gingivostomatitis
gums and mouth

gum operation
gingivectomy
ulotomy

H

hair beading
monilethrix
moniliform
hereditary condition of marked constrictions in the hair

hair brittleness
sclerothrix
trichatrophia
trichorrhexis

hair calcified
tricholith

hair component
keratin
principal component of hair

hair deficiency
hypotrichiasis
hypotrichosis
oligotrichia
oligotrichosis

hair disease
trichitis
trichomycosis
trichopathy

hair in excess
hypertrichosis
polytrichia
excessive growth of hair over all or part of the body

hair follicles inflamed
acne decalvans
folliculitis
perifolliculitis

hair fungus disease
trichomycosis
trichosporosis

hair gray
canities
poliosis

hair growth abnormal
hirsutism
paratrichosis
pilosis
hypertrichosis lanuginosa
on the body of the fetus

hair harsh/dry
sclerothrix
sclerotrichia
xerasia

hair inversion
trichiasis
turning inward of the hair surrounding an opening

hair loss
acomia
for any reason
alopecia
total or partial loss
alopecia aereata
in patches
alopecia cicatrisata
in circular patches due to atrophy of the skin
alopecia senilis
due to aging
alopecia symptomatica
due to systemic or psychogenic causes
alopecia totalis
alopecia universalis
all over the body
atrichia
may be congenital or acquired
madarosis
trichosis
loss of eyelashes/eyebrows

oligotrichia
scarcity of hair
ophiasis
a serpentine form of baldness
phalacrosis
obsolete term for baldness
psilosis
due to a cutaneous disorder

hair of lower abdomen
pubescence
hair that grows at puberty

hair in nose
vibrissa

hair plucking
trichologia
trichology
the science of hair
trichotillomania
uncontrollable desire to pull out hair

hair removing
decalvent
depilate
depilation
depilatory
epilate
epilation
epilatory

hair scarcity
oligotrichia

hair-shaped
filiform

hair smooth/straight
leiotrichous

hair splitting
distrix
schizotrichia

hair-touch sensation
trichoesthesia
experienced when a hair is touched
trichoesthesiometer
instrument to measure the sensation

hair whiteness
leukotrichia
leukotrichous

hairless
glabrous
smooth and bare

hairlike
trichoid

hairy
hirsute
hirsutism
pilar
pilary
pilose

hairy tongue
glossotrichia
trichoglossia
nigrities linguae
black hairy tongue

hallucinatory condition
hallucinosis

hammer bone of ear
malleus

hammer nose
rhinophyma

hand
manus

hand arthritis
chirarthritis

hand burning
erythromelalgia
abnormal burning sensation of hands or
feet

hand dexterity
ambidexter
ambidextrous
individual that uses either hand equally
well

hand excessive number
polycheiria
polychiria

hand joint
articulatio manus

hand joint contraction
acrocontracture
shortening of the muscles in the joints of
hands or feet

hand joint inflammation
chirarthritis

hand lacking
acheiria
achiria
also sense of loss

hand largeness
acrodolichomelia

hand largeness (cont.)
cheiromegaly
chiromegaly
megalocheiria

hand operation
cheiroplasty
chiroplasty

hand smallness
microcheiria
microchiria

hand spasm
acromyotonia
acromyotonus

hand sweat increased
acrohyperhidrosis

hand underdeveloped
perochirus
individual with congenital defect
handless/headless
acephalocheirus
acephalochirus
malformed fetus without hands or head

handwriting study
graphology

hanging breast operation
mammoplasty
mastopexy
mazopexy

hard palate
palatum durum
roof of the mouth

hardening
sclerema
scleroma
sclerosis

hardening of bone
osteosclerosis

hardness measurer
sclerometer

hardness of an organ
scirrhosity

hare's eye
lagophthalmic
lagophthalmos
inability to close the eye

harelip
chiloschisis
cleft lip
congenital opening

harmful
deleteriour
noxious
toxin

harmless
innocuous
innoxious

hatred for children
misopedia
misopedy

hatred for mankind
misanthropy
aversion to people

hatred for marriage
misogamy

hatred for newness
misoneism

hatred for women
misogyny

hay fever
pollenosis
pollinosis
allergic reaction to pollen

head lacking
deranencephalia
deranencephaly

head cold
coryza
acute rhinitis

head largeness
macrocephalia
macrocephaly
megalocephaly

head measurer
cephalometer

head narrowness
stenocephalia
stenocephalic
stenocephalous
stenocephaly

head/neck lacking
atrachelocephalus
fetus with head and neck either lacking
or undeveloped

head pointed
acrocephalia
acrocephalic

acrocephaly
oxycephalic
oxycephaly
turricephaly

head smallness
microcephalia
microcephalism
microcephaly
microcephalus
nanocephalous
nanocaphaly

head to tall
cephalocaudal

head/thorax
cephalothoracic

head-top concave
clinocephaly

headache
cephalalgia
encephalalgia
general term
metopodynia
frontal headache
migraine
vascular cause
psychalalgia
psychalgia
psychalgic
usually caused by depression

headless
acephalus
acephalous

head/arm lacking
abrachiocephalus
abrachiocephaly
acephalobrachius
born without head and arms

head/foot lacking
acephalopodia
acephalopodius
born without head and feet

head/hand lacking
acephalocheirus
acephalochirus
born without head and hands

head/heart lacking
acephalocardia
born without head and heart

head/mouth lacking
acephalostomia

having a mouthlike opening in the upper part of neck/chest

head/spine lacking
acephalorrhachia
born without head and spinal column

head/thorax lacking
acephalothorus
born without head and chest

healing by massage
naprapathy

health anxiety
hypochondriac
hypochondriasis

healthy old age
agerasia

hearing acuteness
hyperacusia
hyperacusis
exceptionally acute sense of hearing

hearing dysfunction
diplacusis

hearing measurer
audiometer
audiometry

heart abnormally situated
bathycardia
ectocardia
exocardia

heart with air
aerendocardia

heart arrest
cardioplegic solution
induced condition

heart assist
counterpulsation
technique for decreasing workload of the heart by using an external pump

heart beat irregular
arrhythmia
cardiataxia
dysrhythmia
tumultus cordis

heart beat rapid
tachycardia

heart beat slow
brachycardia
bradycardia

heart chamber with air/gas
pneumatocardia

heart development
cardiogenesis

heart dilatation
cardiectasis

heart disease
cardiomyopathy
cardiopathy
designating primarily heart muscle disease

heart disease treatment
cardiotherapy

heart displacement
ectocardia
exocardia
cardioptosia
cardioptosis

heart enlargement
auxocardia
bucardia
cardiomegaly
cor bovinum
macrocardius

heart/great vessels
angiocardiopathy

heart hernia
cardiocele
protrusion of the heart through a wound or opening of the diphragm

heart inflammation
carditis
cardiopericarditis
endocarditis

heart lacking
acardia
acardiac
acardiacus
born without heart

heart largeness
cardiomegaly
macrocardia
macrocardius
megalocardia

heart membrane
endocardium
lines the inner cavities of the heart
pericardium
surrounds the heart

heart monitor
cardiography
graphic recording of a physical or functional aspect of the heart

heart operation
cardiectomy
cardiocentesis
cardio-omentopexy
cardiopericardiopexy
cardiopuncture
cardiorrhaphy
cardiomyopexy
cardioplasty
cardiotomy

heart pain
cardialgia
cardiodynia

heart paralysis
cardioplegia
use of chemicals or cold to stop contractions during surgery

heart puncture
cardiocentesis
cardiopuncture

heart on right side
dextrocardia

heart rupture
cardiorrhexis

heart-shaped
cordate
cordiform

heart smallness
microcardia
microcardius

heart softness
cardiomalacia
softening of the muscular substances of the heart

heart stimulant
digitalis
dobutamine
ouabain
strophanthin

heart stroke
angina pectoris

heart study
cardiology

heart suture
cardiorrhaphy

heartburn
pyrosis

heart/head missing
acephalocardius
born without head and heart

heat deprivation
thermosteresis

heat insensibility
thermanalgesia
thermoanalgesia
thermoanesthesia

heat loss
thermolytic
thermolysis
dissipation of bodily heat such as by
evaporation

heat pain
thermalgesia
thermoalgesia

heat-producing
calorifacient

heat production measurer
calorimeter

heat sensitiveness
thermesthesia
thermoesthesia

heating tissues
diathermy
to decrease resistance to passage of radiation, electrical current or ultrasound

heel bone
calcaneus

heel pain
calcaneodynia

hemoglobin deficiency
oligochromemia
insufficient amount of hemoglobin in all
the red blood cells

hemoglobin excess
hemoglobinemia
excessive amount in the blood

hemoglobin measurer
hemoglobinometer

hemoglobin separation
hemolysis

hemoglobin in urine
hemoglobinuria

hemolysis preventer
antihemolytic

hemorrhage control
electrohemostasis

hemorrhage from ear
otorrhagia

hemorrhage from eye
ophthalmorrhagia

hemorrhage of intestine
enterorrhagia

hemorrhage of kidney
nephrorrhagia

hemorrhage of penis
balanorrhagia
inflammation with discharge of pus

hemorrhage of spinal cord
hematomyelia
hemorrhage into the substance of the
spinal cord

hemorrhage of stomach
gastrorrhagia

hemorrhage of veins
phleborrhagia

hemp poisoning
cannabism

heparin in blood
heparinemia

hernia of brain
cephalocele
encephalocele

hernia of choroid
choriocele
coat of the eye

hernia of diaphragm
diaphragmatocele

hernia with fatty tissue
adipocele
lipocele
hernia containing fat

hernia knife
herniotome
surgical instrument

hernia with omentum
epiplocele
epiploenterocele

hernia repair
hernioplasty
herniorrhaphy
herniotomy

hernia of spleen
lienocele

hernia of testes
orchiocele

hernia of umbilicus
omphalocele
protrusion at birth of part of the intestine through the abdominal wall

hernia of vagina
colpocele
vaginocele

heroin
diacetylmorphine

hinge joint
ginglymus

hip bone/socket
os coxae

hip joint
articulatio coxae

hip joint disease
coxarthropathy

hip operation
hemipelvectomy

hip pain
coxalgia
coxodynia

hippuric acid in urine
hippuria
excessive amounts

histamine in blood
histidemia
also reflected in excess urine levels

histidine in urine
histidinuria
also reflected in excess blood levels

histone in urine
histonuria

hives
urticaria

home life aversion
apodemialgia

homogentisic acid in urine
alkaptonuria

homosexuality
lesbianism
sapphism
among females

hook shaped
unciform
uncinate

hookworm disease
ancylostomiasis
necatoriasis
infestation with hookworms

hops
humulus

hops bitter
humulin
lupulin

hormone production
hormonopoiesis

horn component
keratin

horny
keratic
keratinous

horny skin
keratosis
any horny growth(e.g., wart or callus)

horse bone inflammation
peditis

hospital-related
nosocomial

housefly
musca domestica

hoy
phencyclidine (PCP)

human in form
anthropomorphism

humpbacked deformity
gibbosity
kyphosis

hunger in excess
bulimia
resulting from a mental disorder

hyalin in urine
hyalinuria

hydrochloric acid excess
hyperchlorhydria
in the gastric juice

hydrochloric acid low
hypochlorhydria

hydrogen sulfide in blood
hydrothionemia

hydrogen sulfide in urine
hydrothionuria

hydrolysis of proteins
proteolysis
splitting of proteins

hymen inflammation
hymenitis

hymen operation
hymenectomy
hymenotomy

hymen suture
hymenorrhaphy

hypnosis
autohypnosis
autohypnotic
induced by oneself
heterohypnosis
induced by another

hysteria controller
hysterofrenic

hysterical laughter
cachinnation

hysterical paralysis
pseudoplegia

I

idiocy
anoesia
anoia
inability to understand

idiopathic vomiting
autemesia

ileum inflammation
ileitis

ileocolitis
ileum and colon

ileum operation
ileectomy
ileotomy
ileocecostomy
ileocolostomy
ileoileostomy
ileosigmoidostomy
ileostomy

ileum suture
ileorrhaphy

ill health
cachectic
cachexia

illuminated viewer
caveascope
cavernoscope
celoscope
instrument for examining the interior of a
body cavity

image perception in excess
polyopia
polyopsia
seeing more than one image

imaginary odors
cacosmia
parosmia

immunity study
immunology

impairment of senses
dysesthesia
of any sense, especially sense of touch

imperforate cardiac opening
atretogastria

imperforate opening
atresic
atresia
atretic

imperforate pupil
atresia iridis
atretopsia

imperforate pyloric orifice
atretogastria

imperforate urethra
atreturethria

imperforate urinary bladder
atretocystia

impervious to heat
adiathermancy

impregnated ovum
cytula

inability to copy writing
dysantigraphia

Inability to decide
abulia
abulic
    deficiency of will power, initiative or
    drive

Inability to fix attention
aprosexia

inability to form sentences
acataphasia

Inability to locate sensation
atopognosia
atopognosis

Inability for mathematics
acalculia
    inability to calculate

Inability to name objects
anomia
nominal aphasia

Inability to recognize by touch
astereognosis
tactile amnesia
stereoagnosis
stereoanesthesia

Inability to relax
achalasia
    specifically the hollow muscular organs

Inability to arise
ananastasia
    from a sitting position

Inability to sit
acathisia
akathisia
akatizia
    motor restlessness, muscle quivering

Inability to sleep
agrypnia
insomnia

inability to speak
aphasia

Inability to stand

astasic
astatic
    to maintain an erect position
astasia abasia
    to stand or walk

inability to swallow
aphagia

inability to urinate
anuria
anuric

inability to write
agraphia
    loss of ability to write
agraphic
anorthography
    loss of ability to write correctly

inactive
quiescent

Incoherence of speech
allophasis

Incontinence of urine
enuresis
enuretic
uracrasia

incus operation
incudectomy
    of the ear

Indican In urine
indicanuria

Indifferent
adiphoria
    failure to respond to stimuli
pseudodementia
    exaggerated indifference to one's sur-
    roundings

Indigestion
dyspepsia
dyspeptic

Indigo in urine
indigouria
indiguria

indole in urine
indoluria

Indolacetic acid in urine
indolaceturia

Indoxyl in urine
indoxyluria
    secreted as indican

Infant cry
vagitus

infantile paralysis
poliomyelitis

inferiority conscious
micromania

Inflamed adnexa uteri
adnexitis
annexitis
including the tubes, ligaments, ovaries

inflamed amnion
amnionitis

inflamed aorta
aortitis

inflamed appendix
appendicitis

inflamed artery
arteritis

inflamed bone
osteitis
ostitis
myelitis
spinal cord or bone marrow
osteomyelitis
marrow, bone and cartilage
periostitis
connective tissue

Inflamed brain
cerebritis
encephalitis
meningoencephalitis

Inflamed breast
mastitis

Inflamed bronchial glands
bronchoadenitis

Inflamed cheek
melitis

Inflamed ear
otitis
panotitis

Inflamed eye
blepharitis
eyelid
choroiditis
choroid
ophthalmia
ophthalmitis
eye and conjunctiva

panophthalmia
panophthalmitis
entire eyeball structure
scleritis
sclerotitis
eyeball coating
trachoma
granular conjunctivitis

Inflamed Fallopian tube
salpingitis
syringitis
also of Eustachian tube

Inflamed finger
dactylitis

Inflamed foreskin
phimosis
phimotic

Inflamed glands
adenitis

Inflamed gums
gingivitis

Inflamed hair follicles
sycosis

Inflamed intestines
enteritis
any part of the intestinal tract
cecitis
typhlitis
cecum
colitis
colon
enterocolitis
small intestine and colon
enterogastritis
gastroenteritis
intestine and stomach
ileitis
ileum
ileocolitis
ileum and colon
mucoenteritis
mucous membrane of intestine
paratyphlitis
connective tissue near cecum
pericecitis
cecum serosa
perienteritis
intestinal peritoneum
perijejunitis
tissues around the jejunum
proctitis
rectum or anus

inflamed intestines (cont.)
rectocolitis
rectum and colon
seroenteritis
small intestine serous covering
sigmoiditis

inflamed joint
arthritis
periarthritis
around the joint
polyarthritis
several joints

inflamed joint membrane
synovitis

inflamed kidney
nephritis
pyelitis
pelvis of a kidney
pyelonephritis
kidney and its pelvis
pyonephritis
with pus formation

inflamed larynx
laryngitis
laryngopharyngitis
larynx and pharynx
laryngotracheitis
larynx and trachea
laryngotracheobronchitis
larynx, trachea and bronchi

inflamed ligament
syndesmitis

inflamed liver
hepatitis

inflamed lungs
baritosis
due to barium inhalation
kaolinosis
from inhaling kaolin dust
pneumoenteritis
lungs and intestine
pneumonia
pneumonitis
pulmonitis
of the lungs proper

inflamed marrow/bone
osteomyelitis

inflamed mouth
stomatitis

inflamed mucous gland
myxadenitis

Inflamed nail
onychia
onyxitis
nail matrix
paronychia
whitlow
with pus formation

Inflamed nerve
neuritis
mononeuritis
a single nerve
neurochorioretinitis
neurochoroiditis
neuroretinitis
retinal nerves
neuromyelitis
nerves and spinal cord
neuromyositis
nerves and muscles
perineuritis
the perineurial sheath enclosing a bundle of nerves

Inflamed nipple
mammillitis

Inflamed nostril
rhinitis
mucous membranes
rhinoantritis
mucous membrane and sinus
rhinolaryngitis
mucous membrane and larynx
rhinopharyngitis
nose and pharynx

Inflamed nympha
nymphitis
minor lips

inflamed ovaries
oophoritis
ovaritis
oophorosalpingitis
ovariosalpingitis
ovary and oviduct

Inflamed palate
palatitis

Inflamed pancreas
pancreatitis

Inflamed parotid gland
parotitis
the mumps

Inflamed pericardium
pericarditis

Inflamed periosteum
periostitis
membrane covering bones

Inflamed peritoneum
peritonitis
membrane covering abdominal organs

Inflamed pharynx
pharyngitis
pharyngolaryngitis
pharynx and larynx
pharyngorhinitis
with rhinitis
pharyngotonsillitis
with tonsillitis

Inflamed pleura
pleurisy
pleuritis
pleurohepatitis
pleura and liver
pleuropericarditis
with pericarditis

Inflamed prepuce
acroposthitis
posthitis

Inflamed rectum
proctitis

Inflamed retina
retinitis
retinochoroiditis
retina and choroid
retinopapillitis
retina and optic disk

Inflamed skin
dermatitis
acrodermatitis
of an extremity
prurigo
itching and inflammation of the papules
pyoderma
pyodermatitis
with pus
radiodermatitis
caused by radioactivity
toxicodermatitis
caused by poison

Inflamed spinal cord
myelitis
meningomyelitis
spinal cord and its membranes
poliomyelitis
gray matter

radiculitis
spinal nerve root
syringomyelitis
with syringomyelia

Inflamed spleen
splenitis
perisplenitis
membrane covering the spleen

Inflamed stomach
gastritis
enterogastritis
gastroenteritis
stomach and intestine
gastroesophagitis
stomach and esophagus
gastroduodenitis
stomach and duodenum
perigastritis
stomach serosa
pyloritis
pylorus

Inflamed subcutaneous fatty tissue
adipositis
panniculitis

Inflamed synovial membrane
synovitis

Inflamed tendon
tendinitis
tendonitis
tenonitis
tenositis

Inflamed testicles
orchitis

Inflamed thyroid
thyroiditis

Inflamed tongue
glossitis
subglossitis
sublinguitis

Inflamed tonsil
tonsillitis
adenopharyngitis
pharyngotonsillitis
tonsils and pharynx

Inflamed trachea
tracheitis
trachitis
tracheobronchitis
trachea and bronchi
tracheopyosis
purulent inflammation

Inflamed ureter
ureteritis
ureteropyelitis
  ureter and kidney pelvis
ureteropyelonephritis
  ureter, kidney and pelvis
ureteropyosis
  with purulent exudation

Inflamed urethra
urethritis
urethrocystis
urethrotrigonitis
  urethra and bladder

Inflamed uterus
metritis
uteritis
metrolymphangitis
  lymphatic vessels
metroperitonitis
  uterus and peritoneum
metrophlebitis
  veins of the uterus
metrosalpingitis
  uterus and oviducts

Inflamed uvea
uveitis

Inflamed uvula
staphylitis
uvulitis

Inflamed vein
phlebitis
mesophlebitis
  middle coat of the vein
periangitis
  outside tissues

Inflamed vertebra
spondylitis
perispondylitis
  tissues around the vertebrae
spondylopyosis
  accompanied by pus

Inflamed vessel
angiitis
angitis
angiodermatitis
  skin vessels
angiotitis
  ear blood vessels

Inflamed windpipe
tracheitis
trachitis

Inflammation reliever
antiphlogistic
antipyrotic

Inflatable cervix dilator
hystereurynter
  instrument for dilating the uterus

Ingrowing nail
unguis incarnatus

Inguinal pain
bubonalgia
inguinodynia

Inhale/exhale measurer
spirometer

Injury
trauma

Inosital in blood
inosemia
  excess of fibrin in the blood

Inosital in urine
inosituria
inosuria

Insanity over religion
hieromania

Insensibility to pain
analgesia

Insomnia
agrypnia
ahypnia
ahypnosis

Insulin in blood
insulinemia
  excessive amounts

Insulin diminishing
insulinopenic

Insulin formation
insulinogenesis

Insulin tumor
insulinoma
  tumor of the beta cells of the islets of
  Langerhans

Intellectual alertness
prothymia

Intellectual loss
dementia

Interbreeding
amphimixis

intercourse
coitus
copulation
pareunia

intercourse with animals
zooerastia

intercourse painful
dyspareunia

internal hernia
entocele

internal origin
autopathic
autopathy
disease without apparent external cause

internal secretion glands
endocrine glands

internal secretion study
endocrinology

interstitial pregnancy
salpingysterocyesis

intestinal
enteric
enteral

intestinal bloody discharge
hematorrhea

intestinal contraction/motion
peristalsis

intestinal "crawling"
diastalsis
type of downward moving wave in small
intestine during the digestive process

intestinal crusher
splanchnotribe
instrument for crushing a segment of
the intestine

intestinal dilatation
enterectasis

intestinal disease
enteromycosis
fungal disease
enteropathy
any intestinal disease

intestinal gas/air
aerenterectasia
meteorism
tympanites

intestinal hemorrhage

enterorrhagia
enterostaxis

intestinal hernia
enterocele
hernia containing a loop of intestine
enteroepiplocele
hernia of the omentum
enterocystocele
involving intestine and bladder

intestinal inflammation
cecitis
typhlitis
typhlenteritis
of the cecum
diverticulitis
of intestinal sacs
enteritis
in general
enterocolitis
small intestine and colon
enterogastritis
gastroenteritis
intestine and stomach
mucoenteritis
of the mucous membrane
paratyphlitis
of the connective tissue near the cecum
periappendicitis
of tissues around the appendix
pericecitis
of the cecum serosa
perienteritis
of the intestinal peritoneum
perijejunitis
of the tissue around the jejunum
perityphlitis
obsolete term for periappendicitis
seroenteritis
small intestine serous covering
typhlodicliditis
of the ileocecal valve

intestinal irritation
clyster
enema

intestine lacking
anenterous

intestine largeness
enteromegalia
enteromegaly
megaloenteron

intestinal obstruction
splanchnemphraxis
in general

intestinal obstruction (cont.)

volvulus
twisting

intestinal operation

cecectomy
cecocolostomy
cecoileostomy
cecosigmoidostomy
cecostomy
cecotomy
celioenterotomy
typhlectomy
typhlostomy
typhlotomy
involving the cecum
colectomy
colocolostomy
colohepatopexy
coloproctostomy
colosigmoidostomy
colostomy
colotomy
diverticulectomy
enterectomy
enterocolectomy
enterocolostomy
enteroenterostomy
enteropexy
enteroplasty
enterostomy
enterotomy
involving the colon
ileectomy
ileocecostomy
ileocolostomy
ileoileostomy
ileosigmoidostomy
ileostomy
ileotomy
involving the ileum
laparoenterotomy
proctectomy
proctopexy
proctoplasty
proctosigmoidectomy
proctostomy
proctotomy
rectectomy
rectopexy
rectosigmoidectomy
rectostomy
rectotomy
involving the rectum
sigmoidectomy

sigmoidopexy
sigmoidoproctostomy
sigmoidorectostomy
sigmoidosigmoidostomy
sigmoidostomy
sigmoidotomy
involving the sigmoid colon

intestine pain

enteralgia
enterodynia

intestinal paralysis

adynamic ileus
enteroplegia
paralytic ileus

intestinal peristalsis lacking

aperistalsis

intestinal prolapse

coloptosis
enteroptosis

intestinal puncture

enterocentesis
surgical puncture

intestinal rumbling

barborygmus
rugitus

intestinal rupture

enterorrhexis

intestinal sac

diverticulum
may be congenital or acquired

intestinal stone

enterolith

intestinal stricture

enterostenosis

intestinal suture

cecorrhaphy
enterorrhaphy

intestinal toxemia

scatemia
blood poisoning

intestinal toxins

clostridium bacteria

intestinal viewer

enteroscope

intestine worm medicine

anthelmintic
santonin

Involuntary urination
enuresis
nocturnal enuresis
nocturia
nycturia
  bedwetting, usually at night

Iodine sickness
iodism
iododerma

Iris adhesion
synechia
  also applies to any adhesion

Iris angle
angulus iridis

Iris atrophy
iridoleptynsis

Iris eversion
iridectropium

Iris hemorrhage
iridemia

Iris inflammation
iritis
choroidoiritis
iridochoroiditis
  iris and choroid
iridocapsulitis
  iris and capsule
iridocyclitis
  iris and ciliary body
iridoperiphakitis
  iris and part of capsule
scleroiritis
  iris and sclera
sclerokeratoiritis
  iris, sclera and cornea

Iris inversion
iridentropium

Iris knife
corectome
iridectome
  instrument for iris removal

Iris lacking
aniridia
irideremia
  congenital absence

Iris operation
iridoavulsion
iridectomy

iridotomy
iritomy
iritoectomy
iridocyclectomy
iridocystectomy
iridosclerotomy
sclerectoiridectomy

Iris paralysis
iridoparalysis
iridoplegia

Iris prolapse
iridoptosis
  protrusion through a wound or ulcer

Iris ring
annulus iridis

Iris rupture
iridorrhexis

Iris softness
iridomalacia

Iris tremor
hippus
  spasmodic, rhythmical dilation and constriction

Iris thickening
iridauxesis

Iron deficiency
sideropenia

Iron worker disease
siderosis

Isolation hospital
lazaret
lazaretto

Itching
pruritus

Itching reliever
antipruritic

Itching skin
neurodermatitis

J

---

jargon
glossolalia
  unintelligible jargon

jaundice
icteric
icterus

jaundice causing
icterogenic

jaw bone
mandible

jaws equal size
isognathous

jaw force measurer
gnathodynamometer
instrument that records the force exerted in closing jaws

jaw inflammation
gnathitis
also refers to inflammation of the cheek

jaw lacking
agnathia
agnathus
agnathous

jaw largeness
macrognathia
macrognathic
megagnathia

jaws mismatched
anisognathous

jaw muscle
masseter
raises the lower jaw

jaw operation
alveolectomy
alveoloplasty
alveoplasty
alveolotomy
gnathoplasty

jaw projecting
hypognathia
prognathism
prognathic
prognathous

jaw shortness
brachygnathia

jaw smallness
micrognathia

jejunum/ileum
jejunoileal

jejunum inflammation
jejunitis
jejunoileitis
jejunum and ileum

jejunum operation
jejunectomy
jejunocolostomy
jejunoileostomy
jejunojejunostomy
jejunoplasty
jejunostomy
jejunotomy
nestiostomy

joint with air
pneumarthrosis
presence of air in a joint

joint ball-and-socket
enarthrosis

joint disease
arthropathy
osteoarthritis
osteoarthrosis
degenerative disease of the joints

joint drainage
arthrocentesis
arthrostomy

joint flexion measurer
fleximeter
goniometer

joint fusion
arthrodesis
symphysis
synarthrosis

joint gouty deposit
arthrolith
tophus
chalkstone*
*obsolete term

joints of hand contracted
acrocontracture
shortening of muscles in the joints of hands or feet

joint inflammation
arthritic
arthritis
monarthric
monarticular
monoarthritis
pertaining to a single joint

panarthritis
polyarthritis
  of several joints
periarthritis
  of tissues around a joint
synovitis
  of the synovial membrane

joint lubricant
synovia
  clear fluid that functions to lubricate a
  joint

joint mobility reduction
arthroereisis
arthrarisis

joint movement measurer
arthrometer
arthrometry
goniometer
  measurement of the range of movement
  of a joint

joint operation
arthrectomy
arthrotomy
arthrolysis
arthroplasty
arthrostomy
synovectomy
villusectomy

joint pain
arthralgia
arthralgic
arthrodynia
arthrodynic
polyarthralgia

joint pus
pyarthrosis
  suppurative arthritis

joint rigidity
acampsia

joint sensation
arthresthesia

joint stiffness
ankylosis
bony ankylosis
synostosis
true ankylosis

joint suppuration
arthroempyesis

joint viewer
arthroscope

arthroendoscopy
  instrument to view inside joint
arthroscopy
  examining the inside of a joint with an
  endoscope

jumbling words
paraphrasia

K

ketone bodies in blood
ketonemia

ketone bodies in urine
ketonuria
hyperketonuria

kidneys
nephric
nephroid
nephrons
renal
  shape of a kidney

kidney abscess
nephrapostasis

kidney connective tissue
perinephrium
  connective tissue and fat surrounding a
  kidney

kidney cyst
nephrocystosis

kidney dilatation
nephrectasis

kidney disease
nephrasthenia
nephronophthisis
nephropathy
nephrosis
renopathy

kidney displacement
nephrocele
nephrocelon
  hernial displacement of a kidney

kidney function assessment
nephrogram
nephrography
nephrotomogram
nephrotomography
renogram
renography

kidney function lost/diminished
nephratonia
nephratony
renoprival

kidney floating
nephrospasia
nephrospasis
attachment of the organ only by the blood vessels

kidney hardness
nephrosclerosis
nephrosclerotic

kidney hemorrhage
nephremorrhagia
nephrorrhagia
hemorrhage from or into the kidney

kidney inflammation
glomerulonephritis
nephritis
nephrophthisis
nephritides
lithonephritis
nephropyelitis
pyelitis
pyelonephritis
of the kidney pelvis
perinephritis
of tissues around a kidney
pyelocystitis
urinary bladder and the pelvis of a kidney
pyonephritis
accompanied by pus

kidney nourishment
nephrotrophic
nephrotropic
renotrophic
renotrophin
renotropin

kidney operation
nephrectomy
nephrotomy
nephrocapsectomy
nephrocystanastamosis
nephrolithotomy

nephropexy
nephropyeloplasty
nephrostomy
nephroureterectomy
pyelolithotomy
pyeloplasty
pyelostomy
pyelotomy

kidney origination
nephrogenetic
nephrogenic
nephrogenous
renogenic
giving rise to kidney tissue

kidney pain
nephralgia

kidney pelvis distention
hydropyonephrosis

kidney prolapse
nephroptosia
nephroptosis

kidney proximity
adrenal
located near or upon the kidney

kidney shaped
nephroid
reniform

kidney softening
nephromalacia

kidney stone
nephrolith
nephrocalcinosis
nephrolithiasis
pyonephrolithiasis
accompanied by pus

kidney suture
nephrorrhaphy

kidney study/treatment
nephrology

kidney toxin
nephrolysin
antibody that causes destruction of the cells of the kidneys
nephrotoxic
nephrotoxin
cytotoxin specific for cells of the kidney

kidney tumor
nephroadenoma

nephroblastema
nephroblastoma
nephroma
nephroncus

kidney ulceration
nephrelcosis

kidney vessels
glomerulus
renovascular

killing offspring
feticide
before birth
infanticide
after birth

knee inflammation
gonarthritis
gonitis
meniscitis
of the interarticular cartilage

knee-jerk
patellar reflex

knee joint
articulatio genus

knee joint inflammation
gonarthritis
gonarthromeningitis

knee joint operation
gonarthrotomy
incision into the knee joint

knee pain
gonalgia

knee tumor
gonatocele

kneecap
patella

knock-knee
genu valgum
tibia valga

L

labor difficult
dystocia

labor producer
oxytocic
parturifacient
an agent that produces or accelerates
labor

labyrinth inflammation
labyrinthitis

labyrinth operation
labyrinthectomy
labyrinthotomy

lack of alkalinity
acidosis
insufficient amount of alkali/base in the
blood

lack of bile pigment
acholuria
acholuric
in the urine

lack of bile secretion
acholia

lack of heart
acardia
acardius

lack of limbs
ectromelia

lack of mental ability
amentia
dementia

lack of nutrition
cachexia
general wasting seen during a chronic
illness

lack of pigmentation
achromatosis

lack of pupil
acorea

lack of ribs
apleuria

lack of skin pigment
achromasia
achromia

lack of strength
hyposthenia

lack of teeth
adontia
adontism
edentate
edentulous

lack of teeth (cont.)
hypodontia
oligodontia

lack of testes
agenitalism
anorchia
anorchidism
anorchism
having no testes
monorchid
monorchidic
monorchidism
monorchis
monorchism
having only one testis

lack of trunk
acormus
fetus born without a torso

lacrimal duct stone
dacryolith
ophthalmolith
also called a tear stone

lacrimal gland pain
dacryoadenalgia

lacrimal sac protrusion
dacryocele
dacryocystocele

lactation diminisher
antigalactagogue
antigalactic
diminishing or suppressing the secretion
of milk

lactic acid in blood
lactacidemia
lacticacidemia

lactiferous duct inflamed
galactophoritis

lactose in urine
lactosuria

lamina operation
laminectomy
hemilaminectomy
rachiotomy
rachitomy
spondylotomy

languor of organs
atonia
atonicity
atony

weakness of any organ, especially the
muscles

lanolin
adeps lanae hydrosus
wool fat (anhydrous)

large-footed
pachypodous

large hands
cheiromegaly
chiromegaly
megalocheiric
megalochiria

large head
macrocephalia
macrocephaly
macrocephalous
macrocephalus
megacephalus
megalocephalia
megalocephaly
congenital or acquired condition

large heart
cardiomegaly
megacardia
megalocardia

large intestine
enteromegalia
enteromegaly
megaloenteron
abnormal largeness of the intestine

large jaw
megagnathia
macrognathia

large limbs
macromelia
macromelus
megalomelia
abnormal size of one or more of the extremities

large liver
hepatomegaly
megalohepatia

large mouth
macrostomia

large nails
macronychia
megalonychosis
abnormally large fingernails or toenails

large nucleus
macronucleus
meganucleus

large penis
macropenis
macrophallus
megalopenis

large pill
bolus
also large volume of intra-venous fluid
given rapidly

large rectum
megarectum

large sigmoid
macrosigmoid
megasigmoid

large spleen
splenomegaly
splenohepatomegalia
splenohepatomegaly
enlargement of spleen and liver

large stomach
macrogastric
megalogastria
megastria

large teeth
macrodont
macrodontia
megadont
megalodont
megalodontia

large toes
macrodactylia
macrodactylism
macrodactyly
megalodactylia
megalodactylism
megalodactyly
also applies to large fingers

large tongue
macroglossia
megaloglossia
pachyglossia

large writing
macrography
megalographia
writing with very large letters

larva-killer
larvicide

larva second stage
cercaria

larynx artificial
laryngophantom

larynx disease
laryngopathy
any disease of the larynx

larynx dryness
laryngoxerosis

larynx examination
laryngoscopy

larynx falling
laryngoptosis

larynx inflammation
laryngitis
laryngopharyngitis
larynx and pharynx
laryngophthisis
tuberculosis of the larynx
laryngotracheitis
larynx and trachea
laryngotracheobronchitis
larynx, trachea and bronchi
perilaryngitis
tissues surrounding the larynx
pharyngolaryngitis
larynx and pharynx
rhinolaryngitis
larynx and nose mucosa

larynx knife
laryngotome

larynx narrowing
laryngostenosis

larynx obstruction
laryngemphraxis

larynx operation
laryngectomy
laryngofissure
laryngotomy
cricothyroidotomy
intercricothyrotomy
hemilaryngectomy
laryngopharyngectomy
laryngoplasty
laryngostomy
laryngotracheotomy

larynx paralysis
laryngoparalysis

larynx paralysis (cont.)
laryngoplegia
paralysis of the laryngeal muscles

larynx recorder
laryngograph
laryngostroboscope

larynx softening
chondromalacia
laryngomalacia

larynx sounds
laryngophony
voice sounds heard in auscultation of
the larynx

larynx spasm
laryngismus

larynx spasmodic closure
glottidospasm
laryngospasm

larynx specialist
laryngologist
laryngoscopist

larynx study
laryngology
laryngorhinology
larynx and nose

larynx viewer
laryngoscope

laughter
risus

laughter inappropriate
cachinnation
immoderate and loud

lead monoxide
litharge

lead poisoning
plumbism
saturnism

leech
Hirudo medicinalis
leeches used in medicine for bleeding
patients

left-eyed
sinistrocular

left-footed
sinistropedal

left-handed
sinistromanual

left-turning toward
levoversion

leg calf
sura
sural
muscular swelling of the back of the leg
below the knee

leg cramp
systremma

leg excess
polyscelia
polyscelus
fetus born with more than two legs

leg lacking
monoscelous

leg largeness
macroscelia

leg shortness
brachyskelic

leg strength measurer
pedodynamometer
instrument to measure the muscular
strength of the legs

lens bulging
lentiglobus

lens capsule
capsula lentis
phacocyst

lens capsule operation
phacocystectomy

lens displacement
phacocele
hernia of the crystalline lens of the eye

lens measurer
auxometer
axometer
axonometer
lensometer
phacometer*
*obsolete term

lens-shaped
lenticular
lentiform
phacoid

lens small
microlentia
microphakia
spherophakia

lens viewer
phacoscope
dark chamber for observing changes

leprosy hospital
leprosarium
lazaret
lazaretto

leprosy study
leprology

lesbianism
amor lesbicus
sapphism

leucine in urine
leucinuria

leukocyte counter
leukocytometer
glass slide ruled for counting white cells
in a measured volume of blood

leukocyte deficiency
leukocytopenia
leukopenia

leukoma of cornea
exotropia
walleye

levulose in blood
levulosemia
presence of fructose in the circulating
blood

levulose in urine
levulosuria

lewisite
chlorovinyldichloroarsine
poisonous warfare gas

lice
Pediculus

lice infestation
pediculation
pediculosis
presence of the parasites that live in the
hair and feed on the blood

lice-killer
pediculicide

licorice
glycyrrhiza

lie detector
polygraph
psychogalvanometer

life development study
biogenesis
biogeochemistry

lifelessness
abiosis
abiotrophy
absence of life

ligament inflammation
desmitis
syndesmitis

ligament operation
syndesmopexy
syndesmoplasty
syndesmotomy

ligament study
syndesmology

ligament suture
syndesmorrhaphy

ligament-like
desmoid

light decomposing
photolysis
through the action of light
photolyte
product of light decomposition

light measurement
photometry

limb in excess
polymelia
polymelus
presence of supernumerary limbs or
parts

limb lacking
ectromelia
ectromelus
lipomeria
monopodia
monopus

limb largeness
macromelia
macromelus
megalomelia

limbs malformed
melomelus
born with a rudimentary limb attached to
a limb
peromelus
peromelia

limbs malformed (cont.)
peromely
born with malformed or deficient limbs

limb-pertaining
acral

limb sensation lacking
acroagnosis

limb smallness
micromelia
micromelus
nanomelia

limbs unequal
anisomelia
inequality between the two paired limbs

limbless
acolous

liniment
embrocation
rarely used term also meaning the application of

lionlike face
leontiasis

lip biting
cheilophagia
chilophagia

lips/cheeks
buccolabial

lips/chin
labiomental

lip eversion
eclabium

lip fusion/adhesion
syncheilia
synchilia
atresia of the mouth

lip inflammation
cheilitis
chilitis

lips lacking
acheilia
achilia

lip largeness
macrocheilia
macrochilia
abnormally enlarged lips

lip operation

cheilectomy
cheilotomy
cheiloplasty
chiloplasty
cheilostomatoplasty
chilostomatoplasty
labioplasty
rhinocheiloplasty
rhinochiloplasty

lip pain
cheilalgia
chilalgia

lip shortness
brachycheilia
brachychilia

lip silent movement
mussitation
observed in delirium and in semicoma

lip suture
cheilorrhaphy
chilorrhaphy

lip thickness/swelling
pachycheilia
pachychilia

liquid density measurer
densimeter

liquid expeller
hydragogue

liquid tension measurer
stalagmometer
instrument that measures the surface tension of liquids

liquid/gas in tissues
hydropneumatosis
accumulation of liquid and gas

lisping
sigmatism

lithic acid in urine
hyperlithuria
lithuria
excretion of large amounts of uric acid/urates in the urine

liver atrophy
hepatatrophia
hepatatrophy

liver congestion
hepatohemia

liver destruction
hepatonecrosis
death of liver cells
hepatotoic
hepatotoxin
damaging to the liver

liver disease
hepatopathy

liver displacement
hepatoptosis

liver enlargement
hepatomegalia
hepatomegaly
megalohepatia
hepatosplenomegaly
splenohepatomegaly
liver and spleen
hepatonephromegaly
liver and kidneys

liver examination
hepatoscopy

liver hemorrhage
hepatorrhagia

liver hernia
hepatocele

liver inflammation
hepatitis
icterohepatitis
with jaundice
hepatosplenitis
liver and spleen
perihepatitis
peritoneum surrounding the liver
pleurohepatitis
liver and pleura

liver operation
hepatectomy
hepatotomy
hepatocholangioenterostomy
hepatocholangiostomy
hepatocholangiojejunostomy
hepatoduodenostomy
hepatolithectomy
hepatopexy
hepatostomy
hepaticostomy
hepaticoduodenostomy
hepaticoenterostomy
hepaticogastrostomy
hepaticolithotripsy

liver origin
hepatogenic
hepatogenous
formed in the liver

liver pain
hepatalgia
hepatodynia

liver pigmentation
hepatomelanosis
deep pigmentation of the liver

liver proximity
parahepatic

liver rupture
hepatorrhexis

liver softening
hepatomalacia

liver specialist
hepatologist

liver stone
hepatolith
hepatolithiasis

liver study
hepatology

liver suture
hepatorrhaphy

liver tumor
hepatoblastoma
hepatocarcinoma
hepatoma

liver x-ray
hepatography

liverlike
hepatoid

living in air
aerobic
aerophilic
aerophilous
organism that lives in the presence of oxygen

living without oxygen
anaerobic
organism that thrives best in the absence of oxygen

local anemia
hypoemia
ischemia

location abnormal
ectopic

lochial flow
lochiorrhea
lochiorrhagia

lockjaw
tetanus
trismus
painful tonic muscular contractions

long colon
dolichocolon

long-faced
dolichofacial
dolichoprosopic

long-headed
dolichocephalic
dolichocephalism
dolichocephaly
having a disproportionately long head

long-lived
macrobiote
macrobiotic

long-necked
dolichoderus

longevity
macrobiosis

longevity study
macrobiotics
study of the prolongation of life

loop
ansa

loss of appetite
anorexia

loss of body heat
thermolysis

loss of eyelashes
madarosis
milphosis

loss of memory
amnesia

loss of reading ability
alexia
inability to understand written symbols

loss of strength
adynamia
asthenia
debility

loss of taste
ageusia
ageustia

loss of touch/sensation
anesthesia
astereognosis
inability to recognize the form of an object by the touch
acroanesthesia
loss of feeling in the extremities

loss of vocal control
alalia
inability to control speech muscle

loss of voice
anaudia
aphonia

loving animals
zoophilia
zoophilism

loving children
pedophilia
excessive love for small children

loving elderly persons
gerontophilia

loving air
aerophil

low temperature measurer
cryometer

lower abdomen
hypogastrium

lower extremities only
acephalogaster
cojoined twin born with only the pelvis and legs

lower jaw
mandible
mandibula
submaxilla

lower jaw lacking
agnathia
agnathus
hemignathia
hypoagnathus
otocephalus

lower jaw small
hypognatous

lues
  syphilis

lumbar puncture
  rachicentesis

lumbar vertebra/sacrum angle
  sacrovertebral angle

luminous perception
  photopsia
  photopsy
    visual disorder where luminous rays are
    perceived

lump in throat
  globus hystericus
  spheresthesia

lumpy jaw
  actinomycosis
  actinophytosis

lung abscess
  vomica
    obsolete term

lung collapse
  atelectasis

lung covering
  pleura
    the fine membrane covering each lung

lung disease
  bronchopulmonary dysplasia
  C>disorder seen in newborns
  silicosis
    progressive fibrosis due to inhalation of
    silica dust

lung flatulence
  emphysema
    accumulation of gas or air in any of the
    natural cavities

lung fungus disease
  pneumonomycosis
  pneumomycosis *
    *obsolete term

lung gauge
  spirometer
    instrument used to measure lung capac-
    ity
  pneumatometer *
    *obsolete term

lung inflammation
  pneumonia

  pneumonitis
  bagassosis
  bird fancier's lung
  extrinsic allergic alveolitis
  farmer's lung
  pigeon breeder's lung
    hypersensitivity pneumonitis caused by
    repeated exposure to an allergen
  baritosis
    due to barium inhalation
  kaolinosis
    caused by inhaling clay dust
  pneumoconiosis
  pneumonoconiosis
    caused by dust
  pneumonomycosis
    caused by fungi

lung irritation
  byssinosis
  mill fever

lung lacking
  apneumia

lung operation
  lobectomy
  pneumectomy
  pneumonectomy
  pneumonotomy
  pneumotomy
  pulmonectomy
  pneumonopexy
  pneumopexy

lung puncture
  pneumocentesis
  pneumonocentesis
    paracentesis of the lung

lung suture
  pneumonorrhaphy

Lyme disease rash
  erythema chronicum migrans

lymph in blood
  lymphemia

lymph in urine
  chyluria
  lymphuria
    lymph or chyle

lymph cell/node
  lymphoblast
  lymphocele
  lymphocyte

lymph cell/node (cont.)
lymphocyst
lymphonodus

lymph flow/escape
lymphorrhea
from ruptured, torn or cut lymphatic vessels

lymph formation
lymphization
lymphoblast
lymphocerastism
lymphocytopoiesis
lymphogenesis
lymphopoiesis

lymph inflammation
adenitis
of a gland or lymph node
lymphadenitis
lymphangitis
lymphatitis
of a lymph node
lymphangiophlebitis
lymph vessels and veins
periangitis
outside tissues around an artery, vein or lymph vessel
perilymphangitis
tissues around a lymph vessel

lymph lacking
alymphia

lymph node
lymphonodus

lymph node disease
adenopathy
lymphadenopathy
lymphopathy
any disease process affecting the lymph nodes or vessels

lymph node enlargement
hyperadenosis
lymphadema
lymphadenosis
*lymphadenectasia**
*lymphadenia**
*obsolete terms

lymph node/vessel x-ray
lymphadenography
lymphangiography
lymphography

lymph operation
lymphadenectomy

lymphangiectomy
lymphangioplasty
lymphangiotomy
lymphaticostomy
lymphoidectomy
lymphoplasty

lymph tumor
lymphadenoma
lymphoadenoma
lymphocytoma
lymphogranuloma
lymphomyeloma
lymphangiosarcoma
lymphoblastoma
lymphoepithelioma
lymphoma
lymphosarcoma
malignant forms of lymph tumors
lymphangioendothelioma
lymphangioma
lymphomyxoma
nonmalignant forms of lymph tumors

lymph vessel dilatation
lymphangiectasia
lymphangiectasis
lymphangiectatic

lymphatic system study
lymphangiology
lymphatology
lymphology
branch of medical science that pertains to the lymphatic system

M

magnesium/aluminum
magnalium
alloy containing the two metals

magnetism
mesmerism

maidenhead
hymen

malaria study
malariology

male birth
androgenous
giving birth to males

male reproduction
arrhenotocia

male sex disliked
apandria

male sterilization
deferentectomy
gonangiectomy
vasectomy

malnutrition
athrepsia
athrepsy
weakness due to lack of nourishment

malocclusion specialist
orthodontist

malocclusion study
orthodontics

mammary gland overgrowth
hypermastia
polymastia
excessively large mammary glands

mammary gland smallness
hypomastia
hypomazia

mania for one thing
monomania

mania for writing
graphomania

mankind aversion
misanthropy
aversion to people; hatred of mankind

manlike
android
anthropomorphic

many ancestors
polyphletic

marihuana
cannabis

marriage aversion
misogamy

marrow
medulla
any soft, marrow-like structure

marrow cells stoppage
anakmesis

marrow fibrosis
myelofibrosis
myelosclerosis

marrow inflammation
myelitis

marshmallow root
althea

marshy
paludal

mask of pregnancy
chloasma

massage
massotherapy
sciage

massagist
masseur
male

masseuse
female

mastication insufficient
psomophagia
psomophagy
swallow food without sufficient chewing

mastication measurer
phagodynamometer
instrument to measure the force exerted in chewing

mastoid inflammation
mastoiditis

mastoid operation
mastoidectomy
mastoidotomy

maxillary sinus cavity
antronasal

measles
morbelli

measurement of body
anthropometry
art of measuring the human body

meat poisoning
allantiasis
botulism

meatus operation
meatotomy
parotomy

median cerebellar lobe
ala lobuli centralis
the lateral winglike projection of the central lobule of the cerebellum

mediastinum inflammation
mediastinitis
mediastinopericarditis

mediastinum operation
mediastinotomy

melancholia
barythymia

melanin in blood
melanemia

membrane
meninx
   most often seen in pleural form as "meninges" of brain

membrane inflammation
serositis
   of a serous membrane
serosynovitis
   membrane and synovial fluid
synovitis
   of a synovial membrane

membrane in urine
meninguria

memory acuteness
hypermnesia
   extraordinary ability to recall

memory developing
mnemonics

memory divulgement
anamnesis
anamnestic
   information obtained about one's past

memory impairment
dysmnesia
hypomnesia

memory loss
amnesia
amnesic
amnestic
ecmnesia
   ability to recall only recent events

meninges hemorrhage
meningorrhagia

meninges inflammation
leptomeningitis
meningitis

meninges suture
meningeorrhaphy

meningococci in blood
meningococcemia

menses
catamenia
emmenia

menses first appearance
menophania

menses retention
menoschesis
   suppression of menstruation

menstrual disorder
paramenia
xeromenia

menstrual flow deficiency
hypomenorrhea
oligomenorrhea

menstrual flow excessive
hypermenorrhea
menorrhagia

menstrual pain
dysmenorrhea
menorrhalgia
   difficult and painful menstruation

menstrual stoppage
amenorrhea
menopause
menostasia
menostasis

menstruation beginning
menarche
   for the first time

menstruation inducer
emmenagogue

menstruation irregular
menoxenia
paramenia

menstruation lacking
amenia
amenorrhea

menstruation life
menacme
   interval during a woman's lifetime for
   menses

menstruation prolonged
hypermenorrhea
menostaxis

menstruation substitute
  menocelis
    type of vicarious menstruation with
    spots on the skin when menstruation
    fails

mental alertness
  prothymia

mental confusion
  obfuscation
  psychataxia

mental deficiency
  amentia
  ament*
    *obsolete term for a mentally retarded
    person

mental disorder
  neophrenia
  psychoneurosis
  psychoplegia
  psychorrhexis
  psychosis

mental development
  psychogenesis
  psychogeny

mental disease
  psychopathia
  psychopathy
    an old, inexact term referring to a pat-
    tern of inappropriate behavior

mental disease category
  psychonosology
    classification of diseases

mental strain
  psychentonia

mental testing
  psychometrics
  psychometry

mercury
  hydrargyrum

mercury poisoning
  hydrargyria
  hydrargyrism

mesentery fixation
  mesenteriopexy
  mesopexy

mesentery suture

mesenteriorrhaphy
mesorrhaphy
    suture of the layer of peritoneum at-
    tached to the abdominal wall

metabolism measurer
  metabolimeter

metacarpal operation
  metacarpectomy
    excision of one or all of the metacarpal
    bones of the hand

metaphysis inflammation
  metaphysitis

metatarsal operation
  metatarsectomy

metatarsal pain
  metatarsalgia

metatarsal/metacarpal shortness
  brachymetapody

methemoglobin in blood
  methemoglobinemia

methemoglobin in urine
  methemoglobinuria

microbe-killer
  microbicide
    a germicide or antiseptic

microbe study
  microbiology

middle ear
  auris media

midwifery
  obstetrics
  tocology

migraine
  hemicephalalgia
  hemicrania

mild
  benign
  mitis

mild smallpox
  alastrim
    caused by a less virulent strain of virus

milk albumin
  lactalbumin

milk arrester
  antigalactic

milk coagulatory
chymosin
eenase
rennet
rennin
present in the chief cells of the gastric tubules

milk cure
galactotherapy
lactotherapy

milk deficiency
oligogalactia

milk duct dilatation
ampulla lactifera
sinus lactiferi

milk in excess
polygalactia

milk fat measurer
galactometer
lactocrit
lactometer
instrument to determine the specific gravity of milk as an indication of its fat content

milk flow
galactorrhea
lactorrhea

milk flow stoppage
agalorrhea

milk lacking
agalactia
agalactosis
agalactous

milk leg
phlegmasia alba dolens
extreme swelling due to thrombosis of the veins

milk protein
lactoprotein

milk secretion lower
hypogalactia

milk with sugar excess
saccharogalactorrhea

milky diarrhea
chylorrhea
the flow or discharge of chyle

milky urine
chyluria
galacturia

mind
psychic
psychical

mind alertness
eunoia
denoting a normal mental state

mind altering
psychoactive
psychopharmaceutical
psychostimulant
psychotogen
psychogenic
psychotomimetic
psychotropic

mind development/origin
psychogenic
psychogenesis
psychogenetic
of mental origin or causation

mind specialist
psychoanalyst
psychiatrist
psychotherapist

mind stimulant
psychogogic
acting as a stimulant to the emotions

mind study
psychiatry
psychoanalysis
psychodynamics
psychology
psychonomy
psychopathology
psychotherapy

mind treatment
psychotherapy

minor lip inflammation
nymphitis

minute measurer
acribometer
instrument to measure very small objects

miscarriage
abortion

mixable
miscible

molar-shaped
molariform

molecule largeness
macromolecule

monocyte largeness
macromonocyte
an unusually large cell

mood disorder
dysthymia

mood swings
cyclothymia

mortification of tissue
gangrene
necrosis
sphacelation
sphacelism
sphacelous

mother-killer
matricide

motion in excess
acrocinesia
acrocinesis
excessive movement

motion sickness
kinesia

motion study
kinetics

mouth disease
stomatopathy
stomatosis
stomatomycosis
fungal disease

mouth disinfection
stomatocatharsis

mouth dryness
xerostomia

mouth hemorrhage
stomatomenia
stomatorrhagia
stomenorrhagia
bleeding from the gums

mouth inflammation
stomatitis

mouth lacking
astomia
astomatous
astomous
opocephalus
congenital absence

mouth operation
stomatoplasty
stomatotomy

mouth pain
stomatalgia
stomatodynia

mouth proximity
adoral

mouth smallness
microstomia

mouth/teeth study
stomatology
study of the structures, functions and
diseases of the mouth

mouth ulcer
noma
stomatonecrosis
stomatonoma

mouth viewer
stomatoscope

movement difficulty/disorder
dyscinesia
dyskinesia

movement repetition
palicinesia
palikinesia

movement slow
bradykinesia

mucous deficiency
amyxia
amyxorrhea

mucous discharge
blenorrhea
myxorrhea

mucuslike
myxoid

mud treatment
pelopathy
pelotherapy
application of mud, peat, moor or clay to
parts of the body

mumps
parotiditis
parotitis

murderous tendency
hemothymia

muscle cell
myoblast
myocyte

muscle contraction
clonus
alternating with relaxation
myoclonus
shocklike contractions
myodynamia
myodynamics
denotes muscular strength

muscle degeneration
muscular dystrophy

muscle deterioration
amyotrophia
amyotrophy
myoatrophy
myocerosis
myodermia
myolysis
myonecrosis

muscle disease
myonosus
myopathy
any abnormal condition or disease of
muscular tissue

muscle dislocation
myectopia
myectopy

muscle edema
myoedema

muscle fiber sheath
myolemma
sarcolemma

muscle fiber tumor
rhabdomyoma
myoma striocellulare*
*obsolete term

muscle flaccidity
hypotonia

muscle formation
myogenesis

muscle formation lacking
amyoplasia

muscle inflammation
myositis
myocelitis
abdominal muscles

myocellulitis
muscles and cellular tissues
myofibrositis
perimysium
perimyositis
tissues around the muscles
polymyositis
several muscles
pyomyositis
accompanied by pus

muscle measurer
myochronoscope
timing muscle impulse
myodynamometer
determine strength
myograph
timing contractions
myokinesimeter
myometer
myophone
reflexometer
force required to produce movement

muscle operation
myectomy
myoplasty
myotomy
myotenotomy
scalenectomy
scalenotomy
tenomyotomy
tenontomyotomy

muscle origin
myogenetic
myogenic
originating in or starting from muscle

muscle pain
myalgia
myocelialgia
myodynia
myoneuralgia
myosalgia
polymyalgia

muscle paralysis
myoparalysis
myoparesis

muscle quivering
kymatism
myoclonus
myokymia
irregular spasm or twitching of the muscles

muscle rigidity
anochlesia
catalepsy

muscle separation
myodiastasis

muscle softness
myomalacia
pathological softening of muscle tissue

muscle specialist
myologist

muscle study
myology

muscle tumor
leiomyoma
myoblastoma
myocytoma
myoepithelioma
myofibroma
myolemma
myolipoma
myoma
myoneuroma
rhabdomyoma

muscle twitching
myoclonus
chronic spasm of one or a group of muscles
myokyma
myopalmus
irregular twitching of most of the muscles

muscle weakness
myasthenia

muscular atrophy
amyotrophia
amyotrophic
amyotrophy

muscular dystrophy
dystrophia myotonica
myodystrophia
myodystrophy

muscular hypertrophy
myopachynis

muscular impulse failure
adromia
lack of impulse transmission in nerves or muscles

muscular incoordination

amyotaxia
amyotaxy
ataxia

muscular sense lost
muscular anesthesia

muscular strength measurer
dynamometer

muscular tone lacking
amyotonia
myatonia
myatony
abnormal extensibility of a muscle

mushroom poisoning
muscarinism
mycetism
mycetismus

mushroom-shaped
fungiform
fungoid

mushroom study
mycologyi

mushy
pultaceous

musical fascination
melomania

musical recognition loss
amusia
loss of ability to understand music

mustard gas
dichlorodiethylsulfide

mutualism
symbiosis
living together in harmony

myelin destruction
myelinoclasis

myelocytes in blood
myelemia
myelocytosis

myocardium inflammation
myocarditis

myoglobin in blood
myoglobinemia

myoglobin in urine
myoglobinuria

nail
unguis

nail atrophy
onychatrophia
onychatrophy

nail biting
onychophage
onychophagia
onychophagy
one who bites

nail blackness
melanonychia
condition where nails of the fingers or toes turn black

nail breaking
onychoclasis

nail component
keratin

nail curvature
gryposis unguium
onychogryposis
abnormal curvature

nail disease
onychopathy
onychosis

nail displacement
onychoptosis
downward displacement

nail dystrophy
dystrophia unguium

nails in excess
polyunguia
having more than the normal number of nails

nail fungal disease
onychomycosis
tinea ungium

nail hardening
scleronychia
also with thickness

nail hypertrophy
onychauxis

nail inflammation
onychia
onychitis
onyxitis
inflammation of the matrix
onchyia lateralis
paronychia
marginal inflammation accompanied by pus
perionychia
perionyxis
inflammation surrounding the nail

nail ingrowing
onychocryptosis

nails lacking
anonychia
anonychosis

nails largeness
macronychia
megalonychosis

nail in layers
onychoschizia

nail matrix
onychostroma

nail-moon
lunula
the white moon-shaped part at the base of a nail

nail operation
onychectomy
onychotomy

nail smallness
micronychia

nail softness
onychomalacia
abnormal softness

nail splitting
onychorrhexis
schizonychia

nail thickened
pachyonychia

nail thickened/curved
onychogryphosis
onychogryposis

nail whiteness
leukonychia
leukopathia unguis
caused by air beneath the nail

nape of neck
nucha

narcotic craving
narcomania

narrowing
stenosis

narrowing of an opening
arctation
stenosis

narrowness of head
stenocephalia
stenocephalic
stenocephaly

nasal
rhinal

nasal passage dryness
xeromycteria
pertaining to the nose

nasal plug
rhinobyon

nasal proximity
paranasal
located near the nose

nasal voice
rhinolalia
rhinophonia

nasopharynx
epipharynx
pars nasalis pharyngis

nature cure
naturopathy
using physical methods

nausea
sicchasia

navel
omphalos
umbilicus

navel inflammation
omphalitis
inflammation of the umbilicus and surrounding parts

navel operation

omphalectomy
omphalotomy
omphalotripsis

navel region
parumbilical

navel varicosity
varicomphalus

near the mouth
adoral

near a nerve
adnerval
adneural

near the sternum
adsternal

nearsightedness
myope
individual concerned
myopia
the condition

neck-back
nape
nucha
back of the neck

neck cleft
tracheloschisis
congenital fissure

neck/face
cervicofacial

neck/head lacking
atrachelocephalus
fetus with head and neck either missing or not developed

neck pain
trachelodynia

neck spasm
trachelism
trachelismus
spasmodic contraction of the neck muscles

neck stiffness
loxia
torticollis
wryneck

needle-shaped
acicular

nerve activity
neurergic

nerve acupuncture
neuronyxis

nerve antagonist
sympatholytic
adrenergic nerve blocking agent

nerve-bundle sheath
epineurium
envelops a fasciculus of nerves
perineurium
envelops each funiculus of a nerve fiber

nerve cell
axon
neuroblast
neuroblastoma
neurocyte
neuron
neuraxon*
*obsolete term

nerve crushing
neurotripsy

nerve destruction
neurocytolysis
neurolysis

nerve disease
neuropathy
any disease of the nervous system

nerve disease sufferer
neuropath

nerve disease treatment
neuriatria
neuriatry

nerve displacement
neurectopia
neurectopy

nerve energy
neurodynamic

nerve energy lacking
aneuria

nerve exhaustion
neurasthenia
particularly when due to mental strain

nerve fiber divider
leukotome

nerve fibrous sheath
neurilemma
neurolemma

nerve formation
neurogenesis

nerve impulse failure
adromia
absence of impulse transmission in nerves or muscles

nerve inflammation
mononeuritis
affecting only one nerve
neuritis
involving the nerves in general
neurochorioretinitis
chorioretinitis and optic neuritis combined
neurochoroiditis
choroid body and the optic nerve
neurodermatitis
neurodermatosis
skin inflammation where nerves are involved
neuromyelitis
involves spinal cord
neuromyositis
involves nerves and muscles
neuromyelitis optica
optic nerve and white/gray matter of the brain
neuroretinitis
optic nerve and retina
multiple neuritis
polyneuritis
inflammation of several nerves
radiculitis
nerve roots involved
actinoneuritis
radioneuritis
inflammation caused by exposure to x-rays

nerve operation
neurectomy
neuroectomy
neuroplasty
neurotomy
neurotripsy
neurexeresis
neuroanastomosis
radicotomy
rhizotomy
splanchnicectomy
splanchnicotomy

nerve pain
neuralgia
neurodynia
pain in general

polyneuralgia
involving several nerves

nerve proximity
adnerval
adneural

nerve specialist
neurologist
neurosurgeon

nerve stimulant
analeptic
central nervous system stimulant

nerve stretching
neurectasia
neurectasis
neurectasy

nerve study
neurology

nerve suture
neurorrhaphy
neurosuture
joining two parts of a divided nerve

nerve tissue softness
neuromalacia

nerve tumor
neurilemoma
neurinoma
neuroschwannoma
schwannoma
neurocytoma
ganglioneuroma
neurofibroma
neurosarcoma

nerve treatment
neurotherapeutics
neurotherapy
treatment of nervous disorders

nerve/vein network
plexus

network
plexus
reticulum

nettle
urtica

nettle rash
urticaria

neurosis localized
toponeurosis

never borne children
nullipara

newborn measurer
mecometer
instrument for measuring newborn infants

newness aversion
misoneism
dislike of changes

night blindness
nyctalopia

night lover
nyctophilia
scotophilia
condition of giving preference to darkness

night pain
nyctalgia
occurs only at night

nightmare
incubus

nipple erection
thelerthism

nipples in excess
hyperthelia
polythelism
congenital presence of more than usual number

nipple hemorrhage
thelorrhagia

nipple inflammation
mammillitis
thelitis

nipples lacking
athelia

nipple operation
mammilliplasty
theleplasty
plastic surgery of the nipple and areola

nipple pain
thelalgia

nipple smallness
microthelia

nipplelike
papillary

nitrates in urine
nitrituria

nitrogen in blood
hyperazotemia
excessive amount

nitrogen measurer
nitrometer
instrument to determine amount of nitrogen given off in a chemical reaction

nitrogen in urine
hyperazoturia
excessive amount

nodes on bone
Heberden's nodes
tuberculum arthriticum
growths on the end of the phalanges (fingers) seen in osteoarthritis

nodes on hair
monilethrix
disease causing the appearance of nodes

noise pain
odynacusis
discomfort caused by noises

noise-unit
decibel

normal blood pressure
normotensive
normotonic

normal blood volume
normovolemia

normal color
normochromatic

normal calcium in blood
normocalcemia

normal erythrocyte
normocyte
normal cell size

normal erythrocyte color
normochromia

normal glucose in blood
normoglycemia

normal position
normotopia

normal potassium in blood
normokalemia
normal level of potassium in the blood

normal pregnancy
uterogestation

normal temperature
normothermia

normoblast largeness
macroblast
macronormoblast
promegaloblast
pronormoblast

nose acne
rhinophyma
a type appearing on the nose

nose bleeding
epistaxis
rhinorrhagia

nose prominent
rhinokyphosis
refers to the bridge

nose constriction
rhinocleisis
rhinostenosis

nose discharging
rhinorrhea

nose disease
rhinopathy
general term for any disorder of the nose

nose hair
vibrissa

nose hemorrhage
epistaxis
rhinorrhagia

nose inflammation
coryza
inflammation of the mucous membrane
nasopharyngitis
inflammation of the nasal passages and pharynx
pansinuitis
pansinusitis
inflammation of all paranasal tissues
pharyngorhinitis
inflammation of the pharynx and nasal membranes
rhinomycosis
fungal infection
rhinitis
inflammation of the nasal membranes
rhinoantritis
inflammation of the nasal membranes and maxillary sinus
rhinolaryngitis
inflammation of the mucosa and larynx

rhinopharyngitis
inflammation of nose and pharynx
sinusitis
inflammation of the nasal cavities

nose inflator
rhineurynter
elastic bag inflated after insertion into
the nose

nose knife
spokeshave
surgical instrument

nose lacking
arhinia
arrhinia

nose/lips
nasolabial

nose long and thin
leptorrhine

nose measurer
rhinomanometer
rhinomanometry
instrument to measure degree of nasal
obstruction

nose obstruction
rhinocleisis

nose operation
rhinoplasty
rhinotomy
rhinocheiloplasty
septectomy
septotomy
sinusotomy
turbinectomy
turbinotomy

nose pain
rhinalgia
rhinodynia

nose pointed
oxyrhine
having a sharp pointed nose

nose purulent discharge
ozena
rhinitis purulenta

nose running
rhinorrhea
discharge from the nasal mucous membrane

nose shortness

brachyrhinia
shortness of nose in general
brachyrhynchus
shortness of nose and maxilla

nose specialist
rhinologist

nose stone
rhinodacryolith
rhinolith
rhinolite
rhinolithiasis
rhinopharyngolith

nose study
rhinology
laryngorhinology

nose viewer
nasopharyngoscope
instrument to examine nose and pharynx
rhinoscope
instrument to examine nasal passages

nose voice
rhinophonia
voice with nasal quality

nose wing
alinasal

nuclear membrane
karyotheca

numbness
obdormition
due to pressure on the sensory nerve

nutmeg
myristica

nutrition
tropism

nutrition disorder
trophonosis
trophopathy

nutritive
alible

nympha
labium minus

nymph inflammation
nymphitis

nympha operation
nymphectomy
nymphotomy
surgical procedure on the minor lips of
the vulva

nymph swelling
nymphoncus

O

obesity
adiposis
condition of fat accumulation

objects falsely magnified
macroesthesia
sensation that objects are larger than
they are

oblique amputation
loxotomy
in an oblique section

obscenity
coprolalia
coprophrasia
involuntary utterance of obscenities

obscure origin
cryptogenic
refers to source of disease

obstetric tool
vectis

obstruction
emphraxis
of the sweat glands

ocular muscle paralysis
ophthalmoplegia

ohm measurer
ohmmeter

oil gravity measurer
eleometer
oleometer

oily
oleaginous

old age
senium
especially the debility of the aged

old age study
geriatrics

old skin
geroderma
gerodermia

olefiant gas
ethylene

olfactory organs lacking
cyclencephalia
cyclencephaly
cyclocephalia
cyclocephaly
congenital fusion of the two cerebral
hemispheres

omentum
epiploic
omental

omentum hernia
enterepiplocele
enteroepiplocele

omentum lacking
anepiploic

omentum operation
omentectomy
omentopexy
*epiploectomy**
*obsolete term

omentum suture
omentorrhaphy
*epiplorrhaphy**
*obsolete term

one child
primiparous
uniparous
female who has had only one child

one-fingered/toed
monodactylism
monodactyly
a single digit on hand or foot

one-footed
monopodia
monopus
sympus monopus
born with only one foot or leg

one-sided pain
hemialgia

one-track mind
monoideism
monomania
dwelling excessively on a single subject

ooze
transude
liquid through a membrane

open country lover
agromania
having an excessive desire to be isolated or in open country

operation of...
(see under specific site)

opium alkaloids
codeine
morphine
papaverine
thebaine
tritopine

opium tincture
laudanum

opposite therapy
heteropathy
method of treating diseases by creating opposite or different conditions

oppositely situated
antipodal

optical image distortion
anamorphosis
correction by glasses

orbit operation
orbitotomy
of the eye orbit

organ/gland cells
parenchyma
distinguishing cells of a gland or organ

organ correlation
synergy
among different organs of the body

organ displacement
anteversion
dystopia
forward displacement of any organ

organ formation
organogenesis

organ lacking
ectrogeny
loss or congenital absence of all or part of an organ

organ malposition
ectopia
ectopic
ectopy
heterotopia
heterotopic

organ measurer
oncometer
instrument used to measure the size and configuration of organs

organic development
organogenesis
organogeny

organic tissue dissolution
histolysis

orifice muscle
sphincter
surrounding an opening

orifice muscle operation
sphincterectomy
sphincteroplasty
sphincterotomy

origin-equaled
isogenous
having the same origin

orthopedic appliances
orthopraxis
orthopraxy
employment of artificial appliances

osmotic pressure unequal
anisotonic

ossified cancer
osteocarcinoma

ossified fetus
ostembryon
obsolete term for lithopedion

outbreeding
exogamy
cross-fertilization

outgrowth
excrescence

outward appearance
physiognomy
physical characteristics and general appearance

ovarian abscess
pyo-ovarium

ovarian pregnancy
ovariocyesis

ovary development lacking
ovarian agenesis

ovary hardening
sclero-oophoritis

ovary hernia
ovariocele

ovary inflammation
oophoritis
ovaritis
inflammation of the ovary in general
paraoophoritis
perisalpingo-ovaritis
perioophorosalpingitis
inflammation of the tissues around the
ovary and oviduct
perioophoritis
periovaritis
inflammation of the ovary, peritoneum,
and surrounding tissues

ovary operation
oophorectomy
ovariectomy
oophorosalpingectomy
ovariosalpingectomy
oophoroplasty
oophorohysterectomy
ovariohysterectomy
oophorostomy
ovariostomy
ovariotomy
panhysterosalpingo-oophorectomy
salpingo-oophorectomy
salpingo-oothecectomy
salpingoovariectomy

ovary pain
oarialgia
ovarialgia
ovarian neuralgia
ovariodysneuria

ovary puncture
ovariocentesis
also applies to puncture of a cyst

ovary rupture
ovariorrhexis

ovary/testis combined
ovotestis
a form of hermaphroditism

ovary or testis lacking
agonadism
or absence of functions

ovary and tube inflamed
adnexitis
annexitis

ovary tumor
arrhenoblastoma
mesonephroma

ovary and uterine tube
adnexa uteri

ovary varicosity
ovarian varicocele

overdevelopment
hypertrophia
hypertrophy
over development of an organ or body
part not due to tumor

overfeeding
hyperalimentation
hypernutrition
supernutrition

overflowing tears
epiphora
accumulation of tears in the eyes

overlapping
imbrication
layers of tissue in surgical suturing

oviduct hernia
salpingocele
protrusion in general
salpingo-oophorocele
protrusion of an ovary and oviduct

oviduct inflammation
parasalpingitis
inflammation of the tissues surrounding
an oviduct

oviduct operation
panhysterosalpingectomy
hysterosalpingectomy
hysterosalpingooophorectomy
hysterosalpingostomy
oophorosalpingectomy
ovariosalpingectomy
panhysterosalpingooophorectomy

oviduct pus
pyosalpinx
accumulation of pus in an oviduct

ovum elastic envelope
oolemma
zona pellucida

oxalates in blood excessive
oxalemia

oxalic acid in urine
hyperoxaluria

oxaluria
also applies to presence of oxylates

oyster poisoning
ostreotoxism

P

pace measurer
pedometer
podometer
instrument that measures the distance walked

pain of abdominal gas
tympanism
tympanites

pain of Achilles tendon
achillodynia

pain allaying
analgia
analgic
analgesic
analgetic

pain of anus
proctalgia
proctodynia
sphincteralgia
pain at the anus or in the rectum

pain in arm
brachialgia

pain in back
dorsalgia

pain of bladder
cystalgia

pain of body
pantalgia
affecting all parts

pain of bones
ostealgia
osteodynia

pain of breast
mammalgia
mastalgia
mastodynia
mazodynia

pain of burning sensation
causalgia
persistent severe burning sensation of the skin

pain in buttocks
pygalgia

pain of cartilage
xiphodynia
xyphoidalgia

pain in cheek area
carotidynia
carotodynia
pain caused by pressure on the carotid artery

pain of chest
thoracodynia
thoracomyodynia

pain of clitoris
clitoralgia

pain of coccyx
coccyalgia
coccygodynia

pain of cold
cryalgesia
psychralgia
psychroalgia
produced by application of cold

pain, constricting
angina

pain of dental pulp
pulpalgia

pain of ears
otalgia
otodynia
otoneuralgia

pain referred
synalgia
pain away from the injured part

pain of epigastrium
epigastralgia

pain of esophagus
esophagalgia

pain excessive sensitivity
hyperalgesia
    morbid sensitivity to pain

pain of the extremities
melagra
melalgia
acrostealgia
    pain in bones of extremities

pain of eye
ophthalmalgia
ophthalmodynia
ophthalmagra

pain of face
prosoponeuralgia

pain of foot
podalgia
pododynia

pain as girdle sensation
zonesthesia
    sensation similar to that produced by
    the tightness of a girdle

pain of gland
adenalgia
dacryoadenalgia

pain of groin
inguinodynia

pain of head
cephalgia
cephalalgia
cephalodynia
encephalalgia
headache
algopsychalia
phrenalgia
psychalgalia
psychalgia
    usually caused by a depressed condi-
    tion rather than physical causes

pain of heart
cardialgia
cardiodynia

pain of heat
thermalgesia
thermoalgesia
    excessive sensibility to heat

pain of heel
calcaneodynia
talsalgia

pain of hip
coxalgia
coxodynia

pain in inguinal zone
bubonalgia

pain insensitivity
analgesia
analgia
    inability to feel pain in any parts

pain of intestine
enteralgia
enterodynia
gastroenteralgia

pain of joint
arthralgia
arthralgic
arthrodynia
arthrodynic
    severe pain in a joint, especially one not
    inflammatory in nature

pain of kidney
nephralgia

pain of knee
gonalgia
gonagra

pain lacking
anodynia
    absence of pain in a body part

pain of legs
skelalgia

pain of lips
cheilalgia
chilalgia

pain of liver
hepatalgia
hepatodynia

pain measurer
algesimeter
    instrument to measure acuteness of
    pain
dolorimeter
    measures sensitivity to pain
ponograph
    measures progressive fatigue of a con-
    tracting muscle

pain of menstruation
dysmenorrhea
menorrhalgia

pain of metatarsus
metatarsalgia

pain in missing limb
phantom limb
feeling pain in an amputated limb

pain of mouth
stomatalgia
stomatodynia

pain of muscle
myalgia
muscular pain

pain of neck
cervicodynia
trachelodynia
torticollis
wryneck

pain of nerves
neuralgia
neurodynia
polyneuralgia

pain at night
nyctalgia

pain of nipple
thelalgia

pain of noise
odynacusis
hypersensitiveness of the ear

pain of nose
rhinalgia
rhinodynia

pain on one side of body
hemialgia

pain of ovary
oarialgia
ovarialgia
ovarian neuralgia
ovariodysneuria

pain of pharynx
pharyngalgia
pharyngodynia
pain in the region of the throat

pain of pleura
pleuralgia
pleurodynia

pain of pylorus
pyloralgia

pain of rectum
proctalgia
proctodynia
rectalgia

pain reliever
analgesic
anodyne
antineuralgic
relieves pain of a nerve

pain of rheumatism
rheumatalgia

pain of ribs
costalgia
intercostal neuralgia
pleurodynia
subcostalgia

pain of sacrum
sacralgia
sacrodynia

pain of scapula
scapulalgia
pain in the region of the shoulder blades

pain sensitivity
algesia
algesic
algetic

pain sensitivity in excess
hyperalgesia
hyperalgia

pain severe
megalgia

pain of skin
dermatalgia
dermatodynia
erythromelalgia
rodonalgia

pain in sleep
hypnalgia
experienced during sleep

pain source
algogenesia
algogenesis

pain of spleen
splenalgia
splenodynia

pain of stomach
gastralgia
gastroenteralgia
cardialgia
peratodynia

pain from strong light
photalgia
photodynia
  pain experienced when under the intensity of strong light

pain sudden
twinge
  a sudden sharp pain of short duration

pain suffocating
angina
  spasmodic, choking sensation

pain in tarsus of foot
tarsalgia

pain of teeth
dentalgia
odontalgia
odontodynia
toothache
aerodontalgia
  toothache due to high altitude flying

pain of tendon
tenalgia
tenodynia
tenontodynia

pain of thigh
meralgia

pain of tibia
tibialgia

pain of tongue
glossalgia
glossodynia

pain on touching objects
haphalgesia
  pain or unpleasant sensation caused by touch

pain of trachea
trachealgia
trachelodynia

pain of urethra
urethralgia

pain of urinary bladder
cystalgia

pain of urinary tract
urocrisia
urocrisis

pain of urination
dysuria
urodynia
  difficulty or pain when urinating

pain of uterus
hysteralgia
hysterodynia
metralgia
metrodynia
uteralgia

pain of vagina
colpalgia
vaginodynia
vaginismus
vulvismus

pain of vertebrae
spondylalgia
spondylodynia

pain of viscera
visceralgia
  pain in any of the internal organs

painless death
euthanasia

palate cleft
uranoschisis

palate high/narrow
hypsistaphilia

palate inflammation
palatitis

palate operation
palatoplasty
staphylectomy
staphylotomy
uranoplasty
uranostaphyloplasty
uvulectomy

palate paralysis
palatoplegia
  of the soft palate

palate pendulum
uvula
  fleshy conical mass located above the back of the tongue

palate suture
 palatorrhaphy
 staphylorrhaphy
 uranorrhaphy
 uranostaphyloplasty
 uranostaphylorrhaphy

pale urine
 achromaturia
  lacking pigmentation

paleness of skin
 achromia
 achromasia
  due to lack of pigment

palm of hand
 thenar
 vola
 volar

palmar vesicles
 cheiropompholyx
 chiropompholyx
 dyshidria
 dishidrosis
 pompholyx
  blisters that appear on the palms of the
  hands and soles of the feet

palpable vibration
 fremitus

pancreas calculus
 pancreatolith
 pancreolith

pancreas disease
 pancreatopathy
 pancreopathy

pancreas inflammation
 pancreatitis
 peripancreatitis
  inflammation of the tissues surrounding
  the pancreas

pancreas lacking
 apancrea
 apancreatic

pancreas operation
 pancreatectomy
 pancreectomy
 pancreaticoduodenostomy
 pancreatoduodenostomy
 pancreatojejunostomy
 pancreaticolithotomy

pancreatoduodenectomy
 pancreatolithectomy
 pancreatolithotomy
 pancreolithotomy
 pancreatomy
 pancreatotomy

pancreas proximity
 parapancreatic
  near the pancreas

pancreatic extract
 insulin
  Iletin®

pancreatic juice lacking
 achylia pancreatica

panic attack
 unreasoning anxiety
  accompanied by fear

panting
 hyperpnea
 polypnea

paralysis of bladder
 cystoparalysis
 cystoplegia

paralysis of extremities
 acroparalysis

paralysis of eye muscles
 ophthalmoplegia

paralysis of intestines
 adynamic ileus
 enteroplegia
  usually as the result of peritonitis or
  shock

paralysis of legs
 paraparesis
 paraplegia
 paraplegic
 paraplegy

paralysis of limbs
 quadriplegia
 tetraplegia
  paralysis of all four extremities

paralysis of one side of body
 hemiparesis
 hemiplegia
 monoplegia

paralysis on two sides
diplegia
diplegic
affecting equally corresponding parts on both sides of the body

paralysis partial
monoparesis
on one part of the body only

parasite absorber
parasitotropic
substance in the blood that absorbs parasites

parasite affinity
parasitotropism
parasitotropy

parasite in blood
parasitemia

parasite disease
parasitosis
infestation with or any disease caused by parasites

parasite fear
parasitophobia

parasite growth
parasitogenesis

parasite-killer
parasiticide

parasite specialist
parasitologist

parasite study
helminthology
parasitology

parenchyma inflammation
parenchymatitis
inflammation of the specific cells of a gland or organ

parovarium inflammation
parovaritis

parrot fever
psittacosis

part defective or lacking
aplasia
congenital condition

parturition difficult
dystocia
parodynia

parturition normal
eutocia

parturition first time
primipara
primigravida
primiparity
first pregnancy

passage closing
stegnosis

patch/spot
tache

patella operation
patellectomy
removal

patella shaped
patelliform

pathology of extremities
acropathology

pea-shaped
pisiform

peace of mind
ataraxia
calmness or tranquility

Peale pill
phencyclidine (PCP)

peanut oil
arachis oil

peanut oil acid
arachic acid
arachidic acid

pear-shaped
piriform
pyriform

pearl-like
nacreous
resembling mother-of-pearl

peeling off
exfoliation
also denotes scaling off

pelvis measurer
pelvimeter
pelvimetry

pelvis narrowness
leptopellic

pelvis operation
pelvilithotomy

pelviolithotomy
pelviotomy

pelvis viewer
pelviscope
instrument for examining the interior of the pelvis

penis
membrum virile
penile
phallic
phallus

penis deformity
hypospadias
urethra opens on the ventral side of the penis
paraspadias
urethra opens on one side of the penis
phallocampsis
curvature of the erect penis
phallocrypsis
dislocation and retraction

penis discharge
phallorrhea

penis hemorrhage
phallorrhagia

penis inflammation
balanitis
balanoposthitis

penis largeness
macropenis
megalopenis

penis operation
penotomy
phallectomy
phalloplasty
phallotomy

penis pain
phallalgia
phallodynia

penis pulling
peotillomania
manifestation of a nervous disorder

penis shaped
phalloid

penis smallness
micropenis
microphallus

penis tumor/swelling
phalloncus

penis worship
phallicism
phallism

pentose in urine
pentosuria

perception defective
imperception
inability to form a mental picture of an object

perception lacking
agnea
agnosia
inability to recognize by various sensory impressions
auditory agnosia
inability to recognize by sound
optic agnosia
inability to recognize by vision
tactile agnosia
inability to recognize by touch

pericardial sac fluid
pneumohydropericardium
air and fluid in the pericardial sac

pericardium inflammation
pericarditis
inflammation of the pericardium
pleuropericarditis
inflammation of pleura and pericardium
pyopericarditis
inflammation accompanied by pus

pericardium operation
pericardectomy
pericardiectomy
pericardiostomy
pericardiotomy

pericardium puncture
pericardiocentesis

pericardium pus
pyopneumopericardium
pus and gas or air in the pericardium

pericardium suture
pericardiorrhaphy

perineal hernia
perineocele

perineum operation
perineoplasty
perineotomy

perineum suture
perineorrhaphy

perineurium inflammation
perineuritis
inflammation of the connective tissue
surrounding nerve fibers

periodontal inflammation
pericementitis
periodontitis

periosteum inflammation
parosteitis
parostitis

periosteum operation
periosteotomy

peritoneal cavity gas/air
aeroperitoneum
aeroperitonia
pyopneumoperitoneum

peritoneum disease
peritoneopathy
any disease or disorder of the peritoneum

peritoneum inflammation
pachyperitonitis
thickening of the peritoneum due to inflammation
pericolitis
pericolonitis
inflammation of tissues surrounding the
colon
peritonitis
general inflammation
pneumoperitonitis
inflammation plus gas
pyoperitonitis
inflammation plus pus
pyopneumoperitonitis
inflammation plus gas and pus
retroperitonitis
inflammation of the retroperitoneal structures
salpingoperitonitis
inflammation of the tubes and peritoneum

peritoneum operation
peritoneotomy

peritoneum shunt
ascites shunt

peritoneovenous shunt
shunting of ascites fluid from the peritoneal cavity to the jugular vein

persecution delusion
paranoia

perspiration
diaphoresis

perspiration deficiency
hyphidrosis
hypohidrosis
olighidria
oligidria

perspiration lacking
adiaphoresis
anhidrosis

perspiration odor
bromhidrosis
bromidrosis
osmidrosis
ozochrotia
denotes foul smelling perspiration

perspiration preventive
adiaphoretic
anhidrotic

perspiration suppression
anhidrosis
ischidrosis

pesthouse
lazaret
lazaretto
hospital for treatment of contagious diseases

phagocyte destruction
phagocytolysis
phagolysis

phagocyte enhancer
opsonin
substance in the blood making bacteria
more prone to action of phagocytes

phalanges in excess
polyphalangia
polyphalangism

phalanx inflammation
phalangitis

phalanx lacking
hypophalangism
born without one or more bones of finger or toe

phalanx operation
phalangectomy

phalanx shortness
brachyphalangia

pharynx discharge
pharyngorrhea

pharynx disease
pharyngopathy
any abnormal condition of the pharynx

pharynx dryness
pharyngoxerosis

pharynx examination
pharyngoscopy

pharynx inflammation
adenopharyngitis
pharyngotonsillitis
of the pharynx and tonsils
nasopharyngitis
pharyngorhinitis
of the pharynx and nasal passages
pharyngitis
of the pharynx in general
pharyngolaryngitis
of the pharynx and larynx
retropharyngitis
of the tissues behind the pharynx
rhinopharyngitis
of the mucous membrane of the nose
and pharynx

pharynx obstruction
pharyngemphraxis

pharynx operation
pharyngectomy
pharyngoplasty
pharyngotomy

pharynx pain
pharyngalgia
pharyngodynia

pharynx paralysis
pharyngoparalysis
pharyngoplegia

pharynx spasm
pharyngismus
pharyngospasm

pharynx stone
pharyngolith
calculi of the pharynx
rhinopharyngolith
calculi of the nose and pharynx

pharynx stricture
pharyngoperistole
pharyngostenosis

pharynx viewer
nasopharyngoscope
pharyngoscope
instruments used for examining pharynx
and nose

phenetidin in urine
phenetidinuria

phenol poisoning
carbolism

phenol in urine
phenoluria

phenyl-ketone in urine
phenylketonuria

phosphates in urine
phosphaturia

phosphorescent sweat
phosphorhidrosis
phosphoridrosis
excretion of luminous sweat

phosphorescent urine
photuria

phosphorus poisoning
phosphorism

phrase repetition
palilalia
paliphrasia
involuntary repetition of words

pigeon breast
pectus carinatum

pigment-lacking disease
achroderma
alphodermia
any disease resulting from lack of pigmentation
achromatosis
albinism
leukoderma
a condition where the skin lacks pigmentation

pigments in urine
acholuria
acholuric
lacking bile pigment in urine
urochrome
uroletin
yellow pigment in urine

pigments in urine (cont.)
urocyanin
uroglaucin
    bluish-green pigment in urine
urocyanogen
urocyanosis
    blue pigment in urine
urorubin
urofuscohematin
urosein
    red pigment in urine
uromelanin
    black pigment in urine
urophein
    gray pigment in urine
urospectrin
    pigment found in normal urine
indican
uroxanthin
    yellow pigment that turns indigo blue on
    oxidation

piles
hemorrhoids

pine-cone shaped
pineal
piniform

pineal gland operation
pinealectomy
    removal of the gland

pinkeye
conjunctivitis

pinworm in humans
oxyuriasis

placenta inflammation
placentitis

placenta lacking
aplacental

plant eating
herbivorous
phytophagous
    feeds on plants or herbs

plant-fungus disease
schizomycosis
    any disease caused by plant micro-
    organisms

plant juice
succus
    juice extracted for medicinal purposes

plant life
flora

plant poison
phytotoxin
    poisonous protein

plantar vesicles
chiropompholyx
dyshidrosis
pompholyx
    blisters that appear on the soles of the
    feet and palms of the hands

plasma separation
plasmapheresis
    removal of plasma from withdrawn blood
    before return to the donor

plasma substitute
periston

plaster
cataplasm
poultice
    usually applied to the skin after the plas-
    ter has been heated

plastic bone surgery
osteoplasty

plastic cheek surgery
meloplasty

plastic ear surgery
otoplasty

plastic eye surgery
ophthalmoplasty

plastic graft surgery
alloplasty
allotransplantation
    transplanted into the same species
autoplasty
    transplant from one's own body
heteroplasty
heterotransplantation
    transplanted from another species

plastic lip surgery
cheiloplasty
chiloplasty

plastic mouth surgery
stomatoplasty

plastic nose surgery
rhinoplasty

plastic palate surgery
palatoplasty
staphyloplasty
uraniscoplasty
uranoplasty

plastic tissue surgery
uranostaphyloplasty
uranostaphylorrhaphy
zoografting
zooplasty
grafting of animal tissue into the human body

pleasant delusions
habromania
morbid impulse toward gaiety

pleasure diminution
anhedonia

pleura calculus
pleurolith

pleura inflammation
pleurisy
pleuritis
inflammation of the pleura
pleurohepatitis
inflammation of the pleura and liver
pleuropericarditis
inflammation of the pleura and pericardium

pleura operation
pleurectomy
pleuracotomy
pleurotomy
thoracotomy

pleura pain
pleuralgia
pleurodynia

pleural cavity air/gas
pneumothorax

pleural cavity fluid
hydropneumothorax
accumulation of serous fluid and gas

pleural cavity puncture
pleuracentesis
pleurocentesis
thoracentesis

pleural cavity pus
empyema
pyohemothorax
pyopneumothorax
pyothorax

pleurisy/pneumonia
pleuropneumonia

plucking bedclothes
carphology

floccillation
delirious picking during illness considered to be a serious symptom

plucking habit
phaneromania
preoccupation with an external part of the body

plug of cotton
tampon

pneumococci in blood
pneumococcemia

pneumococci in urine
pneumococcusuria

pneumogastric nerve
vagus
nerve located from the cranial cavity to the abdominal organs

pneumonia
pneumonitis
pulmonitis

pneumonia/pleurisy
pleuropneumonia

poem-writing mania
metromania

poikilocytes in blood
poikilocythemia
poikilocytosis
presence of irregularly shaped red blood cells in the peripheral blood

pointed head
acrocephalia
acrocephaly
oxycephaly
turricephaly

poison in blood
septicemia
toxemia
toxicemia

poison fear
toxicophobia
toxiphobia
abnormal fear of poison or being poisoned

poison immunity
mithridatism
immunizing against a poison by gradually increasing the dosage

poison of meat
allantiasis
botulism

poison producing
toxiferous

poison in producing cell
endotoxin
toxin retained in the cell that produces it

polypeptides in blood
polypeptidemia

portal vein dilation
pylephlebectasia
pylephlebectasis

portal vein inflammation
pylephlebitis

portal vein obstruction
pylemphroxis
obstruction of the vein that enters the liver

portal vein relating
pylic

portal vein thrombosis
pylethrombosis

postchildbirth discharge
lochia
the mucus, blood and tissue debris discharged after childbirth

postmortem examination
autopsy
necropsy

pot
marijuana

pouch of testicles
scrotum

powerless
adynamia

pregnancy
cyesis

pregnancy classification
multigravida
multipara
pregnant woman who has previously given birth
multiparity
multiparous
polycyesis
having given birth to several children

primigravida
woman pregnant for the first time

pregnancy convulsions
eclampsia

pregnancy diagnosis
cyesiognosis

pregnancy extrauterine
eccyesis
ectopic pregnancy
paracyesis
development of the fertilized ovum outside the cavity of the uterus

pregnancy prevention
contraception

pregnant
gravid

prepuce constricted
phimosis

prepuce inflammation
acroposthitis
posthitis
foreskin

prepuce lacking
aposthia
congenital condition

pressure sense
baresthesia

pressure sore
decubitus ulcer

preventive treatment
chemoprophylaxis
prophylactic
prophylaxis

prism-shaped
prismatic
prismoid

project obsession
zelotypia
compulsive desire for fostering an enterprise

projecting sharp bone
osseous spicule
acidosteophyte*
*obsolete term

projection inflammation
apophysitis
inflammation of the projection of an organ

projection of an organ
apophysis
protruding outgrowth of organ or bone

prone to infectious disease
anaphylaxis
decreased resistance due to effects of previous attacks

prostate discharge
prostatorrhea

prostate inflammation
prostatitis
inflammation of the gland
extraprostatitis
paraprostatitis
periprostatitis
inflammation of the tissues around the gland
prostatovesiculitis
inflammation of the prostate and the seminal vesicles
utriculitis
inflammation of the prostatic utricle

prostate operation
prostatectomy
prostatolithotomy
prostatotomy

protein accumulation
proteinosis
accumulation in the tissues

protein alteration
biotechnology
recombinant protein

protein in blood
carcinoembryonic antigen
proteinemia

protein conversion
proteolysis
conversion into more simple substances

protein, protective
antibody

protein in urine
proteinuria

protoplasm hereditary cells
mitochondria
small specks found in the protoplasm of certain cells

protoxoid of lead
litharge

protozoa-killer
protozoacide

protrusion of cornea
keratectasia

psycho-process measurer
psychodometry
instrument that measures the speed of the psychic process

psychoanalyzed person
analysand

pterygold canal
Vidian artery
Vidian canal
the internal maxillary artery

puerperal metritis
lochiometritis

pulse clock
sphygmograph
instrument that records pulsation and variations in blood pressure

pulse measurer
pulsimeter
pulsometer
sphygmodynamometer
instrument that measures the force and frequency of the pulse
sphygmochronograph
instrument that registers the pulse related to heart beat

pulse related
sphygmic
sphygmoid

pulse repeated irregularity
allorhythmia
allorhythmic

pulse smallness
microsphygmy
microsphyxia

pulse-wave recorder
kymograph

pulse weakness
acrotism
microsphygmy
microsphyxia
also denotes lack of pulse

puncture with hot needle
ignipuncture

puncture of spine
rachiocentesis

pupil abnormal form
dyscoria

pupil artificial
coremorphosis
formation of an artificial pupil

pupil closure
synizesis

pupil constrictor
miotic

pupil contraction
miosis
mydriatic
myosis*
*obsolete spelling

pupil dilation
corectasia
corectasis
corediastasis
mydriasis
mydriatic

pupil displacement
corectopia

pupil equality
isocoria
two pupils having equal diameter

pupils in excess
polycoria
having more than one pupil in the same orbit

pupil inequality
anisocoria
inequality in diameter

pupils lacking
acorea

pupil measurer
pupillometer
instrument to measure size of the pupil
pupillostatometer
instrument to measure distance between the two pupils
vuerometer
instrument to measure the interpupillary distance

pupil narrowing
stenocoriasis

pupil occlusion
corecleisis
coreclisis

pupil operation
coreoplasty
corepraxy
coreprexy
coroplasty

pupil reflex slow
asthenocoria
slow reaction to a light stimulus

pupil smallness
microcoria

pupil surgical instrument
cortectome

pupillary axis/visual angle
kappa angle

purging
catharsis

purifier
abluent

purines in urine
alloxuria
alloxuric

purple discoloration
livedo reticularis
discoloration of skin caused by dilation of capillaries and venules

purple vision
rhodopsin
erythropsin*
*obsolete term

purpurin in urine
purpurinuria

pus in blood
ichoremia
ichorrhemia

pus containing
purulence
purulency

pus cyst
pyocyst

pus discharge
pyorrhea

pus expectoration
pyoptysis
spitting of pus

pus formation
pyesis
pyogenesis
pyopoiesis
pyosis
suppuration

pus in urine
pyuria

Q

quackery
charlatanism
fraudulent claim to medical knowledge

quartz
silicon dioxide
crystalline form

quicksilver
mercury

quiver
tremor
twitching
involuntary spasmodic movement

R

rabbit eyes
lagophthalmia
lagophthalmos
condition where the eye cannot be
closed entirely

rabbit fever
tularemia

race improvement
euthenics
the science of establishing optimum living conditions

radiant energy measurer
radiomicrometer
detects minute changes in radiant energy
autoradiography
technique to identify tissue binding site

radiant heat, impervious to
adiathermancy

radiant heat measurer
bolometer

radiation therapy
*actinotherapy**
*obsolete term
radiotherapy
sending forth of light, short radio waves,
ultraviolet or x-rays

radioactivity unit
curie
microcurie

rat-bite fever
sodoku

ratlike
murine
also mouse-like

raw flesh eating
omophagia

reaction slow
apathism
delayed response to stimuli

reading impaired
dyslexia

reading slowness
bradylexia

reclining
recumbent

recollection
anamnesis
anamnestic

recovery of strength
analeptic
strengthening, stimulating

rectum examination
proctoscopy
rectoscopy

rectum inflammation
periproctitis
perirectitis

rectum inflammation (cont.)
proctitis
rectitis
  inflammation of the rectum or anus
coloproctitis
rectocolitis
  inflammation of the rectum membrane
  and the colon
proctosigmoiditis
  inflammation of the rectum and sigmoid
  colon

rectum infusion
proctoclysis
  through rectal tube

rectum opening to bladder
anus vesicalis
  absence of normal opening

rectum operation
proctectomy
proctoplasty
proctotomy
rectectomy
rectoplasty
proctocolpoplasty
proctocystoplasty
proctopexy
rectopexy
proctosigmoidectomy
proctostomy
rectosigmoidectomy
rectostomy
proctotomy
sigmoidoproctostomy

rectum pain
proctagra
proctalgia
proctodynia
rectalgia
  pain at the anus or in the rectum

rectum paralysis
proctoparalysis
proctoplegia

rectum prolapse
rectocele
  falling of the rectum into the vagina

rectum spasm
proctospasm

rectum specialist
proctologist

rectum stricture
proctostenosis
  also called rectostenosis

rectum suture
proctorrhaphy
  repair of prolapsed walls

rectum viewer
anoscope
proctoscope
rectoscope
relapse

red blood cell
erythrocyte
reticulocyte

red blood cell clumper
hemagglutinin
  a substance

red blood cell formation
erythropoiesis

red corpuscles dissolution
hematolysis
hemolysis
  causes failure to coagulate

red discoloration
purpura
  purplish or brownish-red discoloration
  from hemorrhage into the tissues

red skin patches
erythema

red vision
erythropsia
  objects appear to be red

reds
secobarbital
  barbiturate

reflex hammer
plessor
plexor
  used to test knee reflex

reflex lacking
areflexia

refractive abnormality
ametropia

relapse
palindromia
palindromic

religious insanity
hieromania
belief of inspiration by a divine power

remedy for epilepsy
antiepileptic

remedy for inflammation
antiphlogistic
antipyrotic

remedy for nightmares
antephialtic

remedy for pain
anodyne
analgesic

remedy for scurvy
antiscorbutic

remedy for vomiting
antemetic
antiemetic

remedy for worms
anthelmintic
santonin
vermifuge
used to expel intestinal worms

remote ancestral traits
atavism
characteristics appearing in an individual

renal pelvis dilatation
pyelectasia

renal pelvis operation
pyeloplasty
pyelostomy
pyelotomy
pyelolithotomy

renal pelvis pus
pyonephrosis

repetition
autoecholalia
continuous repetition of one's own words

reproduction asexual
agamocytogony
agamogony
schizogony

reproductive glands
gonads

resistant to treatment
malignant

respiration
pneusis

respiratory suspension
apnea
apnea vera
when due to decreased carbon dioxide tension
apnea vagal
when due to vagal stimulation

response to contact stimuli
thigmotropism

restlessness
dysphoria

restoration
analeptic
restoring strength

retention in stomach
ischochymia
stagnation of food

retina detachment
amotio retinae

retina examination
retinoscopy
skiascopy

retina image measurer
eikonometer

retina inflammation
retinitis
of the retina
retinochoroiditis
of the choroid and retina
retinopapillitis
of retina and optic disk

retina inner layers
entoretina

retina viewer
retinoscope

rheumatic pain
rheumatalgia

rheumatic study
rheumatology

rhythm defective
dysrhythmia
loss of rhythm, especially an irregularity of heart beat

rhythm lacking
arrhythmia
arrhythmic

rib lacking
apleuria

rib operation
costectomy
costotomy

riblike
costiform

ricelike
riziform

rickets
rachitis
juvenile osteomalacia
in a child

right-eyed
dextrocular
preference in monocular work

right-footed
dextropedal
preference, as in hopping

right-to-left
dextrosinistral

right-side heart
dextrocardia
location on right side

right-twisting
dextrotorsion
as in turning of the eye

ring finger
digitus annularis

ring-shaped
circinate
cricoid

ringing in ears
tinnitus
sound heard in the ear

ringworm
tinea

r-mispronunciation
rhotacism

rod-shaped
bacilliform
baculiform
rhabdoid

rodent killer
rodenticide

roentgen ray measurer
penetrometer
instrument to measure the penetrating power of an x-ray beam

roof-shaped
tactiform

roof-shaped skull
scaphocephalism
tectocephaly

root operation
radicotomy
rhizotomy

rootlike
rhizoid

ropelike
funic
funicular
pertaining to the umbilical cord
restiform
pertaining to nerve fibers

rosalic acid
aurin
corallin
aromatic dye taken from coal tar

rosin
colophony

rumen inflammation
rumenitis

rumination
merycism
regurgitation of food

ruminant stomach
1st-rumen
2nd-reticulum
3rd-omasum
4th-abomasum

running ear
otorrhea

running nose
rhinorrhea

rupture
rhexis
of an organ or vessel

rust of copper
verdigris

S

sac-like
sacciform

sacrum/lumbar vertebra angle
sacrovertebral angle

sacrum operation
sacrectomy
excision of a segment of the lower vertebral column

sacrum pain
sacralgia
sacrodynia

sacrum proximity
parasacral

St. Vitus dance
ballism
ballismus
chorea
monochorea

saliva
spittle

saliva/air swallowing
aerosialophagy
sialoaerophagy
excessive swallowing of air and saliva in the stomach

saliva deficiency
aptyalia
aptyalism
asialia
hypoptyalism
hyposalivation
xerostomia
deficiency or lack of saliva

saliva duct stricture
sialostenosis

saliva flow excessive
hyperptyalism
hypersalivation
polysialia
ptyalism
ptyalorrhea
salivation
sialism

sialismus
sialorrhea

saliva preventer
antisialagogue
antisialic

saliva promoter
ptyalagogue
sialagogic
sialagogue
a substance that enhances the flow of saliva

saliva suppression
sialoschesis

salivary duct inflammation
sialoangitis
sialodochitis

salivary gland
sialaden

salivary gland inflammation
sialadenitis
sialoadenitis

salivary gland operation
sialoadenectomy
sialoadenotomy
sialithotomy
sialolithotomy
sialodochoplasty

salivation
ptyalism
ptyalosis
sialorrhea
sialosis

salt
saline

salt measurer
salimeter
instrument to measure the amount of salt in solutions

saltlike
haloid

sandfly fever
pappataci fever
phlebotomus fever

sandy
arenaceous
psammous
sabulous

satellite cell
amphicyte

saucerlike
patelliform

scale
squama

scaling horny skin
keratolysis
peeling or scaling off the horny layer on skin

scalp disease
favus
kerion
tinea favosa
a type of ringworm usually affecting the scalp

scaly
squamate
squamosa
squamosal
squamous

scaly skin
ichthyosis
pityriasis
a dermatitis marked by scaling

scapula operation
scapulectomy
scapulopexy

scapula pain
scapulalgia
pain in the shoulder blade

scapula pertaining
scapular

scar
cicatrix

scar formation
cicatrization
process of scar formation

scar healing
cicatrize

scar operation
cicatrectomy
cicatricotomy

scar tissue
cheloid
keloid
nodular, lobulated,movable mass of hyperplastic scar tissue

schizophrenia
dementia precox

sciatica
ischialgia
ischiodynia

science of algae
algology
phycology

science of animals
zoology
zoobiology
zoonomy
concerned with the different species of animal life
zootechnics
taming and breeding of animals
zoonosology
zoopathology
classification of diseases of animals

science of arteries
arteriology

science of baths
balneology
science of bathing, as for therapeutic purposes

science of blindness
typhology
study of cause, effects and cure of blindness

science of blood
hematology
hemology

science of blood vessels
angiology
study of blood and lymphatic vessels

science of bones
osteologia
osteology

science of brain
phrenology
an obsolete hypothesis that each form of activity emanates from a separate location in the brain

science of cells
cytology

science of childbirth
obstetrics
tocology

science of children
paidology
pediatrics
pedology

science of climate
climatology
  science dealing with climate
phenology
  study of climate effect on biological
  rhythm of plants and animals

science of deformity
orthopaedics
orthopedics
  dealing with prevention and correction of
  deformities
teratology
  study of congenital malformations and
  abnormal development

science of diseases
etiology
  term for the cause of disease
pathogenesis
pathogeny
  study of origin and development of diseases
pathology
  study of cause, symptoms and results of
  diseases

science of drugs
pharmacology

science of ears
otiatria
otiatrics
otology

science of ears and throat
otolaryngology

science of ears, nose and throat
otorhinolaryngology

science of excretions
eccrinology

science of eyes
ophthalmology

science of feet
chiropody
podiatry

science of female diseases
gynecology
  especially endocrine and reproductive
  functions

science of finger signs
cheirology
chirology
dactylology
  the art of conveying ideas by means of
  the fingers

science of fractures
agmatology

science of fungi
mycology

science of glands
adenology

science of hair
trichology

science of head measuring
cephalometry
  science related to measuring the head
  or skull

science of heart
cardiology

science of heredity
genetics

science of immunity
immunology

science of inanimate
abiology
anorganology
  study of non-living things

science of insects
entomology

science of joints
arthralgia
arthrology
syndesmologia
syndesmology
synosteology

science of light rays
actinology
radiology

science of limb making
prosthetics
  manufacture of artificial parts for the human body

science of liver
hepatology

science of long life
macrobiotics

science of man
anthropogeny
anthropogony
anthropology
study of man's origin and development
somatology
study of the anatomy and physiology of man

science of medicines
pharmacodynamics
study of the effect of medicine on the human body

science of mind
psychology
study of human behavior
psychophysics
study that deals with correlation of mind and matter

science of mouth
stomatology
study of the mouth and its diseases

science of nerves
neurology
study of the nervous system and its disorders

science of nose
rhinology

science of organs
organology
physiology

science of pharynx
pharyngology

science of poisons
toxicology

science of pulse
sphygmology

science of secretions
eccrinology
also applies to excretions
endocrinology
internal secretions

science of sensations
haptics

science of serums
serology
pertaining to antigen and antibody study

science of skin
dermatology

science of stomach
gastrology

science of symptoms
semiology
semiotics
symptomatology

science of treatment
therapeutics
application of remedies for treatment of disease

sclera bulging
sclerectasia
staphyloma
staphylomatous

sclera inflammation
scleritis
sclerotitis
general inflammation
sclerochoroiditis
scleroticochoroiditis
inflammation of the sclera and choroid

sclera knife
sclerotome
surgical instrument for use on the sclera

sclera operation
sclerectomy
scleroplasty
sclerotomy
sclerectoiridectomy
sclerostomy

sclera puncture
scleronyxis

sclera softening
scleromalacia

scoliosis measure
scoliosometry
instrument for measuring the degree of deformity

scotoma measure
scotometry

scraping
abrasion
chemexfoliation
chemical face peeling

scrotal hernia
hydatidocele
orchiocele

scrotum operation
scrotectomy
scrotoplasty

seasickness
naupathia
vomitus marinus

sebaceous cyst
wen

second parturition
secundipara
woman who has borne two children

secretion flow
succorrhea
excessive flow of secretion

secretion high
hypersecretion

secretion low
hyposecretion

secretion of urine
uropoiesis

self-absorption
autism
at the expense of regulation by outward reality
schizophrenia
complex disorder of thinking process and withdrawal

self-analysis
autoanalysis
self-analysis by psychoanalytic method

self-cruelty satisfaction
masochism
finding pleasure in abuses of others

self-hypnotism
autohypnosis
idiohypnotism
self-induced

self-love
autophilia
narcissism

self-starvation
apocarteresis
resulting in death

semen in urine
semenuria
seminuria
spermaturia

seminal deficiency

aspermia
aspermatism

seminal fluid in excess
polyspermia
polyspermism

seminal vesicle inflamed
prostatovesiculitis
vesiculitis

seminal vesicle operation
vesiculectomy
vesiculotomy

senile skin
geroderma
atrophic skin of the aged

sensation defective
hypesthesia
hypoesthesia

sensation lacking
anesthesia
dysesthesia

sensitivity to cold
cryesthesia

sensitivity increased
anaphylaxis

sensitivity measurer
baresthesiometer
instrument to estimate the weight of sensitivity

sensitivity to pain
algesthesia
algesia
algesic
algetic

septum operation
septectomy
septoplasty
septostomy
septotomy
operative procedure on the nasal septum

sequestrum operation
sequestrectomy
sequestrotomy

serum study
serology

severe pain
megalgia

sex chromosome
idiochromosome

sexless
asexual
having no sex or no sexual interest

sexless reproduction
agamogenesis

sexual animal attraction
zoolagnia
sexual attraction to animals

sexual attraction
heterosexuality
for the opposite sex
homosexuality
for the same sex

sexual desire
aphrodisia
aphrodisiomania
eroticism
erotism
erotomania
libido
general terms
kleptolagnia
sexual gratification obtained by theft
necrophilia
necrophilism
sexual impulse for contact with dead
bodies
gynecomania
satyriasis
satyrism
satyromania
strong sexual desire in males
nymphomania
nymphomaniac
strong sexual desire in females
lesbianism
sapphism
tribadism
homosexuality among females
pedophilia
love of children
pederasty
sodomy
anal intercourse
zooerastia
attraction to animals

sexual desire diminisher
anaphrodisiac
antaphrodisiac
medicinal agent that lessens desire

sexual desire impaired
anaphrodisia

sexual desire promoter
erotic

sexual gratification
autoerotism
autosexualism
masturbation
usually by self-manipulation
algolagnia
increased by inflicting pain
coprolagnia
increased by the thought, sight or handling of feces
masochism
increased by receiving pain from others
psycholagny
increased by mental concepts
pyrolagnia
gratification from setting fires
sadism
gratification from inflicting pain on others
sadomasochism
gratification from either inflicting or receiving pain
iconolagny
induced by sculptures or pictures

sexual impotency
idiogamist
impotent except for one or a few of the
opposite sex

sexual intercourse
coitus

sexual perversion
paraphilia
parasexuality

sexual repression
antiorgastic

sexual reproduction
gamogenesis

sexual sensation
hyperhedonia
hyperhedonism

sexually mature
viripotent
obsolete term

shaggy/hairy
hirsute
hirsutism

shaking body
  succussion
    shaking the body to detect the presence of fluid in the thorax

shapeless
  amorphous

sharpness
  acuity
  acuteness

shaving cramp
  xyrospasm

sheath
  theca

shedding
  exfoliation
    detachment of superficial cells from the skin or tissue surface

shin-bone
  tibia
    the largest bone below the knee

shingles
  herpes zoster

shiny skin
  leioderma
    glossy appearance of the skin

shock therapy
  electric shock therapy
  electroconvulsive therapy
  electroshock therapy
    treatment of mental disorder by passage of an electric current through the brain

shortness of breath
  dyspnea
    applies to painful and difficult breathing

shortness of fingers
  brachydactylia
  brachydactyly

shortsightedness
  myopia

shoulder blade
  scapula

shoulder operation
  scapulectomy
  scapulopexy

shoulder pain

  scapulalgia
  scapulodynia

sickle-cell anemia
  meniscocytosis

sicklelike
  falciform
    shaped like a sickle

side-distortion
  rachioscoliosis
  scoliosis
    distortion of the spine to one side

sievelike
  cribrate
  cribriform
  polyporous

sigmoid examination
  sigmoidoscopy

sigmoid inflammation
  sigmoiditis

sigmoid operation
  sigmoidectomy
  sigmoidotomy
  sigmoidopexy
  sigmoidoproctostomy
  sigmoidorectostomy
  sigmoidostomy

sign of death
  rhytidosis
    wrinkles of the cornea

signs/gestures lacking
  animia
    loss of ability to communicate by gestures

silicon dust disease
  anthracosilicosis
    lung disease from inhalation

sinus inflammation
  sinuitis
  sinusitis

sinus operation
  sinuotomy
  sinusotomy

sinusitis
  aerosinusitis
  barosinusitis
    due to difference between internal and external pressures

six children
sextipara
woman who has borne six children
sextuplet
one of six children born from the same parturition

six fingers/toes
hexadactylism
hexadactyly

six pregnancies
sextigravida
pregnant for the sixth time

size cells equal
isocellular

skin aging prematurely
acrogeria
premature wrinkling and looseness of skin on hands and feet

skin allergic disorder
allergodermia

skin atrophy
atrophia cutis
atrophoderma
atrophodermatosis

skin bleeding
dermatorrhagia
blood discharging from skin

skin blue spot
lividity
black and blue spots on skin

skin bone formation
osteodermia
osteosis cutis

skin color lacking
achromasia

skin cyst
dermatocyst

skin darkening
melanoderma
melasma
due to deposition of excess melanin or of metallic substances

skin discoloration
dyschroa
dyschroia
poor complexion
chlorosis
chloranemia

chloroanemia
anemic disorder; green sickness
dermatomyositis
purplish red erythema on the face seen in a progressive muscular disorder

skin disease
dermatopathia
dermatopathy
dermopathy
any disease of the skin
pemphigus
designates a variety of blistering skin diseases
toxicoderma
toxicodermatosis
disease caused by poison

skin disorder
keratolysis
separation or loosening of the horny layer of the epidermis
paresthesia
abnormal sensation such as tingling or burning

skin dryness
fishskin disease
ichthyosis
phrynoderma
xeroderma
xerodermia
xerosis

skin dryness preventer
antixerotic

skin elevation
papule
small, circumcized solid growth
vesicle
containing serum

skin eruption
anthema
generalized, with sudden onset
exanthema
a symptom of an acute viral or coccal disease

skin glossy and smooth
leiodermia

skin grafting
dermatoplasty
dermoplasty
epidermatoplasty

skin hardening
scleroderma

scleriasis
sclerodermatitis

skin healing imperfect
adermogenesis

skin hemorrhage
petechiasis
formation of minute hemorrhagic spots
in the skin

skin indentation measurer
elastometer
device to measure elasticity of the skin

skin inflammation
acrodermatitis
of the skin of an extremity
dermatitis
scytitis
of the skin in general
eczema
generic term for acute or chronic inflam-
matory condition of the skin
erysipelas
caused by a hemolytic strep
prurigo
with itching of the papules
pyoderma
pyodermatitis
accompanied by pus
sclerodermatitis
inflammation with hardening
streptodermatitis
due to streptococci
toxicoderma
toxicodermatitis
caused by poison
tungiasis
caused by the gravid sandflea

skin knife
dermatome
used in surgical procedures

skin lacking
adermia
apellous

skin lesion
keratiasis
keratosis
epidermal lesion with circumscribed
overgrowths of the horny layer
necrobiosis lipoidica
atrophic shiny lesions on the legs, usually seen in diabetes

skin odor offensive

bromidrosis
ozochrotia

skin ointment
thiol
a mixture of petroleum oils used in treating skin disorders

skin operation
dermatoplasty

skin pain
dermatalgia
dermatodynia
erythromelalgia
rodonalgia

skin parasite
dermatozoan
animal parasite of the skin

skin pigment excessive
hyperchromatism
hyperchromia

skin pigment lacking
achromasia
achromia
achromoderma
leukoderma
leukopathia
leukopathy

skin pinching impulse
dermatothlasia
uncontrollable impulse to pinch and
bruise the skin

skin pus disorder
pyoderma
pyodermatitis
pyodermatosis

skin pustules
miliaria pustulosa
periporitis
a form of prickly heat

skin redness
erythema
inflammation due to capillar

skin with scales
ichthyosis
sauriasis

skin sebaceous gland di
steatoderma
steatosis

skin secretion
seborrhea
stearrhea
steatorrhea
due to indigestion of fat

skin sensitization
photoallergy
photosensitization
sensitivity to light caused by certain
drugs or plants

skin smoothness
leiodermia

skin specialist
dermatologist

skin study
dermatology
dermatoglyphics
study of the pattern of ridges of the skin
as a genetic indicator

skin swelling
tumefaction

skin thickness
pachyderma
pachydermia
pachydermatosis
pachydermatous
pachyhymenic
pachylosis
pachymenia
tylosis

skin thin/delicate
leptochroa
leptodermic

~ellow color
~hroia
~nia

congestion

~ase

~ head of the

craniotome
surgical instrument used in perforation
and crushing of the fetal skull
trephine
instrument used to remove a bone disk
from the skull

skull lacking
acrania
acranial
meroacrania
notancephalia
congenital absence of all or part of the
cranium

skull measurer
encephalometer

skull operation
craniectomy
cranioclasia
cranioclasis
craniotomy
cranioplasty

skull proportional
orthocephalic
orthocephalous
height in proportion to length and width

skull-sharer
cephalothoracopagus
monocephalus
monocranius
syncephalus
cojoined fetus

skull smallness
leptocephalous
leptocephalus

skull thickness
pachycephalia
pachycephalic
pachycephalous
pachycephaly

sleep abnormal
parahypnosis
as in hypnotism

sleep disorder
central sleep apnea
sleep apnea syndrome
episodes of cessation of breathing during sleep

sleep preventive
antihypnotic

sleep-talking

somniloquence
somniloquism
somniloquist
somniloquy

sleep unnaturally sound
lethargy

sleeping pain
hypnalgia
pain experienced only during sleep

sleeping sickness
encephalitis

sleeplessness
agrypnia
ahypnia
anhypnosis
insomnia

sleepwalking
somnambulance
somnambulism
somnambulist

slightly swollen
tumefaction
tumescence

slimy
glairy
resembling the white of an egg

sling-shaped
fundiform

slit lamp
biomicroscope

smack
heroin

small arms
microbrachia

small body
dwarfism
microsomia
abnormal smallness of the body

small brain convolutions
microgyria

small breasts
micromazia

small calculi
microlith
microlithiasis
a minute calculus consisting of gravel

small chin
microgenia

small colon
microcolon

small cornea
microcornea

small duct
ductule
ductulus
a small tubular structure giving exit to the secretion of a gland

small ears
microtia

small eyeballs
microphthalmia
microphthalmos
microphthalmus
nanophthalmia
nanophthalmos
nanophthalmus
a rare developmental anomaly

small eyelids
microblepharia
microblepharism
microblepharon

small feet
micropodia
micropus

small fingers/toes
micraodactylia
microdactylous
microdactyly

small genital organs
hypogenitalism
microgenitalism

small hands
microcheiria
microchiria
smallness of the hands

small head
microcephalia
microcephalic
microcephalism
microcephalous
microcephalus
microcephaly

small heart
microcardia
microcardius

small item measurer
acribometer
instrument for meas
jects

small jaw
micrognathia

small lens
microlentia
microphakia
spherophakia
refers to crystalline lens of the eye

small leukoblast
microleukoblast
micromyeloblast
myeloblast

small lips
microcheilia
microchilia

small mouth
microstomia

small myeloblast
micromyeloblast

small nails
micronychia
abnormal smallness of the nails

small nipple
microthelia

small penis
micropenis
microphallus

small pupils
microcoria
miosis
congenital contraction of the pupils

ll red blood cells
rythrocyte

small vision
micropsia
visual disorder causing objects to appear smaller than they are

small voice
microphonia
microphony

smallpox
variola
varioloid

smell acuteness
hyperosmia
macrosmatic
oxyosphresia
an exaggerated or abnormally acute sense of smell

smell deficiency
hyposmia
hyposphresia

smell disorder
dysosmia
parasphresia
parosmia
pseudosmia

smell lacking
anodmia
anosmia

smell measurer
olfactometer
device used to measure the keenness of the sense of smell

smell study
osmics
osmology

snake poisoning
ophidiasis
ophidism

sneezing
ptarmus
sternutation

sneeze producer
ptarmic

snow
cocaine

snow blindness
niphablepsia
niphotyphlosis
chionablepsia*
*obsolete term

ing very small ob-

tooth or

sodium high in blood
hypernatremia
high plasma concentration of sodium ions

sodium low in blood
hyponatremia

sodomy
pederast
pederasty

soft bone tissue
osteogen
tissue that ossifies into bone

soft palate
palatum molle
uvula

soft spot
fontanel
fonticulus
spot in the skull of an infant

softening of...
(see under specific area)

sole
plantar
refers to the sole of the foot

solitude desired
apanthropia
apanthropy

soothing
palliative

sound measurer
phonoautograph
device for recording sound vibrations
phonometer
instrument for measuring the intensity of sound

souring
acescence
ascescent

space
spatium
vacuole

Spanish fly
cantharis
used as an aphrodisiac

sparseness of hair
hypotrichiasis
hypotrichosis
oligotrichia
oligotrichosis

sparseness of teeth
hypodontia
oligodontia

spasm extending
protospasm
spasm that expands to other parts of the body

spasm of fingers
dactylospasm

spasm-rigidity
entasis
rigidity of tonic spasms as in tetanus

speaking fast
agitolalia
agitophasia
excessive rapidity in speech

speaking one word only
monophasia
ability to speak only one word or phrase

specks before eyes
visus muscarum

speech defect
allophasis
incoherency
anaudia
aphonia
loss due to injury or disease
anepia
aphasia
aphrasia
inability to speak
amphoriloquy
speaking with blowing sound
anarthria
articulation defective
aphthongia
aphasia caused by speech muscles controlled by nerves under the tongue
apisthyria
inability to whisper
bradyarthria
bradyglossia
bradylalia
bradylogia
bradyphrasia
slowness in utterance
cataphasia
repetition of the same words or phrases
dyslalia
due to structural defects of the speech organs or to impaired hearing*dyslogia*
also impairment of reasoning power

speech defect (cont.)
laloplegia
inability to speak due to paralysis of muscles
logopathy
any speech defect
mogiphonia
difficulty due to voice strain
monophasia
ability to speak only one word or phrase
neologism
use of new and meaningless words
oxylalia
speaking with excessive speed
paralalia
distortion of sounds
pyknophrasia
thickness of speech

speed in speaking
agitolalia
agitophasia
oxylalia

speed in writing
agitographia
writing with excessive speed, omitting words or letters

speedball
cocaine, heroin
used simultaneously

sperm deficiency
oligospermia
oligospermatism

sperm impotency
necrospermia
condition where the sperm are motionless or dead

sperm involuntary loss
spermatorrhea
*gonacratia**
involuntary discharge without orgasm
*obsolete term

spermatic duct
vas deferens
secretory duct of the testicle

spermatic duct stones
spermolith

sphenoid inflammation
sphenoiditis
inflammation of the sphenoid sinus

sphenoid operation
sphenoidostomy
sphenoidotomy

spider bite disorder
arachnidism
arachnoidism
araneism

spider venom antidote
antiarachnolysin

spinal canal open
holorachischisis
spina bifida
congenital disorder

spinal column pain
rachialgia
rachiodynia
spinalgia
spondylalgia
spondylodynia

spinal cord
medulla spinalis
*myelon**
*obsolete term

spinal cord defective
atelomyelia

spinal cord disease
encephalomyeloradiculopathy
involving the brain, spinal cord and spinal roots
myelopathy
any disease of the spinal cord or myeloid tissues
myeloradiculopathy
involves spinal cord and nerve roots

spinal cord hemorrhage
hematomyelia
myelapoplexy
myelorrhagia

spinal cord hernia
myelocele
myelocystocele
myelomeningocele
meningomyelocele
syringomeningocele
syringomyelocele
defect in closure of the spinal canal with protrusion of cord and membranes

spinal cord inflammation
arachnitis

arachnoiditis
  of the pia mater and arachnoid
cerebrospinal meningitis
  of the meninges and spinal cord
myelitis
  of the bone marrow and spinal cord
meningitis
  general term
meningoencephalomyelitis
  of meninges, brain and spinal cord
meningomyelitis
  of spinal cord and its membranes
myeloneuritis
neuromyelitis
  multiple neuritis with myelitis
myeloradiculitis
  of the spinal cord and nerve roots
endosteitis
endostitis
perimyelitis
  of the pia mater and spinal cord
polioencephalomeningomyelitis
poliomyelencephalitis
poliomyelitis
  of the gray matter and meninges

spinal cord membrane
meninges
  three membranes enveloping the brain
  and spinal cord
pia mater
  the inner membrane
arachnoid
  the center membrane
dura mater
  the outer membrane

spinal cord smallness
micromyelia

spinal cord softness
myelomalacia

spinal curvature
lordosis
rachioscoliosis
scoliosis

spinal fusion
spondylosyndesis

spinal knife
rachiotome
  surgical instrument used in surgery on
  the vertebrae

spinal matter displacement
heterotopia
  congenital displacement of the gray matter

spinal measurer
rachiometer
  instrument for measuring the degree of
  deformity

spinal nerve inflammation
radiculitis

spinal nerve root disease
radiculopathy

spinal nerve root operation
radiectomy
radicotomy
radiculectomy
rhizotomy

spinal operation
cordotomy
laminectomy
rachiotomy

spinal paralysis
myeloparalysis
myeloplegia
rachioplegia

spinal puncture
rachiocentesis
  surgical procedure

spindle-shaped
fusiform

spineless/headless
acephalorrhachia
  born without head and vertebral column

spinelike
acanthoid
spinous

spiral
helical

spirochete destruction
spirocheticide
spirochetolysis
  destructive to the spirochete bacteria

spirochete disease
spirochetosis

spitting
expectorating

spitting blood
hemoptysis

splanchnic nerve operation
splanchnicectomy
splanchnicotomy
splanchnotomy

spleen
lien
lienal
splenic

spleen disease
splenopathy
lienopathy*
  *obsolete term

spleen displacement
splenectopia
splenectopy

spleen enlargement
mezalosplenia
splenectasia
splenomegalia
splenomegaly
splenoma
hepatosplenomegaly
splenohepatomegalia
splenohepatomegaly
  enlargement of both spleen and liver

spleen examination
lienography
splenography

spleen fixation
splenopexia
splenopexy

spleen hernia
lienocele
splenocele

spleen inflammation
splenitis
lienitis*
  *obsolete term

spleen/kidney
lienorenal
splenonephric
splenorenal

spleen operation
splenectomy
splenopexia
splenopexy
splenotomy

spleen pain
splenalgia
splenodynia

spleen softness
lienomalacia
splenomalacia
splenomyelomalacia
  of the spleen and bone marrow

spleen suture
splenorrhaphy

spleen tissue destruction
splenolysis

spleen tumor
splenocele
splenoncus

spontaneous generation
abiogenesis
autogenesis

spore largeness
macrospore
megalospore

spot on cornea
albugo
leukoma
  white spot; cornea opacity

spot/patch
tache

spotted skin
vitiligo
  white patches
piebaldness
  different colored patches
livedo
  black-and-blue spot
xanthoma
  yellow patches
xanthelasma*
  *obsolete term

sprayer
atomizer
nebulizer
vaporizer

staggering gait
titubation

stagnation in stomach
ischochymia
  retention of food

stammering
anarthria

dysarthria
dysphemia
hottentotism
lingual titubation
mogilalia
molilalia
psellism
  stammering or stuttering of speech

stapes operation
stapedectomy
stapediotenotomy

star-shaped
asteroid
stella
stellate
stellula

starch
glycogen
  animal or liver starch

starch digestion
amylohydrolysis
amylolysis

starch formation
amylogenesis

starch liquefier
galactozymase
  a ferment extracted from milk, capable
  of liquefying starch

starch-sugar conversion
amylolysis

starch in urine
amylosuria
amyluria

starchlike
amylaceous

starchy food undigested
amylodyspepsia
  inability to digest

stature shortness
brachymorphic

steal mania
kleptomania
  an irrepressible desire to steal

sterility
barrenness
infecundity

sterilization
asexualization

castration
emasculation
tubal ligation
vasectomy

sternum/clavicle
sternoclavicular

sternum fissure
sternoschisis

sternum lacking
asternia
  congenital absence of the breast bone

sternum operation
sternotomy

sternum pain
sternalgia
sternodynia

sternum proximity
adsternal
  near in location

sticky
viscid

stiffness of joints
ankylosis

stiffness of neck
loxia
torticollis
wryneck

stirrup-bone
stapes
  located in the ear

stomach acidity
chlorhydria

stomach dilatation
gastrectasia
gastrectasis

stomach displacement
gastroptosia
gastroptosis
ventroptosia
ventroptosis
  downward displacement of the stomach

stomach enlargement
gastromegaly
macrogastria
megastria
megalogastria

stomach hemorrhage
gastrorrhagia

stomach hernia
gastrocele

stomach hormone
gastrin

stomach inflammation
gastritis
the stomach in general
gastradenitis
gastroadenitis
the glands of the stomach
perigastritis
the peritoneal coat of the stomach
enterogastritis
gastroenteritis
gastroenterocolitis
gastroileitis
the stomach and intestine
gastroesophagitis
the stomach and esophagus
gastroduodenitis
the stomach and duodenum

stomach juice excessive
gastrorrhea

stomach-light
gastrodiaphane
instrument used to illuminate the inside
of the stomach

stomach mesentery
mesogaster
mesogastrium

stomach operation
celiogastrostomy
celiogastrotomy
gastrectomy
gastroplasty
gastrostomy
gastrotomy
gastrocolostomy
gastrocolotomy
gastroduodenostomy
gastroenteroanastamosis
gastroenteroplasty
gastroenterostomy
gastrojejunostomy
gastropylorectomy

stomach pain
gastralgia
gastrodynia
peratodynia
stomach ache

stomach secretions
gastroblennorrhea
gastrochronorrhea
gastrohydrorrhea
excessive amounts

stomach smallness
microgastria

stomach spasm
gastrospasm

stomach stapling
gastroplication
gastroptyxis

stomach stone
gastrolith

stomach suture
gastroplication
gastrorrhaphy

stomach viewer
esophagoscope
gastroscope
instrument used for examination

stomach washing
gastrolavage

stone in blood vessel
angiolith
arteriolith
phlebolith

stone breaking
lithodialysis
lithotripsy
crushing or solution of a stone usually in
the bladder or urethra

stone formation
lithiasis
lithogenesis
lithogeny

stone in gallbladder
cholecystolithiasis
cholelithiasis
chololithiasis

stone in lacrimal duct
dacryolith
ophthalmolith

stone passed in urine
lithuresis

stone removal

lithectomy
lithotomy
usually refers to surgical procedure for urinary stones

stone in ureter
ureterolith

stonecutter disease
silicatosis
silicosis

stonelike
lithoid

strabismus corrector
chiroscope
instrument used for correction

strabismus downward
hypotropia

straightening teeth
orthodontia
orthodontics
branch of dentistry dealing with correction

strain of voice
mogiphonia
difficulty of speech due to voice strain

strength below normal
hyposthenia

strength lacking
adynamia
asthenia
debility

strength measurer
dynamograph
instrument for recording muscular strength

strengthening
analeptic

stricture cutting
coarctotomy
surgical procedure

stricture of...
(see under specific organ)

striped
striated

strychnine-bearing
ignatia
St. Ignatius' bean
strychnos nux vomica

study of...
(see under specific area)

stuttering
lingual titubation
mogilalia
molilalia
stuttering or stammering in general
psellism
due to harelip or cleft palate

sty, stye
hordeolum

subconscious recall
cryptamnesia
cryptomnesia
recalling something previously forgotten

subcostal pain
subcostalgia
pain under the ribs

subnormal temperature
hypothermia

subtongue inflammation
subglossitis
sublinguitis

sucrose in urine
sucrosuria

sudden
fulminant
onset or course of a pain or disorder

suet
sevum

sugar in blood
hyperglycemia
excessive amounts

sugar measurer
saccharimeter
saccharometer

sugar metabolism
saccharometabolism

sugar pill
placebo
inactive substance

sugar in urine
glycosuria
hyperglycosuria
excessive amounts

suicide
apocarteresis
by self-starvation

sun attraction/rejection
heliotaxis
heliotropism
tendency of plants to lean either towards or away from the sun

sun blindness
photoretinitis
photoretinopathy

sun-caused encephalitis
heliencephalitis

sunburn
erythema solare

sunstroke
siriasis
thermoplegia

superior feeling
egomania
extreme self-appreciation

suppression of discharge
ischesis

suppression of sweat
anhidrosis
ischidrosis

suppression of urine
ischuria

suppuration inhibiter
antipyogenic

surgery of abdomen
celiotomy
ventrotomy
opening of the abdominal cavity

surgery of appendix
appendectomy
appendicectomy

surgery of arm
brachiotomy

surgery of bladder
cystotomy
lithotomy
lithotripsy
lithotrity
vesicotomy

surgery of bones
osteorrhaphy
(see also listings under bones)

surgery of cartilage
chondrotomy

surgery of cyst
cystectomy

surgery of fistula
fistulotomy
syringotomy
incision or surgical enlargement of an abnormal passage

surgery of gallbladder
cholecystectomy
cholecystopexy
cholecystostomy
cholecystotomy

surgery of glands
adenectomy
adenotomy

surgery of goiter
strumectomy

surgery of gonad
gonadectomy
excision of ovary or testis

surgery of hernia
celotomy
herniotomy
herniorrhaphy
kelotomy

surgery of joint
arthrectomy
arthroplasty
arthrostomy
arthrotomy

surgery of kidney
nephrectomy
nephrolithotomy
nephropexy
nephropyeloplasty
nephrostomy
nephrotomy

surgery knife
bistoury
small knife used in surgical procedures

surgery of larynx
laryngectomy
laryngotomy

surgery needle
acus

surgery of nerves
neurectomy
neuroectomy
neurotomy

surgery of nympha
nymphectomy
nymphotomy
removal or incision of the labia minora

surgery of ovary
oophorectomy
oophorcystectomy
oophoropexy
oophoroplasty
oophorostomy
oophorotomy
ovariectomy
ovariostomy
ovariotomy

surgery of pancreas
pancreatectomy
pancreatoduodenectomy
pancreatolithectomy
pancreatolithotomy
pancreatomy

surgery of pharynx
pharyngectomy
pharyngoplasty
pharyngotomy
procedures involving the portion of the
digestive tube between the esophagus
and mouth

surgery of sperm duct
vasectomy
for sterilization

surgery of spine
cordotomy
laminectomy
rachiotomy

surgery of spleen
splenectomy
splenopexia
splenopexy
splenorrhaphy
splenotomy

surgery of sterilization
castration
emasculation
spay
tubal ligation
vasectomy

surgery of tendon
tendinoplasty
tendoplasty
tenectomy
tenontoplasty
tenoplasty

tenotomy
procedures involving the fibrous cords
or bands connecting muscle to bone

surgery of tongue
glossoplasty
glossotomy

surgery of tonsils
tonsillectomy
tonsilotomy

surgery of tooth
odontectomy
involving excision of surrounding bone

surgery of trachea
tracheoplasty
tracheostomy
tracheotomy

surgery of uvula
staphylectomy
staphyloplasty
staphylotomy
uvulectomy
uvolotomy
usually referring to the uvula attached to
the soft palate in the mouth

surgery of veins
phlebectomy
phlebophlebostomy
phleboplasty
phlebotomy
venectomy
venesection
venotomy
venovenostomy

suspended animation
acrotism
asphyxia

suspension of respiration
apnea
temporary absence of breathing

suture of...
(see under specific organ)

swallowing air
aerophagia
aerophagy
pneumophagia

swallowing difficulty
aglutition
aphagia
dysphagia
difficulty or inability to swallow

swallowing difficulty (cont.)
aphagia algera
due to pain

sweat abnormal
dyshidrosis
dysidria
dysidrosis

sweat in armpits
maschalephidrosis
excessive perspiration

sweat blood
hemathidrosis
hematidrosis

sweat causing
hidrotic
sudorific

sweat deficiency
hyphidrosis
hypohidrosis
olighidria
oligidria

sweat excessive
hyperhidrosis
hyperidrosis
hyperephidrosis
polyhidrosis
polyidrosis
sudoresis

sweat glands
eccrine glands
exocrine glands
small glands covering the entire body

sweat glands inefficient
anaphoresis
anhidrosis
diminished activity

sweat gland inflammation
hidradenitis
hidrosadenitis

sweat odor
bromhidrosis
bromidrosis
osmidrosis
foul smelling perspiration

sweat overflow
hidrosis
sudoresis
profuse sweating

sweat phosphorescent
phosphorhidrosis

sweat preventer
antihydriotic
antisudorific

sweat producing
sudarific
sudoriferous
sudoriparous
carrying or producing sweat

sweat suppression
anhidrosis
hidroschesis
ischidrosis

sweat with urine
urhidrosis
uridrosis
excretion of urea or uric acid in the
sweat

sweeten
edulcorate
to purify from salt, acid or any harsh
substance

sweetener
aspartane
noncaloric substance

swell-producing
tumefacient
tumefy

swelling
tumefaction
tumentia
tumescence

sword-shaped
ensiform
xiphoid

symptomatic hand-writing
macrography
megalographia
large handwriting, usually indicating a
nervous disorder

synovial inflammation
synovitis

synovial operation
synovectomy
villusectomy

synovial tumor
synovioma

syphilitic tumor
gumma

syphiloma
    infrequently observed infectuous granu-loma characteristic of syphilis

T

tail lacking
    acaudal
    acaudate

talkativeness
    lalorrhea
    logorrhea
    tachylalia
    tachylogia
    tachyphasia
    tachyphemia
    tachyphrasia
    usually encountered in individuals with mental disorders

talus operation
    astragalectomy

tapeworm
    cestoid
    cestode
    common name for tapeworm

tapeworm disease
    teniasis

tapeworm expeller
    teniacide
    teniafuge

tapeworm head
    scolex

tapeworm infestation
    cestodiasis

tarsal bone
    astragalus
    talus
    the ankle bone
    tarsadenitis
    of the tarsal glands and tarsal plate

tarsal operation
    tarsectomy
    tarsochiloplasty
    tarsoplasia

    tarsoplasty
    tarsotomy

taste abnormal
    dysgeusia
    abnormality in sense of taste

taste acuteness
    hypergeusia
    oxygeusia

taste bud
    caliculus gustatorius
    gustatory bud

taste disorder
    parageusia

taste lacking
    ageusia
    ageustia
    loss or impairment of the sense of taste

taste-pertaining
    gustatory

taste sense
    gustation

taste sense lower
    hypogeusia
    blunting of the sense of taste

tea drinker
    theic

tear flow excessive
    dacryorrhea
    epiphora

tear gland inflammation
    dacryadenitis
    dacryoadenitis

tear gland pain
    dacryoadenalgia

tear-producer
    lacrimator

tear sac
    lacrimal sac

tear passage calculus
    dacryolith
    ophthalmolith
    a concretion in the lacrimal apparatus

tear sac inflammation
    dacryoblennorrhea
    dacryocystoblennorrhea
    dacryocystitis

tear sac knife
lacrimotome
surgical instrument

tear sac operation
dacryocystectomy
dacryocystorhinostomy
dacryocystostomy
lacrimotomy

tear sac protrusion
dacryocele
dacryocystocele

teeth...
(see also listings under tooth)

teeth abnormality
odontatrophia
odontatrophy
odontolaxis
odontoloxy
odontoparallaxis

teeth chattering
odonterism

teeth cleaner
odontosmega

teeth deficiency
hypodontia
oligodontia

teeth disease
odontopathy
disease of the teeth or their sockets

teeth in excess
polydentia
polyodontia
presence of supernumerary teeth

teeth extraction
exodontia

teeth fissure
odontoschism

teeth formation
odontogenesis
odontogeny
odontosis

teeth grinding
bruxism
odontoprisis

teeth improper closure
malocclusion

teeth inflammation
odontitis

odontoneuralgia
facial neuralgia caused by tooth decay
parodontitis
peridentitis
periodontitis
of the tissues around a tooth
operculitis
pericoronitis
of the tissues around the crown of a tooth
pulpitis
of dental pulp

teeth largeness
macrodontia
macrodontism
macrodont
megadont
megalodont

teeth pain
dentalgia
odontalgia
odontodynia
toothache

teeth permanent
monophyodont
having only the permanent set of teeth

teeth similar
homodont

teeth smallness
microdontia
microdontism

teeth straightening
orthodontia
orthodontics
branch of dentistry dealing with correction of irregularities

teeth surgery
odontectomy
odontoplasty
odontotomy

teeth transplanting
allotriodontia
also denotes location of teeth in abnormal places

teeth treatment
dentistry
odontology
odontonosology
odontotherapy

teeth tumor
odontoma

teeth viewer
odontoscope
optical device used in examining teeth

teeth yellow
xanthodont

teething
dentition
odontiasis

tele-influence
automatism
telergy
influence of one individual over the brain of another

temper unrestrained
ecomania
oikomania
particularly in the home environment

temperature elevation
hyperthermia
pyrexia
resulting in fever

temperature evenness
monothermia

temperature measurer
pyrometer
thermometer

temperature subnormal
hypothermia

tendency to murder
hemothymia
a desire to commit murder

tenderness of skin
leptochroa
very thin or delicate skin

tendon fixation
tenodesis

tendon inflammation
peritendinitis
peritenonitis
of tissues surrounding a tendon
thecitis
tenovaginitis
of a tendon sheath
tendosynovitis
tenosynovitis
tendovaginitis
of a tendon and its sheath

tendon knife
tendotome
tenotome
surgical instrument

tendon operation
achillotomy
achillotenotomy
tenectomy
tenodesis
tenonectomy
tenontoplasty
tenoplasty
tenosynovectomy
tenotomy
myotenotomy
tenomyoplasty
tenomyotomy
tenontomyotomy
procedure involving tendon and muscles

tendon pain
tenalgia
tenodynia
tenontodynia

tendon sheath
epitendineum
epitenon
peritenon

tendon suture
tenorrhaphy
tenosuture

tennis elbow
lateral humeral epicondylitis

tension measurer
tensiometer
instrument used to measure the tension of the eyeball, blood vessels, etc.

test tube
in vitro
process or reaction occurring in an artificial environment

terminal proximity
paraterminal

testes in abdomen
cryptorchism
cryptorchidism

testes in excess
polyorchid
polyorchidism

testes in excess (cont.)
polyorchis
polyorchism
  presence of more than two testicles

testes fusion
synorchidism
synorchism
  total or partial within the abdomen or
  scrotum

testis
orchis

testis inflammation
orchiditis
orchitis
orchiepididymitis
epididymo-orchitis

testis operation
cryptorchidectomy
orchidectomy
orchidorrhaphy
orchiectomy
orchiopexy
orchioplasty
orchiotomy
vaso-orchidostomy

testis tumor
orchiocele
sarcocele

tetanic spasm
opisthotonos
opisthotonus
  a spasm that bends the body backward

tetanuslike
tetaniform
tetanoid

therapy by air pressure
aerotherapeutics

therapy by animal extract
organotherapy

therapy by baths
balneotherapeutics
balneotherapy
hydrotherapeutics
  treatment by baths and mineral waters

therapy by bone massage
osteopathy

therapy by climate

climatotherapy
  treatment by changing climate

therapy by colored lights
chromophototherapy
chromotherapy

therapy by drugs
pharmacotherapy

therapy by heat
thermotherapy
  treatment by application of heat

therapy by light rays
lucotherapy
phototherapy
  treatment by either solar or artificial light
  rays

therapy by massage
massotherapy

therapy by mechanics
mechanotherapy

therapy by mind
psychotherapeutics
psychotherapy

therapy by nature
naturopathy
  use of natural forces for healing

therapy by opposite
allopathy
heteropathy
  treatment by creating conditions that are
  opposite or different

therapy by radioactivity
radiotherapy
*actinotherapy**
  *obsolete term

therapy by serum
serum therapy

therapy by sun
heliotherapy
  includes sun bathing

therapy by symptom equal
homeopathy
  application of minute doses of an agent
  that would induce similar symptoms in a
  healthy body

therapy by water
balneotherapy

hydrotherapeutics
hydrotherapy
   treatment by external application
thalassotherapy
   treatment by sea-bathing/traveling

thick-fingered
pachydactilia
pachydactylous
pachydactyly

thicken
inspissation
   thickening as by boiling or by evaporation

thickening in excess
pachynis
   abnormal thickening of a part of the body

thickening of nails
pachyonychia

thickness of ears
pachyotia

thickness of eyelids
pachyblepharon

thickness of lips
pachycheilia
pachychilia

thickness of skin
pachyderma
pachydermatosis
pachydermia
   abnormally thick skin

thickness of skull
pachycephalia
pachycephalic
pachycephalous
pachycephaly

thickness of tongue
macroglossia
pachyglossia

thigh bone
femur
os femoris
   the long bone of the thigh

thigh pain
meralgia

thinness of hair
hypotrichiasis
hypotrichosis

oligotrichia
oligotrichosis

thinness of skin
leptochroa
leptodermic
   abnormally delicate skin

thirst excessive
anadipsia
hydrodipsomania
polydipsia

thirst lacking
adipsia
adipsy

thoracic fluid
hydrothorax
pleurorrhea
serothorax
   accumulation of fluid in the pleural cavity

thorax curved
thoracocyrtosis
   abnormally wide curvature of chest wall

thorax/head
cephalothoracic

thorax operation
pleuracotomy
pleurotomy
thoracoplasty
thoracopneumoplasty
thoracostomy
thoracotomy

thorax pain
thoracalgia
thoracodynia

thorax viewer
thoracoscope

thorax/head lacking
acephalothorus
   congenital absence

thornlike
acanthoid
   spinelike

threadlike
filiform
nematoid
   referring to parasitic worms

three-eared
triotus
   congenital condition

three-eyed
triophthalmos
congenital condition

three-faced
triopodymus
triprosopus
born with three faces on one head

three-fingered
tridigitate

three-headed
tricephalus
born with three heads

three-ingredient medicine
tripharmacon
tripharmacum

three-layered
trilaminar

three-pointed
tricuspid
tricuspidal
tricuspidate

three testes
triorchism
congenital presence of an additional testis

three-toed
tridigitate

throbbing
palpitation

thrush
apatha
aphthoid
Candida albicans
candidiasis
a thrush fungus

thymus disease
thymopathy
any disease of the small organ located in the lower part of the neck

thymus inflammation
thymitis

thymus operation
thymectomy

thyroid activity increased
hyperthyroidism

thyroid activity normal
euthyroidism

thyroid activity reduced
hypothyroidism
thyroprivia

thyroid hormone excess
thyrotoxicosis

thyroid inflammation
thyroadenitis
thyroiditis

thyroid operation
laryngofissure
thyrochondrotomy
thyrocricotomy
thyroidectomy
thyroidotomy
thyroparathyroidectomy
thyrotomy

thyroid protein
thyroglobulin
thyroprotein
produced by the thyroid gland

tibia pain
tibialgia

tic/spasm
myoclonus multiplex
polyclonia

tic sufferer
tiqueur

tick fever
reovirus infection

tick infestation
ixodiasis

tilting
anteversion
anteverted
condition of being tilted forward
retroversion
retroverted
condition of being tilted backward

time-equal
isochronia
occurring at equal intervals of time

tip-pointed
ensiform
mucronate
xiphoid

tissue change
metaplasia

metaplasis
a change in the structure of adult tissues

tissue clotting
electrocoagulation

tissue destruction
fulguration
by means of a high-frequency electric current

tissue development defective
hypoplasia

tissue dissolution
histolysis

tissue grafting
autograft
heterograft
homograft
isograft
zoograft
zooplasty
grafting of tissues taken from an animal

tissue inflammation
cellulitis
inflammation of the connective tissues
pimelitis
inflammation of adipose or connective tissues
myositis
inflammation of fleshy tissues, as muscle
steatitis
inflammation of adipose tissue

tissue knife
histotome
microtome
surgical instrument

tissue layer
stratum

tissue operation
histotomy
microtomy

tissue separated
slough
necrosed tissue separated from the living structure

tissue study
histologic
histological
histology
histophysiology

tissue with urates
uratosis

tissue with urine
urecchysis

tobacco alkaloid
anatabine
nicotine

toes/fingers abnormally long
arachnodactyly
dolichostenomelia

toes/fingers defective
perodactylia
perodactylus
perodactyly

toes/fingers deficiency
adactylia
adactylism
adactylous
adactyly
oligodactylia
oligodactyly
congenital absence of fingers or toes
monodactylism
presence of only one finger or one toe

toes equal length
isodactylism

toes in excess
hyperdactylia
hyperdactylism
hyperdactyly
polydactyly

toes/fingers fused
syndactylia
syndactylism
syndactylous
syndactylus
syndactyly
zygodactyly

toe inflammation
dactylitis
also applies to fingers

toe largeness
macrodactylia
macrodactylism
macrodactyly
megadactyly
megalodactyly
also applies to fingers

toe shortness
brachydactylia

toe shortness (cont.)
brachydactyly
    also applies to fingers

toe slenderness
leptodactylous
    also applies to fingers

toe smallness
microdactylia
microdactylous
microdactyly
    also applies to fingers

toe thickness
pachydactylia
pachydactylous
pachydactyly
    also applies to fingers

tongue
glossa
lingua

tongue alveolar processes
alveolingual
alveololingual

tongue blackness
glossophytia
melanoglossia

tongue burning
glossodynia
glossopyrosis

tongue/cheeks
buccolingual
    pertaining to the tongue and cheeks

tongue cyst
ranula
    cyst under the tongue

tongue disease
glossopathy

tongue displacement
glossoptosia
glossoptosis

tongue with hair
glossotrichia

tongue inflammation
glossitis

tongue inspection
glossoscopy

tongue lacking
aglossia
    refers to congenital absence and to ina-
    bility to speak
aglossostoma
    born without mouth opening

tongue largeness
macroglossia
megaloglossia

tongue membrane
periglottis
    the mucous membrane of the tongue

tongue operation
elinguation
glossectomy
glossoplasty
glossotomy
hemiglossectomy

tongue pain
glossalgia
glossodynia
glossopyrosis

tongue paralysis
glossolysis
glossoplegia

tongue-pertaining
glossal
lingual

tongue pressure measurer
glossodynamometer

tongue register
glossograph
    instrument to measure movements of
    the tongue

tongue shortness
brachyglossal

tongue smallness
microglossia

tongue spasm
glossospasm

tongue split
schistoglossia

tongue study
glossology

tongue suture
glossorrhaphy

tongue swelling
glossocele
glossoncus
    any swelling involving the tongue

tongue thickness
macroglossia
pachyglossia

tongue-tie
ankyloglossia

tonsil inflammation
tonsillitis
adenopharyngitis
pharyngotonsillitis
involving tonsils and pharynx
peritonsillitis
involving tissues surrounding the tonsil

tonsil knife
tonsillotome

tonsil operation
tonsillectomy
tonsillotomy

tonsil stone
tonsillith

tonus lacking
atonia
atonicity
atony

toot
cocaine

tooth...
(see also listings under teeth)

tooth alveolus inflamed
alveolitis

tooth apex locator
apicolocator
instrument used in locating the apex of
a tooth

tooth cement in excess
hypercementosis
formation of excessive amount at the
root base

tooth deposit
tophus
calcium deposit

tooth disease
odontopathy

tooth disease study
dentistry
odontonosology

tooth hemorrhage
odontorrhagia

tooth operation
apicoectomy
odontectomy
odontoplasty
odontotomy
pulpectomy
pulpotomy
radectomy
apicectomy*
*obsolete term

tooth pain
odontalgia
odontodynia
toothache

tooth probe
tine
pointed tool to explore the tooth

tooth root
apex radicus dentis

tooth sets in excess
polyphyodont
formation of more than two sets of teeth

tooth-shaped
dentiform
dentoid
molariform
odontoid

tooth socket alteration
alveoloplasty
alveoplasty

tooth socket hemorrhage
phatnorrhagia

tooth socket incision
alveolotomy

tooth sparseness
oligodontia
having only a few teeth

tooth splitting
odontoschism

tooth straightener
orthodontist
specialist in aligning teeth

tooth toward cheek
buccoversion
where a tooth extends toward the cheek

tooth treatment
odontotherapy

toothache
aerodontalgia
aero-odontalgia
aero-odontodynia
dentalgia
odontalgia
odontalgic
odontodynia
pulpalgia

toothache reliever
antiodontalgic

toper's nose
rhinophyma

torsion measurer
torsiometer
instrument to measure the ocular torsion

torticollis
loxia
wryneck

touch acuteness
hyperaphia
oxyaphia

touch fear
aphephobia
haphephobia

touch inability
dyscheiria
dyschiria
topagnosis
topoanesthesia
inability to determine site of sensibility

touch measurer
esthesiometer
tactometer
instrument to determine the acuteness of the sense of touch

touch recognizable
symbolia
ability to recognize an object by touch

touch sense lacking
anaphia
anhaphia
atactilia

touch sensitivity
hyperaphia
oxyaphia
extreme sensitivity to touch

trachea cleft
tracheoschisis

trachea constriction
tracheostenosis

trachea hemorrhage
tracheorrhagia

trachea hernia
trachelocele
tracheocele
hernia of the trachea mucous membrane

trachea inflammation
tracheitis
trachitis
tracheobronchitis
tracheopyosis

trachea knife
tracheotome
surgical instrument

trachea operation
tracheoplasty
tracheostomy
tracheotomy

trachea pain
cervicodynia
trachealgia
trachelodynia

trachea pus
tracheopyosis
purulent inflammation

tracing descent
matrilineal
through the female side
patrilineal
through the male side

tranquility
euthymia
mental peace; joyfulness

transformation of tissues
metaplasia
metaplasis
change in structure of adult tissues

transition
metabasis
change in the nature or treatment of a disease

transposition
metathesis

treatment by...
(see also therapy by...)

treatment by air
aeropiesotherapy
  using either compressed or rarified air
aerotherapeutics
aerotherapy
  varying pressure or coposition of the air
aerothermotherapy
  by means of hot air

treatment by alkali
alkalitherapy

treatment by blood
hematherapy
hemotherapeutics
hemotherapy
transfusion
  using blood or blood derivatives for
  bleeding disorder or anemia

treatment by causative agent
isopathy

treatment by cold
crymotherapy
cryotherapy

treatment by diet
alimentotherapy

treatment by direct current
galvanotherapy

treatment from distance
teletherapy
  administration of x-ray therapy from a
  distance

treatment by drugs
chemotherapy
pharmacotherapy

treatment by electric light
electrophototherapy

treatment by electricity
electrotherapeutics
electrotherapy

treatment by fever
pyretotherapy
  by induction of fever

treatment by gold
aurotherapy
chrysotherapy
  by use of gold compounds

treatment by hypnotism
hypnotherapy

treatment by liver

hepatotherapy
  by liver or liver extract

treatment by magnets
magnetotherapy

treatment by massage
massotherapy
naprapathy
reflexotherapy

treatment by milk
galactotherapy
lactotherapy

treatment by movements
kinesiatrics
kinesitherapy

treatment by music
melodiotherapy
musicotherapy

treatment by placenta
placentotherapy
  with preparations from animal placentasl

treatment by prayer
theotherapy

treatment by radiation
emanotherapy
radiation therapy
radiotherapeutics
radiotherapy
  with x-rays, radium rays or any other radioactive substance

treatment by reduced fluid
dipsotherapy
fluid restriction

treatment by sea
thalassotherapy
  by sea travel, sea air or sea baths

treatment by spiritual focus
logotherapy

treatment by vapor
vapotherapy

treatment by vibration
seismotherapy
sismotherapy

treatment by water
hydromassage
hydropathy

treatment by work
ergotherapy
by means of physical exercise

tremor of hands/feet
athetosis
involuntary movements

trench mouth
necrotizing ulcerative gingivitis
also known as Vincent's disease

trichina disease
trichinosis

triple vision
triplopia
single object appears as three

triplet
tridymus

tropical ulcer
phagedena tropica

true ribs
costae verae

trunk lacking
acormus
congenital absence

tube
catheter
salpinx

tube feeding
gastrogavage
gastrostogavage
gavage
providing nourishment through a tube
into the stomach

tubes/ovaries inflamed
adnexitis
annexitis

tube pregnancy
salpingocyesis

tuberculosis
consumption
phthisis
obsolete terms

tubular vessel dilatation
ectasia
ectasis
ectatic

tumor

neoplasm
new growth

tumor of blood vessels
angioma

tumor of bone
osteoma
osteophyma
osteophyte

tumor of cartilage
chondroma

tumor cells
oncocytes

tumor of connective tissue
sarcoma
usually highly malignant

tumor destruction
tumoricidal
denoting an agent

tumor dissemination
metastasis

tumor of epithelial cells
carcinoma
epithelioma

tumor of fatty tissue
lipoma

tumor of fibers
fibroma
rhabdomyoma

tumor formation
oncosis

tumor of germ layers
teratoblastoma
teratocarcinoma
teratoma

tumor of glandular tissue
adenocarcinoma
malignant neoplasm
adenoma
usually benign

tumor of jaw
actinomycosis
lumpy jaw

tumor of liver
hepatocarcinoma
hepatoma

tumor of lymph tissue/vessels
angioma

angioma lymphaticum
lymphangioma
lymphoma

tumor of mucous surface
papilloma
villoma

tumor of muscle
myoma
benign neoplasm of muscular tissue

tumor of nerve cells
neuroblastoma

tumor of periosteum
periosteosis
periostosis

tumor of pigment tissue
melanocarcinoma
melanoma

tumor preventor
antineoplastic
preventing development, maturation or spread of neoplastic cells

tumor of striated muscle
rhabdomyoma

tumor of syphilis
gumma
syphiloma

tumor of tendon
tenontophyma
obsolete term

tumor of thyroid
goiter
thyrocele

turbidity measurer
turbidimeter
instrument for determining the degree of cloudiness of a liquid

turpentine poisoning
terebinthism

turpentine tree
terebinth

twin deformities congenital
atlantodidymus
atlodidymus
derodidymus
one body with two heads
cephalothoracopagus
fused head, neck and thorax
craniopagus occipitalis
united at the back of the skull

dicephalus dibrachius
two arms and legs for a double body
dicephalus tetrabrachius
attached from armpits to hips with only two legs
diplopagus
having one or more vital organs in common
dipygus parasiticus
omacephalus
pseudoacephalus
thoracoparacephalus
one fetus poorly developed and dependent
ectopagus
ensomphalus
sternopagus
synthorax
thoracopagus
xiphopagus
united at sternal area
ectopagia
ectopagus
thoracopagus
united at the thorax
epigastrius
ilioxiphopagus
omphalopagus
united at the abdomen
epipygus
pygodidymus
pygopagus
united at the buttocks
cephalopagus
iniopagus
united at the back of the neck
metopagus
united at the forehead
monocephalus
monocranius
syncephalus
having one head and two bodies
notomelus
thoracomelus
additional limbs attached to the back or thorax
diprosopus
two faces on a single skull
paragnathus
polygnathus
prosopagus
prosopopagus
attached to the face of the other twin
hemipagus
prosoposternodidymus

twin deformities congenital (cont.)
prosopothoracopagus
united by the face, chest and upper abdomen
rachiopagus
rachipagus
united back to back
somatopagus
having the trunk in common
thoradelphus
attached as one above the umbilicus
triiniodymus
one body with three heads

twisted
tortuous

twisted neck
loxia
torticollis
wryneck

twisting to one side
laterotorsion

twitching
vellication
of the facial muscles
blepharospasm
blepharospasmus
of the eye or eyelid

two-fingered
didactylism
presence of only two digits on a hand or foot

two-formed
dimorphism
dimorphous
existing in two forms

two-headed
atlantodidymus
atlodymus
bicephalous
derodidymus
dicephalus
diplocephalus

two-horned
bicornate
bicornuate
bicornous

two-jawed
dignathus

two-pronged
bifurcate
bifurcated
having two branches

two sets of teeth
diphyodont
normal in humans

tympanic membrane
membrana tympani
myringa

tympanic ring
anulus tympanicus

tympanum inflammation
myringitis
tympanitis
tympanomatoiditis

tympanum operation
myringectomy
myringodectomy
myringoplasty
myringotomy
tympanectomy
tympanotomy

tyrosine in urine
tyrosinuria

U

ulcer
chancre
ulcus
primary lesion of syphilis

ultrasound diagnosis
Doppler echocardiography
sonography
ultrasonography
use of sound to determine location and measurement of deep structures

umbilical hernia
omphalocele

umbilicus
omphalos

umbilicus bleeding
omphalorrhagia

umbilicus inflammation
 omphalitis
 omphalophlebitis

umbilicus operation
 omphalotomy
 omphalotripsy

umbilicus rupture
 omphalorrhexis

umbilicus ulceration
 omphalelcosis

unborn child
 fetus
  from the eighth week until the moment of birth

uncontrollable temper
 ecomania
 oikomania
  noted in the home environment

under tongue
 hypoglossal
 hypoglossis
 hypoglottis
 subglossal
 sublingual
  surface under the tongue

under tongue cyst
 ptyalocele
 ranula
 sialocele
  salivary gland cyst

underarm perspiration
 maschalyperidrosis
  excessive amounts

unhealthful
 insalubrious

universal antidote
 mithridate
 mithridatism
  immunity against any poisons

unscaling
 desquamation

upper extremities lacking
 omacephalus
  parasitic twin with imperfect head and no arms

upper front
 anterosuperior
  in front and above

upper jawbone
 maxilla

upward turning of eyes
 anaphoria
 anatropia
  particularly when at rest

urachus pus
 pyourachus

urate deposit
 uratosis
  in blood or tissues

urates in blood
 hyperuricemia
 uratemia

urates in urine
 uraturia

urea in blood
 azotemia
 uremia

urea production
 Krebs cycle
  sequence of chemical reactions in the liver that produce urea

urea low in urine
 hypazoturia
 hypoazoturia

ureter calculus
 lithureteria
 ureterolith
 ureterolithiasis

ureter dilation
 ureterectasia

ureter disease
 ureteropathy
  refers to any disease of the ureters

ureter distention
 hydroureter
 ureterohydronephrosis
 uroureter
  abnormal distention from accumulation of urine due to obstruction

ureter fistula
 ureterostoma

ureter hemorrhage
 ureterorrhagia

ureter inflammation
 periureteritis
  of tissues around the ureter

ureter inflammation (cont.)
ureteritis
  of the ureter
ureteropyelitis
  of ureter and kidney pelvis
ureteropyelonephritis
  of ureter, kidney and pelvis
ureteropyosis
  accompanied by pus

ureter largeness
megaloureter
megaureter

ureter operation
ureterectomy
ureterolithotomy
ureterolysis
ureteroplasty
ureterostomy
ureterotomy
ureteroureterostomy
ureterocolostomy
ureteroenterostomy
ureteroileostomy
ureterosigmoidostomy
  involving ureter and intestine
ureterocystostomy
ureteroneocystostomy
ureterovesicostomy
  involving ureter and bladder
ureteronephrectomy
ureteropyeloneostomy
ureteropyelonephrostomy
ureteropyelostomy
  involving ureter and kidney
ureteroproctostomy
  involving ureter and rectum

ureter pain
ureteralgia

ureter pus/mucus
pyoureter
ureterophlegma
ureteropyosis

ureter stricture
ureterostenoma
ureterostenosis

ureter suture
ureterocelorrhaphy
ureterorrhaphy

urethra discharge
urethrorrhea

urethra Inflammation
periurethritis
  of the tissues connecting the urethra
skeneitis
skenitis
  of glands or ducts near the urethra
urethritis
  of the urethra itself
urethrocystitis
  of the urethra and bladder

urethra knife
urethrotome

urethra opening defective
balanic hypospadias
hypospadiasis
hypospadias perinealis
  congenital defect

urethra operation
urethrectomy
urethroplasty
urethrostomy
urethrotomy

urethra pain
urethralgia
urethrodynia

urethra protrusion
urethrocele
  prolapse of the female urethra

urethra proximity
paraurethral

urethra spasm
urethrism
urethrismus
urethrospasm

urethra stricture
urethrostenosis

urethra suture
urethrorrhaphy

urethra viewer
panendoscope
urethrascope
urethroscope
  instrument for examining the urethra

urethral/anal eroticism
amphimixis
  also signifies union of the chromatins

urethral ring
annulus urethralis
musculus sphincter vesicae

urethral stricture tool
electrolyzer
instrument for treatment by electrolysis

uric acid disintegration
uricolysis

uric acid excretion
lithuria
uricosuria

urinary canal
ureter
brings urine from the kidneys to the
bladder
urethra
takes urine out of the bladder

urinary nitrogen
azoturia
excessive amounts

urinary stone expeller
lithagogue

urinate
micturate

urination
emiction
micturition
uresis

urination arrest
anuresis
anuria

urination desire
micturition
also denotes frequent urination

urination in excess
diuresis
hydruria
polyuria

urination frequency
micturition
nocturia
nycturia
pollakiuria
thamuria

urination impossible
acraturesis
due to lack of elasticity of the bladder

urination impulse
uresiesthesia
uriesthesia

urination involuntary
enuresis

incontinence
usually occurring at night or during sleep

urination pain
dysuria
dysury
urodynia

urine with albumin
albuminuria
pseudoalbuminuria

urine with alcohol
alcoholuria

urine with alkalinity
alkalinuria
alkaluria
the passage of alkaline urine

urine with amebas
ameburia

urine with amines
aminuria

urine with amino acids
acidaminuria
aminoaciduria
hyperaminoaciduria

urine with ammonia
ammoniuria

urine by anus
urochesia
passing urine through the anus

urine aromatic odor
uraroma

urine with bacilli
bacilluria

urine with bacteria
bacteriuria
passage of bacteria in the urine

urine with bile salts
biliuria
choleuria
choluria

urine with bilirubin
bilirubinuria

urine with black pigment
melanuria
excretion of a dark-colored urine

urine with blood
hematocyturia
hematuria
hemuresis

urine with blood/chyle
hematochyluria
presence of both in the urine

urine with calcium
calcariuria
calciuria
hypercalciuria
hypercalcinuria
hypercalcuria

urine calculus
urolith
urolithiasis

urine with carbohydrates
carbohydraturia

urine with carbolic acid
carboluria
presence of phenol in the urine

urine with carbons
carbonuria

urine with casts
cylindruria

urine with chlorides
chloriduria
chloruresis

urine with cholesterol
cholesterinuria
cholesteroluria

urine with chyle or lymph
chyluria

urine concentrated
oligohydruria

urine with crystals
crystalluria

urine in a cyst
urinoma
cyst containing urine

urine deficiency
oligohydruria
oliguresia
oliguresis
oliguria

urine with dextrin
dextrinuria

urine with dextrose
glycosuria
glucosuria
*dextrosuria**
*obsolete term

urine with diacetic acid
diacetonuria
diaceturia

urine examination
urinalysis
analysis of the components
urinoscopy
uroscopy
by visual observation

urine in excess
polyuria

urine excretion increased
diuresis
diuretic

urine with fat
adiposuria
lipuria
excretion of lipids in the urine

urine with free myoglobin
myoglobinuria

urine with fructose
fructosuria
levelosuria

urine with globulin
globulinuria

urine with gravel
urocheras
uropsammus
any inorganic or uratic sediment in the
urine

urine gravity low
hyposthenuria
due to inability of kidneys to concentrate
urine

urine gravity measurer
urinometer
urogravimeter
urometer

urine with hematin
urobilin
urofuscohematin
urohematin
urohematoporphyrin
causing presence of red pigment in the
urine

urine with hemoglobin
 hemoglobinuria

urine with hippuric acid
 hippuria
  excretion of abnormally large amounts

urine with histidine
 histidinuria

urine with histone
 histonuria
  observed in certain diseases

urine with homogentisic acid
 alcaptonuria
 alkaptonuria

urine with hyalin
 hyalinuria

urine with hydrogen sulfide
 hydrothionuria

urine incontinence
 enuresis
  occurring usually during sleep

urine with indican
 indicanuria

urine with indigo
 indigouria
 indiguria

urine with indole
 indoluria

urine with indoleacetic acid
 indolaceturia

urine with indoxyl
 indoxyluria

urine infiltration
 urosepsis
  from infiltration of urine into the tissues

urine with inositol
 inosituria
 inosuria

urine interruptions
 urinary stuttering
  involuntary jerky urination

urine with ketone
 hyperketonuria
 ketonuria

urine lacking pigment
 acholuria
 acholuric

urine with lactose
 lactosuria
  excretion of milk sugar in the urine

urine with leucine
 leucinuria

urine with levulose
 levulosuria

urine with lithic acid
 hyperlithuria
 lithuria

urine with lymph
 lymphuria

urine with membrane
 meninguria
  presence of shreds of membrane in
  urine

urine with methemoglobin
 methemoglobinuria

urine with milkiness
 chyluria
 galacturia

urine with nitrates
 nitrituria

urine with nitrogen
 hyperazoturia
  presence of excessive amounts

urine nitrogen lacking
 anazoturia
  also denotes deficiency

urine with oxalic acid
 oxaluria
  also presence of oxalidates

urine paleness
 achromaturia

urine with phenetidin
 phenetidinuria

urine with phenols
 phenoluria

urine with phenyl-ketone
 phenylketonuria

urine with phosphates
 phosphaturia
  presence of excessive amounts

urine phosphorescent
 photuria

urine with protein
proteinuria

urine with purines
alloxuria

urine with purpurin
porphyrinuria

urine with pus
pyuria

urine red
erythruria

urine retention
ischuria
  also denotes suppression

urine with saccharose
saccharosuria
  obsolete term

urine secretion
uropoiesis
  process of urine formation

urine with semen
semenuria
seminuria
spermaturia

urine specific gravity low
hyposthenuria

urine with starch
amyluria

urine with sucrose
sucrosuria

urine sugar
glucosuria
glycosuria
hyperglycosuria
*melituria**
  *obsolete term

urine sugar lacking
aglycosuria

urine in sweat
urhidrosis
uridrosis
  excretion of abnormal quantity of urine
  components in sweat

urine in tissues
urecchysis
uredema
uroedema

urine with tyrosine
tyrosinuria

urine with urates
lithuria
uraturia

urine with xanthine
xanthinuria
xanthiuria
xanthuria
  presence of excessive amounts

urobilin in blood
urobilinemia

urobilin in urine
urobilinuria

uterus
womb

uterus adhesion
hysterolysis
  cutting off the attachment

uterus atony
metratonia
  after childbirth

uterus atrophy
metratrophia
metratrophy

uterus closing
hysterocleisis

uterus discharge
lochia
lochial
lochiometra
metrorrhea

uterus disease
hysteropathy
metropathia
metropathy
  any disorder of the uterus

uterus displacement
metroptosia
metroptosis
*metrectopia**
*metrectopy**
  *obsolete terms

uterus fibroid operation
fibroidectomy
fibromectomy

uterus fixation
hysteropexy
uterofixation
uteropexy

uterus gas distention
physometra

uterus gas/fluid
physohydrometra
accumulation of air and gas

uterus hemorrhage
metrorrhagia
irregular menstrual flow
metrostaxis
slight, persistent flow
metropathia hemorrhagica
abnormal bleeding
polymenorrhea
frequent menstrual periods

uterus hernia
hysterocele

uterus inflammation
metritis
uteritis
of the uterus in general
endometritis
of the inner layer of the uterine wall
metrolymphangitis
of the lymphatic vessels
metroperitonitis
perimetritis
of the uterus and peritoneum
metrophlebitis
of the uterus veins
mesometritis
myometritis
of the muscular tissue
parametritis
of the connecting tissues
perisalpingitis
of the tissues around a tube
pyosalpingitis
pus and inflammation of the uterine tube
pyosalpingo-oophoritis
pus and inflammation of the tube, ovary
and oviduct
salpingo-oophoritis
of the tubes and ovaries
salpingoperitonitis
of tubes and peritoneum
cervicitis
trachelitis
of the neck of the uterus

uterus lacking
ametria

uterus ligament
ligamentum teres uteri
the round ligament
mesometrium
the wide ligament
mesosalpinx
the upper part of the wide ligament surrounding the tube

uterus measurer
hysterometer
uterometer
instrument for measuring the cavity of
the uterus
metrodynamometer
used to measure contractions
parturiometer
measures expulsive force
uretometer
measures the uterus size

uterus operation
celiohysterectomy
celiohysterotomy
hysterectomy
hysteromyomectomy
hysteromyotomy
hystero-oophorectomy
hysteropexy
metroplasty
metrotomy
hysterosalpingectomy
hysterosalpingo-oophorectomy
hysterotrachelectomy
hysterotrachelotomy
hysterocervicotomy
cervicectomy
cervicotomy
trachelectomy
trachelopexia
trachelopexy
tracheloplasty
stomatomy
stomatotomy
surgical incision to facilitate labor

uterus pain
hysteralgia
hysterodynia
metralgia
metrodynia

uterus paralysis
metroparalysis
during or after childbirth

uterus pus
pyometra

uterus rupture
hysterorrhexis
metrorrhexis

uterus softness
metromalacia
metromalacoma
metromalacosis
pathologic softening of the uterine tissues

uterus spasm
uterismus

uterus stone
hysterolith

uterus study
hysterology

uterus suspension
ligamentopexis
ligamentopexy
shortening of the ligaments

uterus suture
hysterorrhaphy
salpingorrhaphy
trachelorrhaphy

uterus tissues
parametrium
connective tissues around the uterus

uterus tube cover
perisalpinx

uterus tube gas/pus
physopyosalpinx

uterus tube operation
salpingectomy
salpingoplasty
salpingotomy
tubectomy
salpingo-oophorectomy
salpingoovariectomy
salpingopexy
salpingostomatomy
salpingostomy

uterus tubes and ovaries
adnexa uteri

uterus tumor
hysteromyoma
benign neoplasm of uterine muscular tissue

uterus varicosity
utero-ovarian varicocele

uterus viewer
hysteroscope
metroscope
uteroscope

utterance slow
bradyarthria
bradyglossia
bradylalia
bradyphasia
slowness of speech

uvea inflammation
uveitis
uveitic
of the iris, ciliary body and choroid of the eye

uvula cleft
bifid uvula
staphyloschisis

uvula elongation
staphyloptosis
uvuloptosis

uvula enlargement
staphyledema

uvula inflammation
peristaphylitis
uvulitis

uvula knife
staphylotome
uvulotome
an instrument for cutting the uvula

uvula operation
palatoplasty
staphylectomy
staphyloplasty
staphylotomy
uvulatomy
uvulectomy
uvolotomy

uvula prolapse
staphyloptosis
uvulaptosis
uvuloptosis

uvula suture
palatorrhaphy
staphylorrhaphy
surgical repair of the uvula
palatopharyngorrhaphy
staphylopharyngorrhaphy
surgical repair of the palate and pharynx

vagina atresia
ankylocolpos

vagina contraction
colpospasm

vagina dilatation
colpectasia
colpectasis
distention in general

vagina discharge
lochia
locial
discharge following childbirth

vagina disease
colpopathy
vaginopathy

vagina distention
aerocolpos
caused by gas or air

vagina dryness
colpoxerosis
of the mucous membrane

vagina examination
colpomicroscopy
study of the cells

vagina fluid removal
culdocentesis

vagina fungus disease
colpitis mycotica
colpomycosis
vaginomycosis

vagina gas
flatus vaginalis
expulsion of gas from the vagina

vagina hemorrhage
colporrhagia

agina hernia
colpocele
vaginocele

vagina Inflammation
colpitis
vaginitis
of the vagina in general

pachyvaginitis
with thickening of the walls
paracolpitis
paravaginitis
pericolpitis
perivaginitis
of the connective tissue around the vagina
colpocystitis
of the vagina and bladder
vulvovaginitis
of the vagina and vulva

vagina laceration
colporrhexis

vagina mucus
hydrocolpocele
hydrocolpos
mucocolpos
accumulation of mucus in the vagina

vagina occlusion
colpatresia
gynatresia

vagina operation
colpectomy
colpocleisis
colpopexy
colpoplasty
colpopoiesis
colpotomy
vaginapexy
vaginectomy
vaginofixation
vaginoplasty
vaginotomy
proctococlytroplasty
proctocolpoplasty
repair of a rectovaginal fistula

vagina pain
colpalgia
colpodynia
vaginism
vaginismus
vaginodynia
vulvismus
spasmodic pain

vagina prolapse
colpoptosia
colpoptosis

vagina proximity
paravaginal

vagina pus
pyocolpos
pyocolpocele

vagina stricture
colpostenosis

vagina suture
colporrhaphy

vagina tissue
paracolpium
the connective tissue

vagina viewer
culdoscope
vaginoscope
instrument for examining the internal
genitalia

valve inflammation
dicliditis
valvulitis

valve knife
valvulotome
surgical instrument

valve operation
valvuloplasty
valvotomy
valvulotomy

vanilla itching
vanillism
skin irritation resulting from contact with
vanilla bean

vaporization
nebulization

variable tension
heterotonia

varicose aneurysm
phlebarteriectasia

varicose inflammation
varicophlebitis
inflammation of a varicose vein

varicose operation
cirsectomy
cirsotomy
varicotomy

varicosity of conjunctiva
varicula
swelling of the veins

vascular system disease
angiopathy

vasomotor disturbance
angioneurosis
vasoneurosis

vein/artery communication
anastamosis

vein congestion
phlebismus

vein dilatation
phelbectasia
varicosis
varix
in general
pylephlebectasia
pylephlebectasis
of the portal vein
phlebismus
due to obstruction

vein displacement
phlebectopia
phlebectopy

vein feeding
phleboclysis
venoclysis
adminsitration of food or drugs

vein hardening
phlebosclerosis
venosclerosis

vein hemorrhage
phleborrhagia

vein inflammation
mesophlebitis
phlebitis
of the middle coat
periangitis
perivasculitis
of the outside coat or tissue
periphlebitis
of the tissues around a vein
peripylephlebitis
pylephlebitis
pylethrombophlebitis
pertaining to the portal vein

vein-nerve network
plexus

vein obstruction
phlebemphraxis
thrombosis of a vein

vein operation
cirsectomy

cirsotomy
phlebectomy
phleboplasty
phlebotomy
phlebophlebostomy
varicocelectomy
varicotomy
venectomy
venesection
venipuncture
venotomy

vein pressure measurer
phlebomanometer

vein rupture
phleborrhexis

vein with salt injection
phleboclysis
injection of saline solution

vein sclerosis
phlebosclerosis
venofibrosis
venosclerosis

vein stone
phlebolite
phlebolith

vein suture
phleborrhaphy

vein twisting
phlebostrepsis
surgical process

venous/arterial
arteriovenous

vermifuge
anthelmintic
helminthalgogue
helminthic
used to expel intestinal worms

vertebra column
rachis

vertebra defect
spondylolysis

vertebra disease
rachiopathy
spondylopathy

vertebra inflammation
perispondylitis
of tissues around the vertebrae
spondylitis
of the vertebrae

spondylopyosis
accompanied by pus

vertebra knife
rachiotome
surgical instrument

vertebra operation
laminectomy
rachiotomy
spondylotomy
vertebrectomy

vertebra pain
spondylalgia

vesical hernia
cystocele

vesical stone crusher
lithoclast
lithotriptor
lithotrite

vesical stone crushing
lithocenosis
litholapaxy
lithotrity
lithotripsy
surgical procedure involving crushing
stones in the bladder

vesical stone viewer
cystoscope
lithoscope

vessel displacement
angiectopia
angioplany
abnormal location

vessel enlargement
angiectasia
angiectasis

vessel inflammation
angiitis
angitis
vasculitis
of the blood or lymphatic vessels
periangitis
perivasculitis
of the sheaths and adventitia

vessel measurer
angiometer
determines vessel diameter or tension

vessel operation
arteriectomy
phlebectomy
venectomy

vessel plastic surgery
angioplasty

vessel viewer
angioscope

vestibule
utricle
utriculus
larger membranous sac in the vestibule
of the labyrinth

vestibule operation
vestibulotomy

vetch/lupine disease
lathyrism
lupinosis
disease caused by eating certain kinds
of vetch or pea species

viewer illuminated
celoscope
optical device for illuminating the interior
of a cavity

vigorous old age
agerasia

vinegar acid measurer
acetimeter
apparatus to determine content of acetic
acid

vinegarlike
acetous

virgin generation
apogamia
apogamy
apomixia
parthenogenesis
nonsexual reproduction

virus in blood stream
viremia

visceral disease virus
cytomegalovirus

viscosity measurer
viscometer
viscosimeter
instrument to determine viscosity of the
blood

viscus collapse
splanchnoptosia
splanchnoptosis
visceroptosis

viscus disease
splanchnopathy

viscus displacement
splanchnodiastasis
splanchnectopia

viscus enlargement
organomegaly
splanchnomegaly
visceromegaly

viscus hardening
splanchnosclerosis

viscus hernia
splanchnocele
protrusion of abdominal viscera

viscus inflammation
perivisceritis

viscus knife
viscerotome
surgical instrument used in autopsy

viscus nerve operation
splanchnicectomy
splanchnicotomy
splanchnotomy

viscus pain
visceralgia

viscus smallness
splanchnomicria

viscus stone
splanchnolith
intestinal calculus

vision in darkness
scotopia
also dark adaptation

vision delusion
pseudoblepsia
pseudoblepsis
pseudopsia

vision dimness
amblyopia
amblyopic

vision impaired
dysopia

vision largeness
macropsia
megalopia
megalopsia

vision measurer
campimeter
haploscope
optometer

vision perverted
parablepsia

vision sensitivity
optesthesia

vision smallness
micropsia
objects appear smaller than they are

vision unequal
aniseikonia
antimetropia
images seen differently by the two eyes

visual image distorted
pseudoblepsia
pseudoblepsis
pseudopsia

visual power fatigue
asthenopia
eyestrain

vitamin deficiency
avitaminosis
hypovitaminosis

vitamin intoxication
hypervitaminosis

vitiated appetite
coprophagy
scatophagy
eating of feces
geophagia
geophagism
geophagy
eating earth
pica
craving for unnatural foods

vitreous body inflammation
hyalitis

vitreous body puncture
hyalonyxis

vitreous humor membrane
hyaloid membrane
membrana vitrea
encloses the vitreous humor of the eye

vocal cord inflammation

chorditis
chorditis vocalis

vocal muscle irritability
hyperphonia
overuse of the voice

voice abnormality
paraphonia

voice impairment
dysphonia
difficulty or pain when speaking

voice loss
alalia
anaudia
aphonia

voice roughness
trachyphonia

voice shrillness
oxyphonia
high pitch of voice

voice strain
mogiphonia

voice weakness
hypophonia
leptophonia
microphonia
microphony
phonasthenia

volume measurement
plethysmography
recording of variations in volume of an organ or part

voluntary motion impaired
dyscinesia
dyskinesia

vomit attempt
retching
vomiturition

vomit inducer
emetic
vomitive
vomitory

vomiting
emesis
anticapatory vomiting
associated with chemotherapy

vomiting blood
hematemesis
vomitus cruentus

vomiting caseous matter
caseation
tyremesis
tyrosis

vomiting in excess
hyperemesis

vomiting excrement
copremesis

vomiting pus
pyemesis

voracious appetite
boulimia
bulimia

vulva incision
episiotomy
to facilitate delivery

vulva inflammation
vulvitis
vulvovaginitis

vulva minor lip
nympha

vulva operation
vulvectomy

vulva/perineum suture
episiorrhaphy

vulva surgical incision
episiotomy
perineotomy
performed at childbirth

walking backward
opisthoporeia

walking difficulty
dysbasia

walking inability
abasia
astasia
inability to maintain erect position
astasia-abasia
inability to stand or walk

walking measurer
pedometer
podometer

walking/standing upright
orthograde

wandering
aberrant
erratic

wanderlust
drapetomania
dromomania
poriomania
uncontrollable desire to leave home

wanting to remember
onomatomania
impulse to dwell upon or recall a word or
name

warm-blooded
hemathermal
hematothermal
homeothermal
homiothermal
homothermal
refers to animals that are warm-blooded

warm/cold sensation
psychroesthesia
experiencing a cold sensation in a warm
part of the body

wart
thymion
verruca
verruga

wart-covered
verrucose
verrucosis

wartlike
verruciform

washing out
lavage
of a hollow cavity or organ

wasting away
atrophic
atrophy
deterioration of flesh and strength

wasting of body
kwashiorkor
limophthisis
seen in African children due to starva-
tion

marasmic
marasmus
symptosis
   due to improper food assimilation
bionecrosis
necrobiosis
   death of cells

water attraction
hydrophilia
   tendency of cells and tissues to attract
   and retain water

water on brain
hydrocephalic
hydrocephalus

water column index
hydrospirometer

water in joints
hydrarthrosis
hydrarthrus
hydrathron
   fluid deposit in the cavity of joints

water magnetism
hydrotropism
   tendency of plants to lean toward or
   away from a moist surface

water massage
hydromassage

water study
limnology

water treatment
aerohydropathy
aerohydrotherapy
affusion

watery eye
epiphora

watery liquid flow
hydrorrhea

wave-length measurer
spectrometer
   instrument for measuring wave length of
   a light ray

weak body
hyposthenia

weak mind
deliquescence
deliquium

weak pulse
acrotism

weak respiration
apnea
   also absence of breathing

weak voice
dysphonia
hypophonia
leptophonia

weaning
ablactation

webbed digits
syndactyly
   most common congenital anomaly of the
   hand

wedge-shaped
cuneate
cuneiform
sphenoid

wedge-shaped head
sphenocephalus
sphenocephaly

weed
marijuana

weight loss
emaciation
   denoting illness

well-being feeling
euphoria
   absence of pain or distress

wheat gum
gluten

wheat protein
glutenin

whiskey nose
rhinophyma

white blood cell
leukoblast
leukocyte

white blood cell deficiency
leukopenia

white blood cell destruction
leukocytolysis
leukolysis
   disintegration of leukocytes

white blood cell excess
leukocytosis

white blood cell formation
leukocytogenesis
leukopoiesis

white blood cell in urine
leukocyturia

white gangrene
leukonecrosis
gangrene with formation of a white slough

white hair
leukotrichia

white spot on skin
leukoderma
leukopathia
leukopathy

white spot on tongue
leukoplakia
disorder characterized by white spots on the tongue

whitlow
felon
paronychia
inflammation near the nail

whooping cough
pertussis

whorl
verticil

will power impaired/lacking
aboulia
abulia
abulic
dysbulia
inability to make decisions

wind measurer
anemometer
determines velocity

winding
tortuous

windpipe
trachea

windpipe viewer
bronchoscope
also used for obtaining specimens for culture

wine-pertaining
vinic
vinous

wine study
enology

wink
nictate

nictation
nictitation
palpebrate

wisdom expert
megalomania
sophomania
belief in one's supreme knowledge

within the abdomen
intraabdominal

within the artery
intra-arterial

within the atria
intraatrial

within the bladder
intracystic
intravesical
also denotes within a cyst

within blood vessels/lymphatics
intravascular

within the bronchi
endobronchial
intrabronchial

within a cartilage
enchondral
endochondral
intracartilaginous

within a cell
intracellular

within the dura mater
intradural
enclosed by the outer covering of the brain

within the ear
intra-aural

within the eyeball
entoptic
intraocular

within the heart
endocardiac
intracardiac
within one of the chambers of the heart

within a joint
intra-articular

within the liver
intrahepatic

within a lobe/lobule
intralobular
of any organ or structure

within the mouth
intrabuccal
intraoral

within the nasal cavity
intranasal

within a nucleus
intranuclear
  of a cell

within the orbit
intraorbital

within the pelvic cavity
intrapelvic

within the peritoneum
intraperitoneal

within the pleural cavity
intrapleural

within the scrotal sac
intrascrotal

within the skin
intracutaneous
intradermal
intradermic
  within the substance of the skin

within the skull
intracranial

within the spinal canal
intraspinal

within the spleen
intrasplanic

within the stomach
intragastric

within the trachea
endotracheal

within a tube
intratubal
  within any tube

within the urinary bladder
intravesical

within the uterus
intrauterine

within the veins
endovenous
intravenous

within a ventricle
intraventricular
  of the brain or heart

without abdominal wall
agenosomus
  congenital deformity

without alimentary canal
agastric

without amnion
anamnionic
anamniotic

without anus aperture
aproctia

without appetite
anorexia

without bile pigment
acholuria
acholuric
  in the urine

without bile secretion
acholia
acholic

without blood lymphocytes
alymphocytosis
  total or partial absence

without brain
pantanencephalia
pantanencephaly
  total absence of any part of the brain

without cerebellum
notanencephalia

without cerebrum/cerebellum
anencephalia
anencephaly

without concentration
aprosexia
  inability to fix attention on a given subject

without cranial vault
holoacrania

without ear pinnae
anotia
anotus

without epiloon/omentum
anepiploic
  lacking the fold of peritoneum passing from the stomach to another abdominal organ

without extremities
acolous

without extremities (cont.)
  amelia
  amelus

without eyes
  anophthalmia
  anophthalmos
  anophthalmus

without face
  aprosopia
    congenital absence

without feet
  apodal
  apodia
  apodous
  apody
  apus

without fetus
  afetal

without fever
  afebrile
  apyretic
  apyrexia
  apyrexial

without fingers
  adactylia
  adctyly
    congenital absence of fingers or toes

without foreskin
  apellous
    circumsized by surgery
  aposthia
    congenital absence

without gestures
  amimia
    loss of ability to communicate by means
    of gestures or signs

without glands
  anadenia
    also denotes deficiency

without glomeruli
  aglomerular

without hair coloring
  canities
    gradual dilution of pigment
  poliosis
    lack of pigmentation

without hands
  acheiria
  achiria

without intestine
  anenterous

without intestinal movement
  aperistalsis

without iris
  aniridia
  irideremia
    total or partial absence

without jaws
  agnathia
  agnathous
  agnathus
    absence of jaws
  hemignathia
    lacking on one side
  tocephalus
  otocephaly
    congenital absence with other deformi-
    ties

without limbs
  lipomeria
    absence of one or more

without lips
  acheilia
  achilia

without lungs
  apneumia

without lymph
  alymphia
    also denotes deficiency

without mammae
  amastia
  amazia
    congenital absence of breasts

without menstruation
  amenia
  amenorrhea
  menostasia
  menostasis

without milk
  agalactia
  agalactosis
  agalactous

without mouth
  astomia
  astomatous
  astomous

without mucous secretion
  amyxia

amyxorrhea
also denotes deficiency of flow

without muscle formation
amyoplasia

without muscle tone
amyotonia
myatonia

without nails
anonychia
anonychosis

without head/neck
atrachelocephalus
congenital absence

without nervous energy
aneuria

without nipples
athelia

without nose
arhinia
arrhinia

without omentum/epiploon
anepiploic

without part of skull
meroacrania

without perception
agnea
auditory agnosia
optic agnosia
tactile agnosia
inability to recognize by the various perceptions

without phalanx
hypophalangism
congenital absence of one or more phalanges

without placenta
aplacental

without prepuce
apellous
circumcised
aposthia
congenital absence

without reflex
areflexia

without rhythm
arrhythmia
arrhythmic

without ribs
apleuria

without sensation
anesthesia
pharmacological or disease-induced

without sense of smell
anosmia
anosmic

without sense of touch
anaphia
anhaphia
atactilia

without signs or gestures
amimia
loss of ability to communicate by signs

without skin
adermia
apellous

without skin pigment
achromoderma
leukoderma

without skull
acrania
acranial
acranius
notancephalia

without sternum
asternia

without strength
adynamia
asthenia
debility

without symptoms
asymptomatic

without tail
acaudal
acaudate

without taste
ageusia
ageustia
loss or impairment of the sense of taste

without teeth
anodontia

without testes
agenitalism
absence of genitals
anorchia

without testes (cont.)
anorchidism
anorchism
    absence of testes

without thirst
adipsia
adipsy

without tongue
aglossia
aglossostomia
    congenital deformity

without tonus
atonia
atony

without upper extremities
omacephalus
    also lacking complete head development

without urinary bladder
acystia

without uterus
ametria

wolf transformation
lycanthropy
    insane delusion believing oneself to be a wolf

woman aversion
misogyny

womb
uterus

wood sugar
xylose

wool fat
adeps lanae
    used in preparation of ointment

wool grease
suint

woolsorter's disease
anthracemia
pneumanthrax

word-blindness
alexia

word-madness
verbomania
    an abnormal flow of speech

word repeating
palilalia
paliphrasia
    repetition of words or phrases

worm killer
vermicide
vermifuge

worm vomiting
helminthemesis

wormlike
vermicular
vermiform

wound breathing
traumatopnea
    passage of air through a wound in the chest wall

wound fluid
ichor

wound study
traumatology
    branch of surgery concerned with injury

woven together
plexus
    interlacing network of nerves, blood or lymphatic vessels

wrinkle
ruga

wrinkle operation
rhytidectomy
rhytidoplasty

wrist bone
capitatum
os magnum
    the largest of the carpal bones

writer's cramp
cheirospasm
chirospasm
dysgraphia
mogigraphia

writing inability
agraphia
absolute agraphia
acoustic agraphia
amnemonic agraphia
atactic agraphia
literal agraphia
logographia
    loss of the ability to write

writin ...**ness**
micr ...*raphy*

wr...**ng speed**
agitographia
writing with excessive speed, omitting
words or letters

wryneck
loxia
torticollis

X

xanthine in urine
xanthinuria
xanthiuria
xanthuria

xiphoid inflammation
xiphoiditis
inflammation of the xiphoid process of
the sternum

x-ray
roentgen

x-ray dermatitis
radiodermatitis

x-ray inflammation
actinoneuritis
radioneuritis
inflammation of the nerves due to x-rays

x-ray measurer
intensimeter
iontoquantimeter
measures intensity or dosage of the x-
rays
qualimeter
quantimeter
obsolete devices
radiometer
roentgenometer
measures quality and penetration of the
x-rays

x-ray picture
computed tomography scan
radiogram
roentgenogram
planigraphy
planography
tomography
use of a curvilinear motion during x-ray
exposure

x-ray specialist
radiologist
roentgenologist

x-ray study
roentgenology

Y

yawning
oscitation

yellow colored
xanthochromatic

yellow jaundice
icteric
icteroid
icterus
yellowish staining of the skin and deeper
tissues

yellow nodule
xanthoma
especially of the skin

yellow skinned
xanthochromia
xanthochroous

yellow teeth
xanthodont

yellow vision
xanthopsia
objects appear yellow

yolk deficiency
oligolecithal

yolk in excess
megalecithal

yolk moderate
medialecithal

youthful
ephebic
hebetic
    pertaining to youth

Eponyms

Ackerman tumor	verrucous carcinoma of the larynx
Addison's disease	chronic adrenocortical insufficiency (caused by atrophy or destruction of the adrenal glands)
Adson syndrome	compression of the brachial plexus leading to sensory disturbance of the upper extremity; also known as Naffziger syndrome
Albright syndrome	hereditary osteodystrophy - pseudohypoparathyroidism; also polycystic fibrous dysplasia
Alport syndrome	hereditary nephritis with nerve deafness and occasional platelet defect and cataract
Alzheimer's disease	dementia presenilis (a general mental deterioration)
Andersen's disease	type 4 glycogenosis (a glycogen storage disease)
Argyll Robertson pupil	does not respond to light, but reacts to accommodation; seen in syphilis, encephalopathy, and diabetes
Arnold Pick syndrome	a perceptive blindness with central atrophy where patient cannot fix reflectively on objects within the gaze
Arthus phenomenon	inflammation resulting from antigen-antibody (IgE) combining in tissues with resultant local reaction and damage
Aschoff nodules	granuloma specific for rheumatic fever
Ashby technique	nonradioisotope technique for determining red cell volume and red cell life span by injecting red cells of a different blood type into the recipient
Babinski sign/test/reflex	test for pyramidal tract disturbance where stroking the lateral aspect of the sole of the foot normally produces plantar flexion of the great toe
Baker cyst	enlargement of the popliteal bursa or herniation of the synovial membrane of the knee joint often associated with degenerative disease of the knee
Bamberger disease	saltatory spasm; polyserositis

Barany syndrome	unilateral headache in the back of the head with recurrent deafness; vertigo, tinnitus, and abnormal pointing test, corrected by stimulating nystagmus
Barany test	caloric test of semicircular canal
Barlow disease	infantile scurvy
Barraquer-Simons disease	progressive lipodystrophy
Barrett ulcer	esophageal ulcer
Barrett's syndrome	chronic peptic ulcer of the lower esophagus
Basedow disease	thyrotoxicosis
Basedow syndrome	myeloneuropathy, not due to vitamin B_{12} deficiency
Beck triad	low arterial pressure, high venous pressure, and absent apex beat; cardiac tamponade
Beevor sign	upward displacement of umbilicus due to paralysis of lower rectus abdominis
Bekhterev-Mendel reflex	tapping the dorsum of the foot normally causes extension of the second and fifth toes; flexion indicates a pyramidal lesion
Bell's palsy	paralysis of the facial muscles supplied by the seventh cranial nerve
Bence-Jones protein	abnormal protein found in the urine of patients with multiple myeloma; consists of monoclonal light chains of the gamma globulin molecules
Benedict solution	copper sulfate solution used to test for glycosuria
Bennett fracture	fracture of the base of the first metacarpal
Berger disease	glomerulonephritis with mesangial IgA deposition
Bernard syndrome	see Horner syndrome
Besnier-Boeck disease	sarcoidosis
Bing sign	extension of the great toe following a pricking of the dorsum of the toe or foot with a pin, seen in pyramidal tract lesions
Blumberg sign	rebound tenderness indicating peritoneal inflammation
Bouchard nodes	seen in gout and osteoarthritis in the proximal interphalangeal joints
Bright's disease	used to denote kidney disease; actually nephritis with albuminuria and edema
Buerger's disease	thromboangiitis obliterans (inflammation of the wall and connective tissue surrounding medium-sized arteries and veins)
Burnett's syndrome	milk-alkali syndrome (a chronic kidney disorder)

Calve disease	osteochondrosis of the vertebrae
Cannon syndrome	increase in adrenaline secretion during emotional stress, resulting in palpitations and sweating
Caplan's syndrome	progressive massive necrosis of the lung, seen with rheumatoid arthritis
Charcot's triad	intention tremor, nystagmus, and scanning speech seen in brain stem involvement in multiple sclerosis
Charcot-Marie-Tooth disease	peroneal muscular atrophy (of the leg muscles near the fibula)
Christensen-Krabble disease	progressive cerebral poliodystrophy
Christmas disease	hemophilia B; sex-linked recessive hereditary bleeding disorder
Colles' fracture	fracture of the lower end of the radius with displacement of the bone
Concato's disease	polyserositis
Conn's syndrome	primary aldosteronism (over-secretion of the hormone)
Costen syndrome	dental malocclusion with associated neurologic headache
Creutzfeldt-Jakob disease	"mad cow" disease; spastic pseudosclerosis with spinal degeneration
Crohn's disease	regional enteritis (inflammation of the intestine)
Cushing's syndrome	pituitary basophilism (disorder of basophilic blood cells)
DaCosta syndrome	circulatory neurasthenia
Darling disease	histoplasmosis
DeQuervain's disease	subacute thyroiditis
Deutschländer's disease	tumor of metatarsal bone
Diamond-Blackfan syndrome	congenital hypoplastic anemia characterized by progressive anemia with sparing of white cells and platelets
Di Guglielmo's disease	acute or chronic erythroleukemia
Down's syndrome	mongolism
Dressler's syndrome	complications developing several days to weeks following a myocardial infarction; postmyocardial infarction syndrome
Dubin-Johnson syndrome	chronic idiopathic jaundice
Duchenne's syndrome	anterior spinal paralysis with neuritis

Duhring's disease	dermatitis herpetiformis
Dupuytren's disease	plantar fibromatosis (abnormal growth of fibrous tissue on the sole of the foot)
Eales disease	recurrent retinal and vitreous hemorrhage of unknown etiology
Ebstein's disease	congenital heart disorder with tricuspid valve displacement into the right ventricle
Ehlers-Danlos syndrome	hyperelasticity of the skin, easy bruising, and joint extensibility usually due to faulty collagen synthesis
Engelmann disease	progressive diaphyseal dysplasia
Epstein's disease	diphtheroid; an infection suggesting diphtheria
Epstein syndrome	nephrotic syndrome; edema, proteinuria, hypoalbuminemia, and hyperlipidemia
Epstein-Barr virus	a herpetovirus found in lymphoma and mononucleosis
Erb's palsy	progressive bulbar paralysis involving the muscles of the upper arm
Erb-Charcot disease	spastic diplegia (paralysis of corresponding parts on both sides of the body)
Erb-Goldflam disease	myasthenia gravis
Ewing's sarcoma	a malignant tumor of the bone marrow seen in children
Fanconi's syndrome	renal tubular dysfunction
Farber disease	disseminated lipogranulomatosis giving nodular plaques in the skin
Felty's syndrome	rheumatoid arthritis with splenomegaly and leukopenia
Filatov disease	infectious mononucleosis
Fisher syndrome	ophthalmoplegia, ataxia, and loss of tendon reflexes
Foix-Alajouanine syndrome	subacute necrotizing myelopathy, often associated with thrombophlebitis or vascular malformation of the spinal cord
Folling's disease	phenylketonuria
Forbes disease	type 3 glycogenosis; a glycogen storage disease
Friedreich disease	paramyoclonus multiplex
Fröhlich syndrome	adiposogenital dystrophy; pituitary tumor with obesity and sexual infantilism
Gamstorp disease	periodic paralysis, usually with hyperkalemia
Gardner syndrome	variant of congenital polyposis of the colon
Gasser syndrome	acute transient aplasia of erythropoietic tissue in young children; also acute hemolytic uremic (HUR) syndrome in children

Gehrig disease	amyotrophic lateral sclerosis
Gélineau disease	narcolepsy
Gerhardt disease	erythromelalgia
Gerhardt syndrome	bilateral abductor paralysis of the larynx
Gierke's disease	type 1 glycogenosis; a glycogen storage disorder
Goldflam disease	myasthenia gravis (a chronic, progressive muscular weakness)
Goodpasture syndrome	acute glomerulonephritis with hemoptysis intrapulmonary hemorrhage, and anemia
Grave's disease	toxic goiter; hyperthyroidism
Guillain-Barré syndrome	acute idiopathic polyneuritis (simultaneous inflammation of a large number of the spinal nerves)
Gull disease	myxedema; hypothyroidism
Hamman-Rich syndrome	idiopathic diffuse interstitial pulmonary fibrosis
Hammond disease	congenital athetosis
Hansen's disease	leprosy (a chronic granulomatous infection of the skin)
Harley disease	paroxysmal hemoglobinuria
Hashimoto's disease	lymphadenoid goiter; thyroiditis
Hirschsprung disease	dilation of the colon causing obstruction at the rectum with resultant constipation and growth retardation
Hodgkin's disease	anemia lymphatica; also a term for lymphoma
Hoppe-Goldflam disease	myasthenia gravis
Huchard disease	essential hypertension
Jakob-Creutzfeldt disease	progressive encephalopathy believed caused by a slow virus
Kahler disease	multiple myeloma
Kasabach-Merritt syndrome	hemangioma-thrombocytopenia syndrome
Kawasaki syndrome	febrile illness of unknown etiology occurring mainly in children under five years
Kimmelstiel-Wilson disease	glomerulosclerosis (scarring within the kidney glomeruli)
Klein-Levin syndrome	periodic attacks of sleep and hunger with amnesia for periods of the attacks, related to narcolepsy
Kohler disease	aseptic necrosis of the navicular bone
Larsen-Johansson disease	osteochondrosis involving the apex of the patella
Legg-Calve-Perthes disease	epiphyseal aseptic necrosis of the upper end of the femur

Legionnaire's disease	*Legionella pneumophilia* infection
Little disease	spastic paraplegia
Lyme disease	*L. borreliosis* (inflammatory disorder transmitted by the tick)
Mallory-Weiss syndrome	hematemesis due to a tear in the esophagus following forceful vomiting
Marie-Strümpell disease	ankylosing spondylitis (arthritis of the spine)
McArdle's disease	type 5 glycogenosis; accumulation of glycogen in muscle
Meniere's disease	endolymphatic hydrops (excessive accumulation of fluid in the inner ear)
Meyer's disease	adenoids (chronic inflammation of the pharyngeal tonsil)
Monge disease	mountain sickness
Morgagni's disease	also known as Stokes-Adams syndrome
Oguchi's disease	hereditary night blindness
Oppenheim-Ziehan disease	dystonia musculorum deformans
Ortner syndrome	left vocal cord paralysis associated with enlarged left atrium in mitral stenosis
Osler's disease	erythremia (increase in size of bone marrow and blood volume)
Osler-Vaquez' disease	erythremia; polycythemia rubra vera
Paget's disease	osteitis deformans (generalized skeletal disorder with thickening and softening of bone)
Parkinson's disease	shaking/trembling palsy
Pick's disease	multiple polyserositis (with ascites, hepatomegaly, peritonitis, and pleural effusion); also cerebral atrophy of frontal and temporal lobes resulting in senile dementia
Plummer's disease	hyperthyroidism with a nodular goiter
Pompe's disease	type 2 glycogenosis; accumulation of glycogen in heart, muscle, liver, and nervous system
Pott's disease	tuberculous spondylitis (inflammation of the vertebra)
Pott's fracture	fracture of the lower end of the fibula with outward displacement of the foot
Purtscher syndrome	sudden blindness following severe trauma or prolonged exposure with exhaustion and shock
Rasmussen's syndrome	a type of progressive encephalopathy seen in juveniles
Raynaud's disease	idiopathic, paroxysmal, bilateral cyanosis of the digits

Reye's syndrome	postinfectious syndrome of liver, kidney, and brain damage seen in children
Rokitansky disease	postnecrotic cirrhosis of the liver
Rust disease	tuberculous spondylitis of the cervical region
St. Giles disease	leprosy
St. Vitus' dance	ballism; ballismus (jerking or shaking movements)
St. Zachary disease	mutism
Sanders disease/ syndrome	epidemic keratoconjunctivitis
Saunders disease	acute gastritis in infants due to excessive carbohydrate in the diet
Simmonds disease	hypopituitarism
Sjögren's syndrome	group of symptoms associated with rheumatoid arthritis seen in menopausal women
Steele-Richardson-Olszewski syndrome	progressive supranuclear paralysis
Stein-Leventhal syndrome	hirsutism, amenorrhea, enlarged polycystic ovary
Stevens-Johnson syndrome	erythema multiforme (acute skin eruptions, sometimes due to drug allergy)
Still's disease	juvenile-type rheumatoid arthritis
Stokes-Adams syndrome	slow or absent pulse, vertigo, syncope, and convulsions, usually as the result of heart block
Vaquez' disease	erythremia; polycythemia rubra vera
Vincent's disease	necrotizing ulcerative gingivitis (inflammation of the gums)
von Gierke's disease	type 1 glycogenosis; glycogen accumulation in liver and kidney
Wilks disease	subacute glomerulonephritis; subcutaneous tuberculosis
Zollinger-Ellison syndrome	peptic ulceration with gastric hypersecretion

Medical Abbreviations

A	alive; ambulatory; apical; artery; assessment
A_2	aortic second sound
AA	amino acid; achievement age; active assistance; arm ankle (pulse ratio); authorized absence; auto accident; Alcoholics anonymous
AAA	abdominal aortic aneurysmectomy/aneurysm
AAC	antibiotic agent-associated colitis
AAFP	American Academy of Family Physicians
AAL	anterior axillary line
AAMA	American Association of Medical Assistants
AAN	analgesic-associated nephropathy; analgesic abuse nephropathy; attending physician's admission notes
AAO × 3	awake and oriented to time, place and person
AAP	assessment adjustment pass; American Academy of Pediatrics
AAPA	American Academy of Physician Assistants
AAPC	antibiotic acquired pseudomembranous colitis
AAROM	active assistive range of motion
AAS	atlanto axis subluxation
AAV	adeno-associated virus
AAVV	accumulated alveolar ventilatory volume
Ab	abortion; antibody
A & B	apnea and bradycardia
ABC	airway, breathing, circulation; absolute band counts; artificial beta cells
ABCDE	botulism toxoid pentavalent
Abd	abdomen; abdominal
ABDCT	atrial bolus dynamic computer tomography
ABE	acute bacterial endocarditis
ABG	arterial blood gases
ABI	atherothrombotic brain infarction
ABL	allograft bound lymphocytes
ABLB	alternate binaural loudness balance

ABMT	autologous bone marrow transplantation
ABN	abnormality
Abnor.	abnormal
ABR	absolute bed rest; auditory brain (evoked) responses
ABS	at bedside; admitting blood sugar; absorption
ABT	aminopyrine breath test
ABW	actual body weight
Abx	antibiotics
AC	acute; before meals; acromio-clavicular; air conduction; air conditioned; assist control; abdominal circumference; anchored catheter
A/C	anterior chamber (of the eye)
ACA	anterior cerebral artery; acrodermatitis chronicum atrophicans; acute or chronic alcholism
ACB	antibody-coated bacteria
AC & BC	air and bone conduction
ACBE	air contrast barium enema
ACC	accommodation; adenoid cystic carcinomas; administrative control center
ACD	anterior chest diameter; anterior chamber diameter; anemia of chronic disease; absolute cardiac dullness
ACEI	angiotensin-converting enzyme inhibitor
ACH	adrenal cortical hormone
ACI	aftercare instructions
ACL	anterior cruciate ligament
ACLS	advanced cardiac life support
ACPP-PF	acid phosphatase prostatic fluid
ACT	automated coagulation time; allergen challenge test
Act Ex	active exercise
ACOA	adult children of alcoholics
ACS	American Cancer Society; American College of Surgeons
ACTH	adrenocorticotropic hormone
ACTSEB	anterior chamber tube shunt encircling band
ACV	atrial/carotid/ventricular
A & D	admission and discharge
AD	Alzheimer's disease; right ear; accident dispensary
ADA	American Diabetes Association; American Dental Association
ADAU	adolescent drug abuse unit
ADCC	antibody-dependent cellular cytotoxicity
ADD	attention deficit disorder; adduction
ADDU	alcohol and drug dependence unit
ADEM	acute disseminating encephalomyelitis
ADH	antidiuretic hormone

ADHD	attention deficit hyperactivity disorder
ADL	activities of daily living
ad lib	as desired; at liberty
ADM	admission
adol	adolescent
ADPKD	autosomal dominant polycystic kidney
ADR	adverse drug reaction; acute dystonic reaction
ADP	adenosine diphosphate
ADS	anonymous donor's sperm; anatomical dead space
ADT	anticipate discharge tomorrow
ADX	adrenalectomy
AE	above elbow; air entry
AEC	at earliest convenience
AED	automated external defibrillator
AEG	air encephalogram
AER	acoustic evoked response; auditory evoked response
Aer. M	aerosol mask
Aer. T	aerosol tent
AES	anti-embolic stocking
AF	atrial fibrillation; acid-fast; amniotic fluid; anterior fontanel
AFB	acid-fast bacilli; aorto-femoral bypass
AFC	air filled cushions
A. fib	atrial fibrillation
AFO	ankle-foot orthosis
AFP	alpha-fetoprotein
AFV	amniotic fluid volume
AFVSS	afebrile, vital signs stable
A/G	albumin to globulin ratio
Ag	antigen
AG	anti-gravity; anion gap
AGA	acute gonococcal arthritis; appropriate for gestational age
AGD	agar gel diffusion
AGE	angle of greatest extension
AGF	angle of greatest flexion
AGG	agammaglobulinemia
aggl.	agglutination
AGL	acute granulocytic leukemia
AGN	acute glomerulonephritis
AGNB	aerobic gram-negative bacilli
AGPT	agar-gel precipitation test
AGS	adrenogenital syndrome
AH	airway hyperresponsiveness
AHA	autoimmune hemolytic anemia; American Heart/Hospital Association

AHC	acute hemorrhagic conjunctivitis; acute hemorrhagic cystitis
AHD	autoimmune hemolytic disease
AHF	antihemophilic factor
AHG	antihemophilic globulin
AHM	ambulatory Holter monitoring
AHT	autoantibodies to human thyroglobulin
AI	aortic insufficiency; artificial insemination; allergy index
A & I	allergy and immunology department
AI-Ab	anti-insulin antibody
AICA	anterior inferior communicating artery; anterior inferior cerebellar artery
AICD	automatic implantable cardioverter/defibrillator
AID	artificial insemination donor; automatic implantable defibrillator
AIDS	acquired immune deficiency syndrome
AIE	acute inclusion body encephalitis
AIF	aortic-iliac-femoral
AIH	artificial insemination with husband's sperm
AIHA	autoimmune hemolytic anemia
AILD	angioimmunoblastic lymphadenopathy
AIMS	abnormal involuntary movement scale; arthritis impact measure scale
AIN	acute interstitial nephritis
AINS	anti-inflammatory nonsteroidal
AION	anterior ischemic optic neuropathy
AIP	acute intermittent porphyria
AIR	accelerate idioventricular rhythm
AIVR	accelerated idioventricular rhythm
AJ	ankle jerk
AK	above knee
AKA	above knee amputation; alcoholic ketoacidosis; all known allergies
ALAT	alanine transaminase (alanine aminotransferase; SGPT)
Alb	albumin
ALC	acute lethal catatonia; alcohol
ALC R	alcohol rub
ALD	alcoholic liver disease; adrenoleukodystrophy
ALDOST	adosterone
ALFT	abnormal liver function tests
ALG	antilymphocyte globulin
alk	alkaline
ALK-P	alkaline phosphatase
ALL	acute lymphocytic leukemia

ALM	acral lentiginous melanoma
ALMI	anterolateral myocardial infarction
ALP	alkaline phosphatase
ALS	amyotrophic lateral sclerosis; acute lateral sclerosis; advanced life support
ALT	alanine aminotransferase (SGPT); Argon laser trabeculoplasty
ALWMI	anterolateral wall myocardial infarct
AM	myopic astigmatism; amalgam; morning
AMA	against medical advice; antimitochondrial antibody; American Medical Association
AMAP	as much as possible
A-MAT	amorphous material
Amb	ambulate; ambulatory
AMC	arm muscle circumference
AMD	age-related macular degeneration
AMegL	acute megokaryoblastic leukemia
AMG	acoustic myography
AMI	acute myocardial infarction
AML	acute myelogenous leukemia
AMM	agnogenic myeloid metaplasia
AMMOL	acute myelomonoblastic leukemia
amnio	amniocentesis
AMOL	acute monoblastic leukemia
AMP	amputation; ampule
A-M pr	Austin-Moore prosthesis
AMR	alternating motor rates
AMS	acute mountain sickness; amylase
AMV	assisted mechanical ventilation
AMSIT	A—appearance; M—mood; S—sensorium; I—intelligence; T—thought process (portion of the mental status examination)
amt	amount
AMY	amylase
ANA	antinuclear antibody; American Nurses/Neurologic Association
ANAD	anorexia nervosa and associated disorders
ANC	absolute neutrophil count
AND	anterior nasal discharge
anes	anesthesia
ANF	antinuclear factor; atrial natriuretic factor
ANG	angiogram
ANLL	acute nonlymphoblastic leukemia
ANOVA	analysis of variance

ANP	atrial natriuretic peptide
ANS	autonomic nervous system; answer
ant	anterior
ante	before
A & O	alert and oriented
AOA	American Optometric Association
AOAP	as often as possible
AOB	alcohol on breath
ao-il	aorta-iliac
AOC	area of concern
AODM	adult onset diabetes mellitus
AOM	acute otitis media
AOP	aortic pressure
A & O × 3	awake and oriented to person, place, and time
A & O × 4	awake and oriented to person, place, time and date
AOSD	adult onset Still's disease
A & P	auscultation and percussion; anterior and posterior; assessment and plans
AP	anterior-posterior; antepartum; apical pulse; abdominal-peritoneal; appendicitis
A$_2$ > P$_2$	second aortic sound greater than second pulmonic sound
APB	atrial premature beat; abductor pollicis brevis
APC	atrial premature contraction
APCD	adult polycystic disease
APD	automated peritoneal dialysis; atrial premature depolarization
APE	acute psychotic episode
APKD	adult onset polycystic kidney disease
APL	acute promyelocytic leukemia; abductor pollicis longus; accelerated painless labor; chorionic gonadotropin
appr	approximate
appt	appointment
APR	abdominoperineal resection
APTT	activated partial thromboplastin time
AQ	achievement quotient
aq	water
aq dist	distilled water
AR	aortic regurgitation
A & R	advised and released
A-R	apical-radial (pulse)
ARB	any reliable brand
ARC	AIDS-related complex; anomalous retinal correspondence
ARD	adult respiratory distress; acute respiratory disease; antibiotic removal device

ARDMS	American Registry of Diagnostic Medical Sonographers
ARDS	adult respiratory distress syndrome
ARF	acute renal failure; acute rheumatic fever; acute respiratory failure
ARLD	alcohol-related liver disease
ARM	artificial rupture of membranes
ARMD	age-related macular degeneration
AROM	active range of motion; artificial rupture of membranes
ARS	antirabies serum
ART	arterial; automated reagin test (for syphilis)
ARV	AIDS-related virus
AS	aortic stenosis; arteriosclerosis; anal sphincter; left ear; activated sleep; ankylosing spondylitis
ASA I	healthy patient with localized pathological process
ASA II	patient with mild to moderate systemic disease
ASA III	patient with severe systemic disease limiting activity but not incapacitating
ASA IV	patient with incapacitating systemic disease
ASA V	moribund patient not expected to live (American Society of Anesthesiologist classifications)
ASAA	acquired severe aplastic anemia
ASAP	as soon as possible
ASAT	aspartate transaminase (aspartate aminotransferase) (SGOT)
ASB	anesthesia standby; asymptomatic bacteriuria
ASC	altered state of consciousness; ambulatory surgery center
ASCP	American Society of Clinical Pathologists
ASCVD	arteriosclerotic cardiovascular disease
ASD	atrial septal defect
ASE	acute stress erosion
ASH	asymmetric septal hypertrophy
ASHD	arteriosclerotic heart disease
ASIS	anterior superior iliac spine
ASL	airway surface liquid
AsM	myopic astigmatism
ASMI	anteroseptal myocardial infarction
ASO	antistreptolysin-O titer; arteriosclerosis obliterans
ASOT	antistreptolysin-O titer
ASP	acute suppurative parotitis
ASS	anterior superior supine
AST	aspartic acid transaminase; astigmatism
ASTZ	antistreptozyme test
ASU	acute stroke unit
ASVD	arteriosclerotic vessel disease

AT	applanation tonometry; atraumatic; antithrombin
ATB	antibiotic
ATC	around the clock
ATD	autoimmune thyroid disease; antithyroid drug
AtFib	atrial fibrillation
ATG	antithymocyte globulin
ATgA	antithyroglobulin antibodies
ATHR	angina threshold heart rate
ATL	Achilles tendon lengthening; atypical lymphocytes; adult T-cell leukemia
ATLS	advanced trauma life support
ATN	acute tubular necrosis
ATNC	atraumatic normocephalic
aTNM	autopsy staging of cancer
ATNR	asymmetrical tonic neck reflux
ATPS	ambient temperature and pressure; saturated with water vapor
ATR	Achilles tendon reflex; atrial
ATT	arginine tolerance test
AU	allergenic units; both ears
AUC	area under the curve
AV	arteriovenous; atrioventricular; auditory-visual
AVA	arteriovenous anastomosis
AVD	apparent volume of distribution
AVF	arteriovenous fistula
AVH	acute viral hepatitis
AVM	atriovenous malformation
AVN	atrioventricular node; arteriovenous nicking; avascular necrosis
AVR	aortic valve replacement
AVS	atriovenous shunt
AVSS	afebrile, vital signs stable
AVT	atypical ventricular tachycardia
A & W	alive and well
A waves	atrial contraction waves
AWI	anterior wall infarct
AWOL	absent without leave
ax	axillary
A-Z test	Aschheim-Zondek test; diagnostic test for pregnancy
B	bacillus; bands; bloody; black; both; buccal
Ba	barium
BA	backache; bile acid; blood alcohol; Bourns assist
BAC	blood alcohol content; buccoaxiocervical

BAD	bipolar affective disorder
BaE	barium enema
BAE	bronchial artery embolization
BAEP	brain stem auditory evoked potential
BAER	brain stem auditory evoked response
BAL	blood alcohol level; bronchoalveolar lavage
BAO	basal acid output
BAP	blood agar plate
baso.	basophil
BAVP	balloon aortic valvuloplasty
BB	bed bath; bowel or bladder; breakthrough bleeding; blood bank; blow bottle
BBA	born before arrival
BBB	bundle branch block; blood brain barrier
BBBB	bilateral bundle branch block
BBD	benign breast disease; biparietal diameter
BBM	banked breast milk
BBS	bilateral breath sounds
BBT	basal body temperature
BBVM	brush border vesicle membrane
BC	birth control; blood culture; bone conduction; Bourn control; bed and chair
BCA	balloon catheter angioplasty; basal cell atypia; brachiocephalic artery
BCAA	branched-chain amino acids
BCC	basal cell carcinoma
BCD	basal cell dysplasia
BCE	basal cell epithelioma
B cell	large lymphocyte
BCG	bacillus Calmette-Guérin vaccine
BCL	basic cycle length
BCP	birth control pills
BCS	battered child syndrome; Budd-Chiari syndrome
BD	birth defect; brain dead; bronchial drainage
BDAE	Boston Diagnostic Aphasia Examination
BDI SF	Beck's Depression Index—Short Form
BDR	background diabetic retinopathy
BE	barium enema; below elbow; bacterial endocarditis; base excess; bread equivalent
BEAM	brain electrical activity mapping
BEC	bacterial endocarditis
BEE	basal energy expenditure
BEI	butanol-extractable iodine
BEP	brainstem evoked potentials

BF	black female
BFO	balance forearm orthosis
BFP	biologic false positive
BFT	bentonite flocculation test
BFUE	erythroid burst-forming unit
BG	blood glucose
BGC	basal ganglion calcification
BGM	blood glucose monitoring
BHI	biosynthetic human insulin
BHN	bridging hepatic necrosis
BHR	bronchial hyperresponsiveness
BHS	beta-hemolytic streptococci
BI	bladder irritation; bowel impaction; bioelectric impedance
BIB	brought in by
BID	twice daily
BIG 6	analysis of 6 serum components
BIH	bilateral inguinal hernia; benign intracranial hypertension
bil	bilateral
BILAT SLC	bilateral short leg cast
BILAT SXO	bilateral salpingo-oophorectomy
bili	bilirubin
BILI-C	conjugated bilirubin
BIMA	bilateral internal mammary arteries
BIW	twice a week
BJ	bone and joint
BJE	bones, joints, and examination
BJM	bones, joines, and muscles
BJ protein	Bence-Jones protein
BK	below knee
BKA	below knee amputation
Bkg	background
BLB	Boothby-Lovelace-Bulbulian (oxygen mask)
bl cult	blood culture
BLE	both lower extremities
BLESS	bath, laxative, enema, shampoo, and shower
BLOBS	bladder obstruction
BLS	basic life support
B.L. unit	Bessey-Lowry unit
BM	basal metabolism; black male; bone marrow; bowel movement; breast milk
BMA	bone marrow aspirate
BMC	bone marrow cells
BMI	body mass index
BMJ	bones, muscles, joints

BMR	basal metabolic rate
BMT	bone marrow transplant; bilateral myringotomy tubes
BMTU	bone marrow transplant unit
BNO	bladder neck obstruction
BNR	bladder neck retraction
BO	body odor; bowel obstruction; behavior objective
BOA	born on arrival; born out of asepsis
BOM	bilateral otitis media
BOO	bladder outlet obstruction
BOT	base of tongue
BOW	bag of water
BP	blood pressure; bed pan; British Pharmacopeia
BPD	biparietal diameter; bronchopulmonary dysplasia
BPF	bronchopleural fistula
BPG	bypass graft
BPH	benign prostatic hypertrophy
BPM	breaths per minute; beats per minute
BPPV	benign paroxysmal positional vertigo
BPRS	Brief Psychiatric Rate Scale
BPSD	bronchopulmonary segmental drainage
BPV	benign paroxysmal vertigo
Bq	becquerel
BR	bathroom; bedrest; Benzing retrograde
BRAO	branch retinal artery occlusion
BRATT	bananas, rice, applesauce, tea, and toast
BRB	blood-retinal barrier
BRBPR	bright red blood per rectum
BRJ	brachial radialis jerk
BRM	biological response modifiers
BRP	bathroom privileges
BS	blood sugar; bowel sounds; breath sounds; bedside; before sleep
B & S	Bartholin and Skene (glands)
BSA	body surface area
BSB	body surface burned
BSC	bedside commode
BSE	breast self-examination; bovine spongiform encephalopathy
BSER	brainstem evoked responses
BSGA	beta streptococcus group A
BSO	bilateral salpingo-oophorectomy
BSOM	bilateral serous otitis media
BSPM	body surface potential mapping
BSS	balanced salt solution; black silk sutures

BSU	Bartholin, Skene's, urethra
BT	bladder tumor; brain tumor; breast tumor; blood transfusion; bedtime; bituberous
BTB	breakthrough bleeding
BTFS	breast tumor frozen section
BTL	bilateral tubal ligation
BTPS	body temperature pressure saturated
BTR	bladder tumor recheck
BU	Bodansky unit
BUE	both upper extremities
BUN	blood urea nitrogen
BUR	backup rate (ventilator)
BUS	Bartholin, urethral and Skene's glands
BVL	bilateral vas ligation
BW	birth weight; body weight; body water
BWCS	bagged white cell study
BWFI	bacteriostatic water for injection
BWS	battered woman syndrome
Bx	biopsy
C	carbohydrate; Celsius; hundred; cyanosis; clubbing
C1	first cervical vertebra
C1 to C9	precursor molecules of the complement system
C-II	controlled substance, class 2
CA	cardiac arrest; carcinoma; carotid artery; chronologic age; coronary artery
C & A	Clinitest and Acetest
CAA	crystalline amino acids
CAB	coronary artery bypass
CABG	coronary artery bypass graft
CaBI	calcium bone index
CABS	cornonary artery bypass surgery
CACI	computer-assisted continuous infusion
CAD	cornonary artery disease
CAE	cellulose acetate electrophoresis
CAFT	Clinitron® air fluidized therapy
CAH	chronic active hepatitis; chronic aggressive hepatitis; congenital adrenal hyperplasia
CAL	calories; callus; chronic airflow limitation
CALD	chronic active liver disease
CALGB	Cancer and Leukemia Group B
CALLA	common acute lymphoblastic leukemia antigen
cAMP	cyclic adenosine monophosphate
CAN	cord around neck

CAO	chronic airway obstruction
CAP	capsule; compound action potentials
CAPD	chronic/continuous ambulatory peritoneal dialysis
CAR	cardiac ambulation routine
CARB	carbohydrate
CAS	carotide artery stenosis
CAT	computed axial tomography; children's apperception test; cataract
cath	catheter; catheterization
CAVB	complete atrioventricular block
CAVC	common atrioventricular canal
CAVH	continuous arteriovenous hemofiltration
CB	code blue; chronic bronchitis; cesarean birth; chair and bed
C & B	crown and bridge
CBA	chronic bronchitis and asthma
CBC	complete blood count
CBD	common bile duct; closed bladder drainage; cannabidiol
CBF	cerebral blood flow
CBFS	cerebral blood flow studies
CBFV	cerebral blood flow velocity
CBG	capillary blood glucose
CBI	continuous bladder irrigation
CBN	chronic benign neutropenia
CBR	complete bedrest; chronic bedrest; carotid bodies resected
CBS	chronic brain syndrome
CC	chief complaint; cubic centimeter; critical condition; creatinine clearance; cerebral concussion; chronic complainer; clean catch (urine); cord compression
CCA	common carotid artery
CCAP	capsule cartilage articular preservation
CC & C	colony count and culture
CCE	clubbing, cyanosis, and edema
CCF	compound comminuted fracture; crystal-induced chemostatic factor
CCG	Children's Cancer Group
CCHD	cyanotic congenital heart disease
CCI	chronic coronary insufficiency
CCMSU	clean catch midstream urine
CCNS	cell cycle nonspecific
C-collar	cervical collar
CCPD	continuous cycling/cyclical peritoneal dialysis
CCR	continuous complete remission
CCRU	critical care recovery unit
CCS	cell cycle specific; Cooperative Care Suite

CCT	congenitally corrected transposition
CCTGA	congenitally corrected transposition of the great arteries
CCTV	closed circuit television
CCU	coronary care unit
CCUP	colpocystourethropexy
CCX	complications
CD	Crohn's disease; cesarean delivery; continuous drainage
C/D	cup to disc ratio
C & D	cytoscopy and dilatation; curettage and desiccation
CDA	congenital dyserythropoietic anemia
CDAI	Crohn's Disease Activity Index
CDB	cough, deep breathe
CDC	Cancer Detection Center; Centers for Disease Control; calculated day of confinement
CDE	common duct exploration
CDH	congenital dysplasia of the hip; chronic daily headache
CDLE	chronic discoid lupus erythematosus
CDS	chronic dieting syndrome
cdyn	dynamic compliance
CE	cardiac enlargement; contrast echocardiology; central episiotomy; continuing education
CEA	carotid endarterectomy; carcinoembryonic antigen
CECT	contrast enhancement computed tomography
CEI	continuous extravascular infusion
CEP	congenital erythropoietic porphyria; countercurrent electrophoresis
CEPH	cephalic
CEPH Floc	cephalin flocculation
CE & R	central episiotomy and repair
CERA	cortical evoked response audiometry
CERV	cervical
CES	cognitive environmental stimulation
CF	cystic fibrosis; Caucasian female; complement fixation; cardiac failure; cancer-free; count fingers; Christmas factor; contractile force
CFA	common femoral artery; complete Freund's adjuvant
CFIDS	chronic fatigue and immune dysfunction syndrome
CFM	close fitting mask
CFP	cystic fibrosis protein
CFS	cancer family syndrome; chronic fatigue syndrome
CFT	complement fixation test
CF test	complement fixation test
CFU	colony forming units
CFU-S	colony forming unit—spleen

CG	cholecystogram
CGB	chronic gastrointestinal bleeding
CGD	chronic granulomatous disease
CGI	Clinical Global Impression (scale)
CGL	chronic granulocytic leukemia; with correction/with glasses
CGN	chronic glomerulonephritis
CGTT	cortisol glucose tolerance test
CH	child; chronic; chest; crown-heel; convalescent hospital; cluster headache
CHAI	continuous hepatic artery infusion
CHB	complete heart block
CHD	congenital heart disease; childhood diseases
CHF	congestive heart failure; Crimean hemorrhagic fever
CHFV	combined high frequency of ventilation
CHI	closed head injury
CHO	carbohydrate
chol	cholesterol
chr	chronic
CHRS	congenital hereditary retinoschisis
CHS	Chédiak-Higashi syndrome
CHU	closed head unit
CI	cardiac index; cesium implant; complete iridectomy
Ci	curie(s)
CIA	chronic idiopathic anhidrosis
CIAED	collagen-induced autoimmune ear disease
CIB	cytomegalic inclusion bodies
CIBD	chronic inflammatory bowel disease
CIC	circulating immune complexes
CICE	combined intracapsular cataract extraction
CICU	cardiac intensive care unit
CID	cytomegalic inclusion disease
CIDP	chronic inflammatory demyelinating polyradineuropathy
CIDS	continuous insulin delivery system; cellular immunodeficiency syndrome
CIE	counterimmunoelectrophoresis; crossed immunoelectrophoresis
CIN	chronic interstitial nephritis; cervical intraepithelial neoplasia
Circ	circumcision; circumference; circulation
CIS	carcinoma *in situ*
CIU	chronic idiopathic urticaria
CJD	Creutzfeldt-Jakob disease
Ck	check; creatinine kinase
CK-MB	a creatine kinase isoenzyme

cl	cloudy
CL	critical list
CLA	community living arrangements
clav	clavicle
CLBBB	complete left bundle branch block
CLC	cork leather and celastic (orthotic)
CLD	chronic lung disease
CLF	cholesterol-lecithin flocculation
CLH	chronic lobular hepatitis
CLL	chronic lymphocytic leukemia
CLLE	columnar-lined lower esophagus
cl liq	clear liquid
CLO	cod liver oil; close
CL & P	cleft lip and palate
ClH	hepatic clearance
CLT	chronic lymphocytic thyroiditis
Cl VOID	clean voided specimen
clysis	hypodermoclysis
cm	centimeter
CM	Caucasian male; costal margin; continuous murmur; contrast media; centimeter; cochlear microphonics; culture media; common migraine
CMA	certified medical assistant
CMBBT	cervical mucous basal body temperature
CMC	chronic mucocutaneous moniliasis
CME	continuing medical education; cystoid macular edema
CMG	cystometrogram
CMHC	Community Mental Health Center
CMHN	Community Mental Health Nurse
CMI	cell-mediated immunity; Cornell Medical Index
CMJ	carpometacarpal joint
CMK	congenital multicystic kidney
CML	cell-mediated lympholysis; chronic myelogenous leukemia
CMM	cutaneous malignant melanoma
CMRNG	chromosomally resistant *Neisseria gonorrhoeae*
$CMRO_2$	cerebral metabolic rate for oxygen
CMS	circulation motion sensation
CMSUA	clean midstream urinalysis
CMT	chiropractic manipulative treatment
CMV	cytomegalovirus; cool mist vaporizer; controlled mechanical ventilation
CN	cranial nerve
CNA	chart not available
CNH	central neurogenic hyperpnea

CNP	continuous negative pressure ventilation
CNS	central nervous system; clinical nurse specialist
C/O	complains of; complaints; under care of
CO	cardiac output; carbon monoxide
Co	cobalt
CO$_2$	carbon dioxide
CoA	coarctation of the aorta
COAD	chronic obstructive airway disease; chronic obstructive arterial disease
COAG	chronic open angle glaucoma
COC	combination oral contraceptive
COD	cause of death
COEPS	cortically originating extrapyramidal symptoms
COG	cognitive function tests; Central Oncology Group
COH	carbohydrate
Coke	Coca-Cola
Collyr	eye wash
col/ml	colonies per milliliter
COLD	chronic obstructive lung disease
COLD A	cold agglutinin titer
COMP	complications; compound
conc	concentrated
CONG	congenital
COPD	chronic obstructive pulmonary disease
COPE	chronic obstructive pulmonary emphysema
cor	coronary
CORF	comprehensive outpatient rehabilitation facility
COT	content of thought
COTX	cast off to X-ray
COU	cardiac observation unit
CP	cerebral palsy; cleft palate; creatine phosphokinase; chest pain; chronic pain; chondromalacia patella
C & P	cystoscopy and pyelography
CPA	costophrenic angle; cardiopulmonary arrest; cerebellar pontile angle
CPAF	chlorpropamide-alcohol flush
CPAP	continuous positive airway pressure
CPB	cardiopulmonary bypass
CPBA	competitive protein-binding assay
CPC	clinicopathologic conference; cerebral palsy clinic
CPCR	cardiopulmonary-cerebral resuscitation
CPD	chorioretinopathy and pituitary dysfunction; cephalopelvic disproportion; chronic peritoneal dialysis
CPDD	calcium pyrophosphate deposition disease

CPE	chronic pulmonary emphysema; cardiogenic pulmonary edema
CPGN	chronic progressive glomerulonephritis
CPH	chronic persistent hepatitis
CPI	constitutionally psychopathia inferior
CPID	chronic pelvic inflammatory disease
CPK	creatinine phosphokinase
CPKD	childhood polycystic kidney disease
CPM	central pontine myelinolysis; continuous passive motion; continue present management; counts per minute
CPmax	peak serum concentration
CPmin	trough serum concentration
CPN	chronic pyelonephritis
CPP	cerebral perfusion pressure
CPPB	continuous positive pressure breathing
CPPV	continuous positive pressure ventilation
CPR	cardiopulmonary resuscitation
CPS	complex partial seizures
CPT	chest physiotherapy
CPTH	chronic posttraumatic headache
Cr	creatinine
CR	cardiorespiratory; controlled release; cardiac rehabilitation; colon resection; closed reduction; complete remission
CRA	central retinal artery
CRAO	central retinal artery occlusion
CRBBB	complete right bundle branch block
CRC	colorectal cancer
CrCl	creatinine clearance
CRD	chronic renal disease
CREST	calcinosis, Raynaud's phenomenon, esophageal dysmotility, sclerodactyly and telangiectasia
CRF	chronic renal failure; corticotropin-releasing factor
CRI	chronic renal insufficiency
CRIE	crossed radioimmuno-electrophoresis
crit	hematocrit
CRL	crown rump length
CRO	cathode ray oscilloscope
CRP	C-reactive protein
CRPF	choroquine-resistant plasmodium falciparum
CRST	calcification, Raynaud's phenomenon, scleroderma, and telangiectasia
CRT	copper reduction test; cathode ray tube; central reaction time; cadaver renal transplant
CrTr	crutch training

CRTX	cast removed take X-ray
CRUMBS	continuous remove, unobtrusive monitoring of biobehavioral systems
CRVO	central retinal vein occulsion
CS	coronary sclerosis; central supply; clinical stage; conjunctiva-sclera; consciousness; cat scratch
C & S	culture and sensitivity
C/S	cesarean section; culture and sensitivity
CSBF	coronary sinus blood flow
CSC	cornea, sclera, conjunctiva
CS & CC	culture, sensitivity, and colony count
CSD	cat scratch disease
CSE	cross section echocardiography
C sect	cesarean section
CSF	cerebrospinal fluid; colony-stimulating factor
C-Sh	chair shower
CSH	carotid sinus hypersensitivity
CSICU	cardiac surgery intensive care unit
CSH	continuous subcutaneous insulin infusion
CS IV	clinical stage 4
CSLU	chronic status leg ulcer
CSM	circulation, sensation, movement; cerebrospinal meningitis
CSOM	chronic serous otitis media
CSP	cellulose sodium phosphate
CSR	Cheyne-Stokes respiration; central supply room; corrective septorhinoplasty
CST	convulsive shock therapy; contraction stress test; cosyntropin stimulation test; certified surgical technologist
CSU	cardiac surveillance unit; cardiovascular surgery unit
CT	computed tomography; circulation time; coagulation time; clotting time; corneal thickness; cervical traction; Coomb's test; cardiothoracic; coated tablet
Cta	catamenia (menses)
CTA	clear to auscultation
CTB	ceased to breathe
CT & DB	cough, turn, and deep breathe
CTD	chest tube drainage; cumulative trauma disorder
CTF	Colorado tick fever
CTL	cytotoxic T lymphocytes
CT/MPR	computed tomography with multiplanar reconstructions
cTNM	clinical-diagnostic staging of cancer
CTP	comprehensive treatment plan
CTR	carpal tunnel release
CTS	carpal tunnel syndrome

CTSP	called to see patient
CTW	central terminal of Wilson
CTXN	contraception
CTZ	chemoreceptor trigger zone
Cu	copper
CU	cause unknown
CUC	chronic ulcerative colitis
CUD	cause undetermined
CUG	cystourethrogram
CUS	chronic undifferentiated schizophrenia
CUSA	Cavitron® ultrasonic aspirator
CV	cardiovascular; cell/closing volume
CVA	cerebrovascular accident; costovertebral angle
CVAT	costovertebral angle tenderness
CVC	central venous catheter
CVD	collagen vascular disease
CVI	cerebrovascular insufficiency; continuous venous infusion
CVID	common variable immune deficiency
CVO	central vein occlusion; conjugate diameter of pelvic inlet
CVP	central venous pressure
CVRI	coronary vascular resistance index
CVS	clean voided specimen; cardiovascular system; chorionic villus sampling
CVUG	cysto-void urethrogram
C/W	consistent with; crutch walking
CWE	cottonwool exudates
CWMS	color, warmth, movement sensation
CWP	coal worker's pneumoconiosis
CWS	cotton wool spots
Cx	cervix; culture; cancel
CsMT	cervical motion tenderness
CXR	chest X ray
CYSTO	cystoscopy; cystogram
CZI	crystalline zinc insulin
D	diarrhea; day; divorced; distal; dead; right; diopter
D1, D2	dorsal vertebra #1, #2
DA	direct admission
DAD	drug administration device
DAF	decay-accelerating factor
DAI	diffuse axonal injury
DAH	disordered action of the heart
DAL	drug analysis laboratory
DANA	drug-induced antinuclear antibodies

DAPT	draw-a-person test
DAT	direct agglutination test; diet as tolerated; dementia of the Alzheimer type
DAW	dispense as written
DAWN	Drug Abuse Warning Network
dB	decibel
DB	date of birth
DB & C	deep breathing and coughing
DBE	deep breathing exercise
DBIL	direct bilirubin
DBP	diastolic blood pressure
DBS	diminished breath sounds
D & C	dilation and curettage
DC, d/c	discontinue; discharge; decrease; diagonal conjugate; Doctor of Chiropractic
DCH	delayed cutaneous hypersensitivity
DCO	diffusing capacity of carbon monoxide
DCR	delayed cutaneous reaction
DCSA	double contrast shoulder arthrography
DCT	direct (antiglobulin) Coombs test; deep chest therapy
DCTM	delay computer tomographic myelography
DD	differential diagnosis; down drain; dependent drainage; dry dressing; Duchenne's dystrophy
D & D	diarrhea and dehydration
DDD	degenerative disc disease; dense deposit (renal) disease
DDS	dialysis disequilibrium syndrome; Doctor of Dental Surgery
DDST	Denver Development Screening Test
DDx	differential diagnosis
D & E	dilation and evacuation
DEC	decrease
decub	decubitus
DEF	decayed, extracted, or filled
degen	degenerative
del	delivery, delivered
DEP ST SEG	depressed ST segment
DER	disulfiram-ethanol reaction
DES	disequilibrium syndrome; diffuse esophageal spasm
DEV	duck embryo vaccine; deviation
DEVR	dominant exudative vitreoretinopathy
dex.	dexter (right)
DEXA	dual energy X-ray absorpiometry
DF	decayed and filled
DFD	defined formula diets

DFE	distal femoral epiphysis
DFMC	daily fetal movement count
DFR	diabetic floor routine
DFU	dead fetus in uterus
DGI	disseminated gonococcal infection
DGM	ductal glandular mastectomy
DH	developmental history; diaphragmatic hernia; delayed hypersensitivity
DHBV	duck hepatitis B virus
DHF	dengue hemorrhagic fever
DHHS	Department of Health and Human Services
DHL	diffuse histiocytic lymphoma
DHS	duration of hospital stay
DI	diabetes insipidus; detrusor instability
diag	diagnosis
Diath SW	diathermy short wave
DIC	Drug Information Center; disseminated intravascular coagulation
DIE	die in emergency department
DIFF	differential blood count
DIJOA	dominantly inherited juvenile optic atrophy
dil	dilute
DILD	diffuse infiltrative lung disease
DILE	drug-induced lupus erythematosus
dim	diminish
DIMOAD	diabetes insipidus, diabetes mellitus, optic atrophy, and deafness
DIP	distal interphalangeal; desquamative interstitial pneumonia; drip infusion pyelogram
dis	dislocation
DIS	Diagnostic Interview Schedule questionnaire
disch	discharge
DISH	diffuse idiopathic skeletal hyperostosis
dist	distilled
DIV	double inlet ventricle
DIVA	digital intravenous angiography
DJD	degenerative joint disease
DK	diabetic ketoacidosis; dark
DKA	diabetic ketoacidosis
dl	deciliter
DL	danger list; deciliter; direct laryngoscopy; diagnostic laparoscopy
DLE	discoid lupus erythematosus
DLIS	digitalis-like immunoreactive substance

DLMP	date of last menstrual period
DLNMP	date of last normal menstrual period
DM	diabetes mellitus; diastolic murmur; dermatomyositis
DMARD	disease-modifying antirheumatic drug
DMD	Duchenne's muscular dystrophy
DME	durable medical equipment
DMF	decayed, missing, or filled
DMKA	diabetes mellitus ketoacidosis
DMOOC	diabetes mellitus out of control
DMX	diathermy, massage, and exercise
DN	down
DNI	do not intubate
DNKA	did not keep appointment
DNP	do not publish
DNR	do not resuscitate/report
DNS	do not show; deviated nasal septum; dysplastic nevus syndrome
DO	right eye; Doctor of Osteopathy
DOA	dead on arrival; date of admission
DOA-DRA	dead on arrival, despite resuscitative attempts
DOB	date of birth; doctor's order book
DOC	drug of choice; died of other causes
DOE	dyspnea on exertion
DOI	date of injury
DOLV	double outlet left ventricle
DORV	double outlet right ventricle
DORx	date of treatment
DOT	Doppler ophthalmic test; died on table
DP	dorsalis pedis (pulse); diastolic pressure
DPC	discharge planning coordinator; delayed primary closure
DPDL	diffuse poorly differentiated lymphocytic lymphoma
DPM	disintegrations per minute; Doctor of Podiatric Medicine
DPN	diabetic peripheral neuropathy
DPT	diphtheria, pertussis, tetanus
DPV	delayed pressure urticaria
DR	delivery room; diabetic retinopathy
DREZ	dorsal root entry zone
DRG	diagnosis-related groups
DRSG	dressing
DS	discharge summary; Down's syndrome; double strength; disoriented; dextrose stick
DSA	digital subtraction angiography
DSAP	disseminated superficial actinic porokeratosis
DSD	dry sterile dressing; discharge summary dictated

dsg	dressing
DSI	deep shock insulin
DSIAR	double-stapled ileoanal reservoir
DSM	drink skim milk; *Diagnostic & Statistical Manual*
DSS	dengue shock syndrome
DST	dexamethasone suppression test; donor specific transfusion
DT	delirium tremens; discharge tomorrow
DTD #30	dispense 30 such doses
DTH	delayed-type hypersensitivity
DTR	deep tendon reflexes
DTs	delirium tremens
DTS	donor specific transfusion
DTT	diphtheria tetanus toxoid
DTV	due to void
DTX	detoxification
DU	duodenal ulcer; duroxide uptake; diabetic urine; diagnosis undetermined
DUB	dysfunctional uterine bleeding
DUE	drug use evaluation
DUI	driving under the influence
DUR	drug utilization review
DVD	dissociated vertical deviation
DVIU	direct vision internal urethrotomy
DVR	double valve replacement
DVT	deep vein thrombosis
DW	dextrose in water; distilled water; deionized water
DWDL	diffuse, well-differentiated lymphocytic lymphoma
Dx	diagnosis
Dz	disease; dozen
E	edema
4E	4 plus edema
E > A	say EEE, comes out as A,A,A, upon auscultation of lung, showing consolidation
EAA	electrothermal atomic absorption
EAC	external auditory canal
EAHF	eczema, allergy, hay fever
EAM	external auditory meatus
EAR	early asthmatic response
EAST	external rotation, abduction stress test
EAT	ectopic atrial tachycardia
EB	epidermolysis bullosa
EBL	estimated blood loss
EBV	Epstein-Barr virus

EC	enteric coated; eyes closed; extracellular
ECBD	exploration of common bile duct
ECC	emergency cardiac care docervical curettage
ECCE	extracapsular cataract extraction
ECD	endocardial cushion defect
ECEMG	evoked compound electromyography
ECF	extracellular fluid; extended care facility; eosinophilic chemotactic factor
ECG	electrocardiogram
ECHO	echocardiogram
ECL	extent of cerebral lesion; extracapillary lesions
ECM	erythema chronicum migrans
ECMO	extracorporeal membrane oxygenation
ECN	extended care nursery
ECR	emergency chemical restraint
ECRL	extensor carpi radialis longus
ECT	electroconvulsive therapy; enhanced computer tomography; emission computed tomography
ECU	extensor carpi ulnaris
ECW	extracellular water
ED	emergency department; epidural
ED50	median effective dose
EDC	estimated date of confinement; estimated date of conception; end diastolic counts; digitorum communis
EDD	expected date of delivery
EDF	extension, derotation, flexion
EDM	early diastolic murmur
EDS	Ehlers-Danlos syndrome
EDV	end-diastolic volume
EE	equine encephalitis; end to end
EEE	Eastern equine encephalomyelitis; edema, erythema, and exudate
EEG	electroencephalogram
EENT	eyes, ears, nose, throat
EF	extended-field (radiotherapy); endurance factor; ejection fraction
EFAD	essential fatty acid deficiency
EFE	endocardial fibroelastosis
EFM	external fetal monitoring
EFW	estimated fetal weight
EGA	estimated gestational age
EGBUS	external genitalia, Bartholin, urethral, Skene's glands
EGD	esophagogastroduodenoscopy
EGF	epidermal growth factor

EGTA	esophageal gastric tube airway
EH	essential hypertension; enlarged heart; extramedullary hematopoiesis
EHB	elevate head of bed
EHF	epidemic hemorrhagic fever
E & I	endocrine and infertility
EIA	exercise-induced asthma; enzyme immunoassay
EIAB	extracranial-intracranial arterial bypass
EIB	exercise-induced bronchospasm
EID	electronic infusion device
EIF	eukaryotic initiation factor
EIS	endoscopic injection scleropathy
EJ	external jugular; elbow jerk
EKC	epidemic keratoconjunctivitis
EKG	electrocardiogram
EKY	electrokymogram
E-L	external lids
ELF	elective low forceps
ELH	endolymphatic hydrops
ELISA	enzyme-linked immunosorbent assay
elix	elixir
ELOP	estimated length of program
ELP	electrophoresis
EM	electron microscope; ejection murmur; erythema multiforme
EMB	endomyocardial biopsy
EMC	encephalomyocarditis
EMD	electromechanical dissociation
EMF	erythrocyte maturation factor; evaporated milk formula; electromotive force
EMG	electromyography; essential monoclonal gammopathy
EMIC	emergency maternity and infant care
E-MICR	electron microscopy
EMIT	enzyme multiplied immunoassay technique
EMR	emergency mechanical restraint; empty, measure and record; educable mentally retarded
EMS	emergency medical services/ systems
EMT	emergency medical technician
EMV	eye, motor, verbal
EMW	electromagnetic waves
ENA	extractable nuclear antigen
ENDO	endotracheal
ENG	electronystagmography
ENL	erythema nodosum leprosum

ENP	extractable nucleoprotein
ENT	ears, nose, throat
EO	eyes open
EOA	examine, opinion, and advice; esophageal obturator airway
EOG	electro-oculogram; Ethrane®, oxygen, and gas
EOM	extraocular movement; extraocular muscles
EOMI	extraocular muscles intact
EORA	elderly onset rheumatoid arthritis
eos	eosinophil
EP	endogenous pyrogen; electrophysiologic
EPA	eicosapentaenoic acid
EPB	extensor pollicis brevis
EPIS	episiotomy
epith	epithelial
EPL	extensor pollicis longus
EPM	electronic pacemaker
EPO	recombinant human erythropoietin
EPP	erythropoietic protoporphyria
EPR	electrophrenic respiration; emergency physical restraint
EPS	electrophysiologic study; extrapyramidal syndrome/symptoms
EPT®	early pregnancy test
EPTS	existed prior to service
ER	emergency room; estrogen receptor; external rotation
ERA	evoked response audiometry; estrogen receptor assay
ERCP	endoscopic retrograde cholangiopancreatography
ERFC	erythrocyte rosette forming cells
ERG	electroretinogram
ERL	effective refractory length
ERP	estrogen receptor protein; endoscopic retrograde pancreatography
ERPF	effective renal plasma flow
ERPS	event-related potentials
ERT	estrogen replacement therapy
ERV	expiratory reserve volume
ESAP	evoked sensory (nerve) action potentiation
ESC	end systolic counts
ESM	ejection systolic murmur
ESP	end systolic pressure
ESR	erythrocyte sedimentation rate; electric skin resistance
ESRD	end-stage renal disease
ess	essential
EST	electroshock therapy
ESWL	extracorporeal shockwave lithotripsy

ET	endotracheal; esotropia; eustachian tube; ejection time; exercise treadmill
et	and
et al	and others
ETF	eustachian tubal function
ETO	estimated time of ovulation
ETS	environmental tobacco smoke
ETT	endotracheal tube; exercise tolerance test
EU	excretory urography
EUA	examine under anesthesia
EUS	endoscopic ultrasonography
EVAC	evacuation
eval	evaluate
EWB	estrogen withdrawal bleeding
EWSCLs	extended-wear soft contact lenses
exam	examination
EXP	exploration; experienced
exp lap	exploratory laparotomy
ext	extract; external
ext rot	external rotation
EX U	excretory urogram
F	Fahrenheit; female; flow; facial; firm; French
F1	offspring from first generation
F2	offspring from second generation
FA	folic acid; femoral artery
FAAP	family assessment adjustment pass
FAC	fractional area concentration
FACH	forceps to after-coming head
FACS	Fellow of the American College of Surgeons
FAD	Family Assessment Device
FAI	functional assessment inventory
FALL	fallopian
FAM	family
FANA	fluorescent antinuclear antibody
FAP	fibrillating action potential; familial amyloid polyneuropathy; familial adenomatous polyposis
FAS	fetal alcohol syndrome
FAST	functional assessment staging (of Alzheimer's disease); fluoro-allegro sorbent test; fetal acoustical stimulation test
FAT	fluorescent antibody test
FB	fasting blood sugar; foreign body; finger breadth
FBG	fasting blood glucose

FBM	fetal breathing movements
FBN	fibronectin
FBP	fetal biophysical profile
FBS	fasting blood sugar; fetal bovine serum
FBU	fingers below umbilicus
FBW	fasting blood work
FC	Foley catheter; finger counting; fever, chills
F + C	flare and cells
F & C	foam and condom
F cath	Foley catheter
FCC	follicular center cells; familial colonic cancer; fracture compound comminuted
FCDB	fibrocystic disease of the breast
FCH	familial combined hyperlipidemia
FCMC	family-centered maternity care
FCMD	Fukuyama's congenital muscular dystrophy
FCMN	family-centered maternity nursing
FCP	flow cytometric platelet crossmatching
FCR	flexor carpi radialis
FCRB	flexor carpi radialis brevis
FCSNVD	fever, chills, sweating, nausea, vomiting, diarrhea
FCU	flexor carpi ulnaris
FD	focal distance; familial dysautonomia
F & D	fixed and dilated
FDA	fronto-dextra anterior
FDIU	fetal death in utero
FDP	fibrin-degradation products; flexor digitorum profundus
FDS	flexor digitorum superficials; for duration of stay
Fe	iron; female
FEC	forced expiratory capacity
FEF	forced expiratory flow
FEL	familial erythrophagocytic lymphohistiocytosis
FEM	femoral
Fem-pop	femoral popliteal (bypass)
FEN	fluid, electrolytes, nutrition
FENa	fractional extraction of sodium
FEP	free erythrocyte protoporphyrin
FEV	forced expiratory volume
FF	filtration fraction; fundus firm; flat feet; fat free; force fluids
FFA	free fatty acid
F factor	fertility/sex factor
FFP	fresh frozen plasma
FFT	fast-Fourier transforms

FGF	fibroblast growth factor
FH	family history; fetal heart; fundal height
FHF	fulminant hepatic failure
FHH	familial hypocalciuric hypercalcemia
FHI	Fuchs heterochromic iridocyclitis
FHR	fetal heart rate
FHS	fetal heart sounds; fetal hydantoin syndrome
FHT	fetal heart tone
FiCO$_2$	fraction of inspired carbon dioxide
FIM	functional independent measure
FiO$_2$	fraction of inspired oxygen
FL	fluid
FLK	funny looking kid
FLS	flashing lights and/or scotoma
FM	fetal movements; face mask
F & M	firm and midline (uterus)
FMC	fetal movement count
FMD	foot and mouth disease
FME	full mouth extraction
FMF	forced midexpiratory flow; familial Mediterranean fever
FMG	foreign medical graduate; fine mesh gauze
FMH	family medical history; fibromuscular hyperplasia
FMP	fasting metabolic panel
FMX	full mouth X ray
FN	false negative; finger-to-nose
FNAB	fine-needle aspiration biopsy
FNAC	fine-needle aspiration cytology
FNCJ	find needle catheter jejunostomy
FNH	focal nodular hyperplasia; febrile nonhemolytic reaction
FNR	false negative rate
FNS	functional neuromuscular stimulation
FOB	foot of bed; fiberoptic bronchoscope; father of baby
FOBT	fecal occult blood test
FOC	father of child
FOD	free of disease
FOI	flight of ideas
FOOB	fell out of bed
FP	family planning; family practice; frozen plasma; flat plate; false positive
FPAL	full-term, premature, abortion, living
FPB	flexor pollicis brevis
FPD	feto-pelvic disproportion; fixed partial denture
FPG	fasting plasma glucose
FPIA	fluorescence-polarization immunoassay

FPL	flexor pollicis longus
FPNA	first-pass nuclear angiocardiography
FR	flow rate
F & R	flow and rhythm (pulse)
FRC	functional residual capacity
FRJM	full range of joint motion
FROM	full range of movement
FS	frozen section; flexible sigmoidoscopy
FSB	fetal scalp blood
FSBM	full-strength breast milk
FSE	fetal scalp electrode
FSG	focal and segmental
FSGS	focal and segmental glomerulosclerosis
FSH	follicle stimulating hormone; facioscapulohumeral
FSHMD	facioscapulohumeral muscular dystrophy
FSHRF	follicle stimulating hormone releasing factor
FSP	fibrin split products
FT	full term
FTA	fluorescent treponemal/titer antibody
FTD	failure to descend
FTI	free thyroxine index
FTLFC	full-term living female child
FTLMC	full-term living male child
FTN	finger-to-nose; full-term nursery
FTND	full-term normal delivery
FTP	failure to progress
FTR	for the record
FTSG	full-thickness skin graft
FTT	failure to thrive
F & U	flanks and upper quadrants
F/U	followup; fundus at umbilicus
FUB	functional uterine bleeding
FUN	followup note
FUO	fever of undetermined origin
FVC	forced vital capacity
FVH	focal vascular headache
FVL	flow volume loop
FWB	full weight bearing
FWS	fetal warfarin syndrome
FWW	front wheel walker
Fx	fracture; fractional urine
Fx-dis	fracture-dislocation
FXN	function
FXR	fracture

G	gauge
G1–4	grade 1–4
GA	gastric analysis; general appearance; general anesthesia; gestational age
GABA	gamma-aminobutyric acid
GABHS	group A beta hemolytic streptococci
GAD	generalized anxiety disorder
GAF	Global Assessment of Functioning (Scale)
GAS	general adaptation syndrome
GAT	group adjustment therapy
GB	gallbladder
GBM	glomerular basement membrane
GBP	gastric bypass
GBS	gallbladder series; Guillain-Barré syndrome; group B streptococci
GC	gonococci (gonorrhea); geriatric chair
G − C	gram-negative cocci
G + C	gram-positive cocci
GCA	giant cell arteritis
GCDFP	gross cystic disease fluid protein
GCIIS	glucose control insulin infusion system
GCS	Glasgow coma scale
GCT	giant cell tumor
GD	Graves disease
G & D	growth and development
GDF	gel diffusion precipitin
GDM	gestational diabetes mellitus
GE	gastroenteritis
GEP	gastroenteropancreatic
GER	gastroesophageal reflux
GERD	gastroesophageal reflux disease
GETA	general endotracheal anesthesia
GF	grandfather; gluten-free; gastric fistula
GFR	glomerular filtration rate
GG	gamma globulin
GGE	generalized glandular enlargement
GGT	gamma glutamyl transpeptidase
GGTP	gamma glutamyl transpeptidase
GH	growth hormone; glycosylated hemoglobin
GHb	glycosylated hemoglobin
GHD	growth hormone deficiency
GHQ	general health questionnaire
GI	gastrointestinal; granuloma inguinale
GIB	gastric ileal bypass

GIC	general immunocompetence
GIFT	gamete intrafallopian treatment
GIP	giant cell interstitial pneumonia; gastric inhibitory peptide
GIS	gastrointestinal series
GIT	gastrointestinal tract
GJ	gastrojejunostomy
GL	greatest length
GLA	gingivolinguoaxial
GLNH	giant lymph node hyperplasia
GM	gram; grandmother
GMC	general medicine clinic
GMTs	geometric mean antibody titers
GN	glomerulonephritis; gram-negative; graduate nurse
GnRH	gonadotropin-releasing hormone
GOT	glucose oxidase test
GP	general practitioner; gutta percha
G/P	gravida/para
GPC	gram-positive cocci; giant papillary conjunctivitis
G6PD	glucose-6-phosphate dehydrogenase
GPMAL	gravida, para, multiple births, abortions, and live births
GPN	graduate practical nurse
gr	grain
G− R	gram-negative rods
G+ R	gram-positive rods
grav	gravid (pregnant)
GRD	gastroesophageal reflux disease
GRN	granules
GSC	Glasgow coma scale
GSD	glycogen storage disease •
GSD-1	glycogen storage disease, type 1
GSE	grip strong and equal; gluten sensitive enteropathy
GSI	genuine stress incontinence
GSP	general survey panel
GSPN	greater superficial petrosal neurectomy
GSR	galvanic skin resistance
GSW	gunshot wound
GT	gastrotomy tube; gait training
GTN	gestational trophoblastic neoplasms
GTT	glucose tolerance test; drop
GU	genitourinary
GUS	genitourinary sphincter; genitourinary system
GVF	good visual fields
GVHD	graft-versus-host disease
G & W	glycerin and water

GW	glucose in water
GWA	gunshot wound of the abdomen
GWT	gunshot wound of the throat
GXT	graded exercise testing
GYN	gynecology
H	hypodermic; hydrogen; hour; husband
H2	histamine
HA	headache; hyperalimentation; hypothalamic amenorrhea; hearing aid; hemolytic anemia; hospital admission; hepatitis, type A; hemagglutination assay
HAA	hepatitis-associated antigen
HAE	hereditary angioedema; hepatic artery embolization; hearing aid evaluation
HAI	hepatic arterial infusion
HAL	hyperalimentation
HAN	heroin associated nephropathy
HANE	heredity angioneurotic edema
HAPS	hepatic arterial perfusion scintigraphy
HAQ	Headache/Health Assessment Questionnaire
HAS	hyperalimentation solution
HASHD	hypertensive arteriosclerotic heart disease
HAT	head, arms, and trunk
HAV	hepatitis A virus; hallux abducto valgus
HB	hemoglobin; heart block; hepatitis, type B; hold breakfast
HBBW	hold breakfast blood work
HBD	has been drinking
HBGM	home blood glucose monitoring
HBI	hemibody irradiation
HBIG	hepatitis B immune globulin
HbAIc	glycosylated hemoglobin
HBF	hepatic blood flow
HBO	hyperbaric oxygen
HBP	high blood pressure
HBS	Health Behavior Scale
HBsAg	hepatitis B surface antigen
HBV	hepatitis B virus; hepatitis B vaccine; honeybee venom
HC	home care; head circumference; heel cord; house call; Hickman catheter
HCA	health care aide
HCC	hepatocellular carcinoma
HCFA	Health Care Financing Administration
HCG	human chorionic gonadotropin
HCL	hair cell leukemia

HCLs	hard contact lenses
HCM	health care maintenance; hypertropic cardiomyopathy
HCP	hereditary coprophemia
HCT	hematocrit; histamine challenge test
HCV	hepatitis C virus
HCVD	hypertensive cardiovascular disease
HD	Hodgkin's disease; Huntington's disease; hearing distance; hemodialysis; heloma mole; hip disarticulation; high dose
HDC	high-dose chemotherapy
HDCV	human diploid cell vaccine
HDL	high-density lipoprotein
HDLW	hearing distance for watch in left ear
HDRW	hearing distance for watch in right ear
HDN	hemolytic disease of the newborn
HDPAA	heparin-dependent, platelet-associated antibody
HDRS	Hamilton Depression Rate Scale
HDV	hepatitis D virus
H & E	hemorrhage and exudate; hematoxylin and eosin
HEENT	head, eyes, ears, nose, and throat
HEK	human embryonic kidney
HEL	human embryonic lung
hemi	hemiplegia
HEMPAS	hereditary erythrocytic multinuclearity with positive acidified serum test
HEP	histamine equivalent prick; hepatic
HES	hypereosinophilic syndrome
HEV	hepatitis E virus
HF	heart failure
HFD	high forceps delivery
HFHL	high frequency hearing loss
Hbg	hemoglobin
HGH	human growth hormone
HH	hiatal hernia; hypogonadotropic hypogonadism; home health; hard of hearing
H & H	hematocrit and hemoglobin
HHC	home health care
HHD	hypertensive heart disease
HHFM	high-humidity face mask
HHN	hand-held nebulizer
HHNK	hyperglycemic hyperosmolar nonketotic (coma)
HHT	hereditary hemorrhagic telangiectasis
HHV-6	human herpes virus 6
HI	hemagglutination inhibition; head injury

HIA	hemagglutination inhibition antibody
HIB	haemophilus influenzae type B (vaccine)
HID	headache, insomnia, depression
HIE	hypoxic-ischemic encephalopathy
HIF	higher integrative functions
HIL	hypoxic-ischemic lesion
HIR	head injury routine
HIS	Health Intention Scale
Histo	histoplasmin skin test
HIT	heparin-induced thrombocytopenia; histamine inhalation test
HIV	human immunodeficiency virus
HIVD	herniated intervertebral disc
HJR	hepato-jugular reflex
H–K	hand to knee
HKAFO	hip-knee-ankle-foot orthosis
HKO	hip-knee orthosis
HL	heparin lock; harelip; hairline; hearing level; Hickman line
HLA	human lymphocyte/leukocyte antigen
HLD	herniated lumbar disc
HLHS	hypoplastic left heart syndrome
HLV	hypoplastic left ventricle
HM	hand motion
HMD	hyaline membrane disease
HMG	human menopausal gonadotropin
HMI	healed myocardial infarction
HMO	health maintenance organization
HMP	hot moist packs
HMR	histiocytic medullary reticulosis
HMX	heat massage exercise
HN	high nitrogen
H & N	head and neck
HNP	herniated nucleus pulposus
hnRNA	heterogeneous nuclear ribonucleic acid
HNV	has not voided
HO	house officer
H/O	history of
H2O	water
HOB	head of bed
HOB UPSOB	head of bed up for shortness of breath
HOC	Health Officer Certificate
HOCM	hypertrophic obstructive cardiomyopathy
HOG	halothane, oxygen, and gas (nitrous oxide)
HOH	hard of hearing

HOPI	history of present illness
HP	hemiplegia; hemipelvectomy; hot packs
H & P	history and physical
HPA	human papilloma virus; hypothalamic-pituitary-adrenal (axis)
HPF	high-power field
HPFH	hereditary persistence of fetal hemoglobin
HPI	history of present illness
HPL	human placenta lactogen
HPLC	high-pressure (performance) liquid chromatography
HPG	human pituitary gonadotropin
HPL	hyperpexia; human placental lactogen
HPM	hemiplegic migraine
HPN	home parenteral nutrition
HPO	hypertrophic pulmonary osteoarthropathy; hydrophilic ointment
HPT	hyperparathyroidism
HPZ	high-pressure zone
HR	heart rate; hour; hallux rigidus; hospital record; Harrington rod
HRA	histamine releasing activity
HRLA	human retrovirus-like agent
HRS	hepatorenal syndrome
HRT	hormone replacement therapy
HS	bedtime; hereditary spherocytosis; heel spur; heel stick; herpes simplex; Hartmann's (lactated Ringer's) solution
H > S	heel to shin
HSA	human serum albumin; hypersomnia-sleep apnea; health systems agency
HSBG	heel stick blood gas
HSE	herpes simplex encephalitis
HSG	hysterosalpingogram
HSM	hepato-splenomegaly; holosystolic murmur
HSP	Henoch-Schönlein purpura
HSR	heated serum reagin
HSSE	high soap suds enema
HSV	herpes simplex virus
HT	hypertension; hypermetropia; height; heart; hammertoe; hyperopia; Hubbard tank
ht aer	heated aerosol
HTAT	human tetanus antitoxin
HTC	hypertensive crisis
HTF	house tube feeding
HTL	human thymic leukemia

HTLC	human T-cell leukemia virus
HTLV III	human T-cell lymphotrophic virus type III
HTN	hypertension
HTP	House-Tree-Person test
HTR	acute hemolytic transfusion reaction
HTVD	hypertensive vascular disease
HUIFM	human leukocyte interferon meloy
HUR	hemolytic uremic syndrome
HUS	hemolytic uremic syndrome
HV	hallux valgus; has voided
H & V	hemigastrectomy and vagotomy
HW	heparin well; housewife
hwb	hot water bottle
Hx	history; hospitalization
Hz	Hertz
HZ	herpes zoster
HZO	herpes zoster ophthalmicus
I	independent; impression; incisal; one
IA	intra-amniotic
IAA	interrupted aortic arch
IABC	intra-aortic balloon counterpulsation
IABP	intra-aortic balloon pump
IAC	internal auditory canal
IAC-CPR	interposed abdominal compressions-cardiopulmonary resuscitation
IACP	intra-aortic counterpulsation
IADH	inappropriate antidiuretic hormone
IA DSA	intra-arterial subtraction arteriography
IAHA	immune adherence hemagglutination
IAI	intra-abdominal infection
IAM	internal auditory meatus
IAN	intern admission note
IAP	intermittent acute porphyria
IASD	interatrial septal defect
IAT	indirect antiglobulin test
IB	isolation bed
IBC	iron binding capacity
IBD	inflammatory bowel disease
IBI	intermittent bladder irrigation
ibid	at the same place
IBNR	incurred but not reported
IBS	irritable bowel syndrome
IBW	ideal body weight

IC	irritable colon; intercostal; intracranial; individual counseling; inspiratory capacity
ICA	internal carotid artery; islet cell antibodies
ICBT	intercostobronchial trunk
ICCE	intracapsular cataract extraction
ICCU	intermediate coronary care unit
ICD	instantaneous cardiac death
ICD 9 CM	International Classification of Diseases, 9th Revision, Clinical Modification
ICF	intracellular fluid; intermediate care facility
ICG	indocyanine green
ICH	intracranial hemorrhage
ICM	intracostal margin
ICN	intensive care nursery
ICP	intracranial pressure
ICPP	intubated continuous positive pressure
ICS	intracostal space
ICSH	interstitial cell-stimulating hormone
ICT	intensive conventional therapy; inflammation of connective tissue
ICU	intensive care unit
ICVH	ischemic cerebrovascular headache
ICW	intercellular water
ID	intradermal; initial dose, infectious disease; identification; immunodiffusion; identify
I & D	incision and drainage
IDE	Investigational Device Exemption
IDDM	insulin-dependent diabetes mellitus
IDDS	implantable drug delivery system
IDFC	immature dead female child
IDM	infant of a diabetic mother
IDMC	immature dead male child
IDS	Infectious Disease Service
IDV	intermittent demand ventilation
IEC	inpatient exercise center
IEF	iso-electric focusing
IEM	immune electron microscopy
IEP	individualized education program; immunoelectrophoresis
IF	intrinsic factor; immunofluorescence; involved field
IFA	indirect fluorescent antibody test
IFE	immunofixation electrophoresis
IgA	immunoglobulin A
IgD	immunoglobulin D
IgE	immunoglobulin E

IGF	insulin-like growth factor
IgG	immunoglobulin G; immune gammaglobulin
IGIV	immune globulin intravenous
IgM	immunoglobulin M
IGR	intrauterine growth retardation
IGT	impaired glucose tolerance
IH	infectious hepatitis; inguinal hernia; indirect hemagglutination
IHA	immune hemagglutination assay
IHC	immobilization hypercalcemia
IHD	ischemic heart disease; intrahepatic duct
IHH	idiopathic hypogonadotropic hypogonadism
IHS	Idiopathic Headache Score
IHs	iris hamartomas
IHSS	idiopathic hypertrophic subaortic stenosis
IHT	insulin hypoglycemia test
IICP	increased intracranial pressure
IICU	infant intensive care unit
IIT	intensive insulin therapy
IJ	internal jugular; ileojejunal
IL	independent living
ILD	ischemic leg disease
ILFC	immature living female child
ILM	internal limiting membrane
ILMC	immature living male child
ILMI	inferolateral myocardial infarct
IM	intramuscular; infectious mononucleosis; intermetatarsal; internal medicine
IMA	inferior mesenteric artery; internal mammary artery
IMAG	internal mammary artery graft
IMB	intermenstrual bleeding
IMF	intermaxillary fixation
IMG	internal medicine group (practice)
IMH	indirect microhemagglutination (test)
IMI	inferior myocardial infarction; imipramine
IMIG	intramuscular immunoglobulin
IMN	internal mammary (lymph) node
IMP	impression; impacted
IMV	intermittent mandatory ventilation
IN	interstitial nephritis
INB	intermittent nebulized beta-agonists
INC	incomplete; incontinent; inside-the-needle catheter
IND	investigational new drug
INDM	infant of nondiabetic mother

INF	inferior; infusion; infant; infected
ING	inguinal
inj	injection; injury
INS	insurance
INST	instrumental delivery
int	internal
int-rot	internal rotation
inver	inversion
I & O	intake and output
IO	intraocular pressure; inferior oblique; initial opening
IOC	intern on call; intraoperative cholangiogram
IOD	interorbital distance
IOF	intraocular fluid
IOFB	intraocular foreign body
IOH	idiopathic orthostatic hypotension
IOL	intraocular lens
ION	ischemic optic neuropathy
IOP	intraocular pressure
IORT	intraoperative radiation therapy
IOS	intraoperative sonography
IOV	initial office visit
IP	intraperitoneal
IPA	invasive pulmonary aspergillosis; individual practice association
IPCD	infantile polycystic disease
IPD	immediate pigment darkening; intermittent peritoneal dialysis
IPFD	intrapartum fetal distress
IPG	impedance plethysmography; individually polymerized grass
IPJ	interphalangeal joint
IPK	intractable plantar keratosis
IPMI	inferoposterior myocardial infarct
IPN	infantile periarteritis nodosa; intern's progress note
IPP	inflatable penile prosthesis
IPPA	inspection, palpation, percussion, and auscultation
IPPB	intermittent positive pressure breathing
IPPV	intermittent positive pressure ventilation
IPV	inactivated polio vaccine
IQ	intelligence quotient
IR	internal rotation; infrared
IRBBB	incomplete right bundle branch block
IRMA	intraretinal microvascular abnormalities
IRR	intrarenal reflux
IRV	inspiratory reserve volume

IS	intercostal space; incentive spirometer; induced sputum
ISB	incentive spirometry breathing
ISCs	irreversible sickle cells
ISG	immune serum globulin
ISH	isolated systolic hypertension
ISMA	infantile spinal muscular atrophy
ISS	Injury Severity Score
IST	insulin sensitivity test; insulin shock therapy
ISW	interstitial water
IT	intrathecal; inhalation therapy; intertuberous
ITCP	idiopathic thrombocytopenia purpura
ITE	insufficient therapeutic effect
ITP	idiopathic thrombocytopenic purpura; interim treatment plan
ITVAD	indwelling transcutaneous vascular access device
IU	international unit
IUCD	intrauterine contraceptive device
IUD	intrauterine device; intrauterine death
IUFD	intrauterine fetal death
IUGR	intrauterine growth retardation
IUP	intrauterine pregnancy
IUPD	intrauterine pregnancy delivered
IV	intravenous
IVC	intravenous cholangiogram; inferior vena cava; intraventricular catheter
IVD	intervertebral disk; intravenous drip
IVDA	intravenous drug abuse
IVF	*in vitro* fertilization; intravenous fluid
IVFE	intravenous fat emulsion
IVF-ET	*in vitro* fertilization, embryo transfer
IVGTT	intravenous glucose tolerance test
IVH	intravenous hyperalimentation; intraventricular hemorrhage
IVIG	intravenous immunoglobulin
IVLBW	infant of very low birth weight
IVP	intravenous pyelogram; intravenous push
IVPB	intravenous piggyback
IVR	idioventricular rhythm
IVS	intraventricular septum
IVSD	intraventricular septal defect
IVSP	intravenous syringe pump
IVT	intravenous transfusion
IVU	intravenous urography
IWL	insensible water loss
IWMI	inferior wall myocardial infarct

J	joint
JAMG	juvenile autoimmune myasthenia gravis
JC	junior clinicians
JDMS	juvenile dermatomyositis
JE	Japanese encephalitis
JF	joint fluid
JI	jejunoileal
JIB	jejunoileal bypass
JJ	jaw jerk
JMS	junior medical student
JODM	juvenile onset diabetes mellitus
JP	Jobst pump; Jackson-Pratt (drain)
JRA	juvenile rheumatoid arthritis
JSPN	junior student progress note
jt	joint
juv	juvenile
JVD	jugular venous distention
JVP	jugular venous pulse; jugular venous pressure
JVPT	jugular venous pulse tracing
KA	ketoacidosis
KAFO	knee-ankle-foot orthosis
KAO	knee-ankle orthosis
KAS	Katz Adjustment Scale
KBM	a below-knee prosthesis
K Cal	kilocalorie
KCS	keratoconjunctivitis sicca
KD	Kawasaki's disease; knee disarticulation; Keto Diastex®
KDA	known drug allergies
KDDM	kidney disease of diabetes mellitus
KF	kidney function
KFD	Kyasanur Forrest disease
kg	kilogram
K24H	potassium, urine 24 hour
KI	karyopyknotic index
KID	keratitis, ichthyosis, deafness
KILO	kilogram
KISS	saturated solution of potassium iodide
KJ	knee jerk
KK	knee kick
KLH	keyhole limpet hemocyanin (antibody)
KNO	keep needle open
KO	keep open
KP	keratoprecipitate; hot pack

KS	ketosteroids; Kaposi's sarcoma
17-KS	17-ketosteroids
KTU	kidney transplant unit
KUB	kidney, ureter, bladder
KVO	keep vein open
KW	Kimmelstiel-Wilson (disease); Keith-Wagener (ophthalmoscopic finding)
K-wire	Kirschner wire
L	left; liter; lumbar; lingual; lymphocyte; fifty
L2	second lumbar vertebra
LA	left atrium; local anesthesia; long acting; left arm; Latin American
L + A	light and accommodation
lab	laboratory
LAC	laceration; long arm cast
LAD	left anterior descending; left axis deviation
LAD-MIN	left axis deviation minimal
LAE	left atrial enlargement
LAF	lymphocyte-activating factor; laminar air flow; Latin American female
LAG	lymphangiogram
LAH	left atrial hypertrophy
LAL	left axillary line; limulus amebocyte lysate
LAM	Latin American male
LAN	lymphadenopathy
LAO	left anterior oblique
LAP	laparotomy; laparoscopy; left arterial pressure; leukocyte; leucine amino peptidase
LAPMS	long arm posterior molded splint
LAR	late asthmatic response
LAT	left anterior thigh; lateral
LATS	long-acting thyroid stimulator
LAV	lymphadenopathy associated virus
LAVH	laparoscopic-assisted vaginal hysteroscopy
LB	low back; left buttock; large bowel; left breast; pound
LBB	left breast biopsy
LBBB	left bundle branch block
LBCD	left border of cardiac dullness
LBD	left border dullness
LBF	*Lactobacillus bulgaricus* factor
LBM	lean body mass; loose bowel movement
LBO	large bowel obstruction
LBP	low back pain; low blood pressure

LBT	lupus band test
LBV	left brachial vein
LBW	low birth weight; lean body weight
LC	living children; low calorie
LCA	left coronary artery; Leber's congenital amaurosis
LCCA	leukocytoclastic angitis; left common carotid artery
LCCS	low cervical Cesarean section
LCD	liquor carbonis detergens (coal tar solution); localized collagen dystrophy
LCGU	local cerebral glucose utilization
LCH	local city hospital
LCLC	large cell lung carcinoma
LCM	left costal margin; lymphocytic choriomeningitis
LCR	late cutaneous reaction
LCS	low constant suction; low continuous suction
LCT	long chain triglyceride; low cervical transverse; lymphocytotoxicity
LCV	low cervical vertical
LCX	left circumflex coronary artery
LD	lethal dose; loading dose; liver disease; labor and delivery
LDA	left dorsoanterior position
LDB	Legionnaires' disease bacterium
LDDS	local dentist
LDH	lactic dehydrogenase
LDL	low-density lipoprotein
LDP	left dorsoposterior position
LDV	laser Doppler velocimetry
LE	lupus erythematosus; lower extremities; left eye
LED	lupus erythematosus disseminatus
LEEP	loop electrocautery excision procedure
LEHPZ	lower esophageal high-pressure zone
L-ERX	leukoerythroblastic reaction
LES	lower esophageal sphincter; local excitatory state
LESP	lower esophageal sphincter pressure
LET	linear energy transfer
LF	low forceps; left foot
LFA	left fronto-anterior; low friction arthroplasty
LFC	living female child
LFD	low fat diet; low forceps delivery; lactose free diet
LFP	left frontoposterior
LFS	liver function studies
LFT	liver function test; left frontotransverse; latex flocculation test
lg	large; left gluteus

LG	lymph glands
LGA	large for gestational age
LGL	Lown-Ganong-Levine (syndrome)
LGV	lymphogranuloma venereum
LH	luteinizing hormone; left hyperphoria; left hand
LHF	left heart failure
LHL	left hemisphere lesions
LHP	left hemiparesis
LHR	leukocyte histamine release
LHRH	luteinizing hormone-releasing hormone
LHT	left hypertropia
LIB	left in bottle
LIC	left iliac crest; left internal carotid
LICA	left internal carotid artery
LIF	left iliac fossa; liver inhibitory factor
lig	ligament
LIH	left inguinal hernia
LIMA	left internal mammary artery (graft)
LIP	lymphocytic interstitial pneumonia
LIQ	lower inner quadrant; liquid
LIS	low intermittent suction
LISREL	(computer program that performs structural equation modeling)
LISS	low ionic strength saline
LK	left kidney
LKKS	liver, kidneys, spleen
LKS	liver, kidneys, spleen
LL	large lymphocyte; lumbar length; lymphoblastic lymphoma; left leg; lower lip
LLB	long leg brace
LLC	long leg case
LLE	left lower extremity
LLETZ	large loop excision of transformation zone (of cervix)
LL-GXT	low-level graded exercise test
LLL	left lower lobe; left lower lid
LLO	Legionella-like organism
LLQ	left lower quadrant
LLS	lazy leukocyte syndrome
LLSB	left lower sternal border
LLT	left lateral thigh
LMA	left mento-anterior; liver membrane autoantibody
LMB	Laurence-Moon-Biedl syndrome
LMC	living male child
LMCA	left main coronary artery

LMD	low molecular weight dextran
LMEE	left middle ear exploration
L/min	liters per minute
LML	left medial lateral/lobe
LMM	lentigo maligna melanoma
LMP	last menstrual period; left mentoposterior
LMT	left mentotransverse
LMWD	low molecular weight dextran
LN	lymph nodes
LND	lymph node dissection
LNMP	last normal menstrual period
LO	lateral oblique
LOA	left occiput anterior; leave of absence
LOC	loss of consciousness; level of consciousness; level of care; laxative of choice; local
LOD	line of duty
LOM	limitation of motion; left otitis media
LoNa	low sodium
LOP	left occiput posterior; leave on pass
LOQ	lower outer quadrant
LORS	Level of Rehabilitation Scale
LOS	length of stay
LOT	left occiput transverse
LOV	loss of vision
loz	lozenge
LP	lumbar puncture; light perception
LPC	laser photocoagulation
LPD	luteal phase defect
LPF	low power field
LPH	left posterior hemiblock
LPN	licensed practical nurse
LPO	left posterior oblique; light perception only
LPP	lipoprotein lipase
LR	light reflex; labor room; left-right
L > R	left to right
LRD	living renal donor
LRND	left radical neck dissection
LRQ	lower right quadrant
L-S	lumbo-sacral
L/S	lecithin-sphingomyelin ratio
LSA	left sacrum anterior; lipid-bound sialic acid; lymphosarcoma
LSB	left sternal border
LS BPS	laparoscopic bilateral partial salpingectomy

LSD	low-salt diet
LSE	local side effects
LSF	low saturated fat
LSKM	liver-spleen-kidney-megalgia
LSM	late systolic murmur
LSO	left salpingo-oophorectomy
LSP	left sacrum posterior; liver-specific (membrane) lipoprotein
L/S ratio	lecithin/sphingomyelin ratio
LSS	liver-spleen scan
LST	left sacrum transverse
LSTL	laparoscopic tubal ligation
LT	light; left; left thigh; lumbar traction; Levin tube; leukotrienes
LTB	laparoscopic tubal banding; laryngotracheobronchitis
LTC	long-term care; left to count; lean tissue compartment
LTCF	long-term care facility
LTCS	low transverse cesarean section
LTGA	left transposition of great artery
LTL	laparoscopic tubal ligation
LTT	lymphocyte transformation test
L & U	lower and upper
LUE	left upper extremity
LUL	left upper lobe
LUQ	left upper quadrant
LUSB	left upper sternal border
LV	left ventricle
LVA	left ventricular aneurysm
LVAD	left ventricular assist device
LVE	left ventricular enlargement
LVEDP	left ventricular end diastolic pressure
LVEDV	left ventricular end diastolic volume
LVEF	left ventricular ejection fraction
LVF	left ventricular failure
LVFP	left ventricular filling pressure
LVH	left ventricular hypertrophy
LVL	left vastus lateralis
LVMM	left ventricular muscle mass
LVN	licensed vocational nurse
LVP	left ventricular pressure; large volume parenteral
LVPW	left ventricular posterior wall
LVSWI	left ventricular stroke work index
LVV	left ventricular volume
L & W	living and well
LWCT	Lee-White clotting time

LYG	lymphomatoid granulomatosis
lymphs	lymphocytes
lytes	electrolytes
M	murmur; meter; minimum; medial, myopia; monocytes; male; molar; married; thousand
M1	first mitral sound
M2	square meters (body surface)
MA	mental age; medical assistance; milliamps; menstrual age; Miller-Abbott (tube)
M/A	mood and/or affect
MAA	macroaggregates of albumin
MAB	monoclonal antibody
MABP	mean arterial blood pressure
MAC	maximum allowable concentration; midarm circumference; minimum alveolar concentration; mycobacterium avium complex
MAE	moves all extremities
MAEEW	moves all extremities equally well
MAFAs	movement-associated fetal (heart rate) accelerations
MAHA	microangiopathic hemolytic anemia
MAI	mycobacterium avium-intracellular
MAL	midaxillary line
MALT	mucosa-associated lymphoid tissue
MAMC	mid-arm muscle circumference
mammo	mammography
MAOI	monoamine oxidase inhibitor
mand	mandibular
MAP	mean arterial pressure
MAS	meconium aspiration syndrome; mobile arm support
MAST	military antishock trousers
MAT	multifocal atrial tachycardia
max	maximal; maxillary
M-BACOD	a drug combination protocol
MBC	maximum breathing capacity; minimal bacteriocidal concentration
MB-CK	a creatinine kinase isoenzyme
MBD	minimal brain damage; minimal brain dysfunction
MBI	methylene blue installation
MBM	mother's breast milk
MC	mixed cellularity; metatarso-cuneiform
MCA	middle cerebral aneurysm; middle cerebral artery; motorcycle accident; monoclonal antibodies
MCC	midstream clean-catch

MCCU	midstream clean-catch urine
MCD	minimal change disease
mcg	microgram
MCGN	minimal change glomerular nephritis
MCH	mean corpuscular hemoglobin; muscle contraction headache
MCHC	mean corpuscular hemoglobin concentration
MCL	midclavicular line; midcostal line
MCLNS	mucocutaneous lymph node syndrome
MCP	metacarpophalangeal joint
MCS	microculture and sensitivity
MCSA	minimal cross-sectional area
MCT	medium chain triglyceride; mean circulation time
MCTD	mixed connective tissue disease
MCV	mean corpuscular/cell volume
MD	medical doctor; mental deficiency; muscular dystrophy; manic depression
MDA	manual dilation of the anus; micrometastases detection assay
MDC	medial dorsal cutaneous (nerve); major diagnostic category
MDD	manic-depressive disorder; major depressive disorder
MDF	myocardial depressant factor
MDI	multiple daily injection; metered dose inhaler
MDII	multiple daily insulin injection
MDM	mid-diastolic murmur; minor determinant mix
MDR	minimum daily requirement
MDS	maternal deprivation syndrome; minimum data set
MDTP	multidisciplinary treatment plan
ME	macula edema; medical examiner; middle ear
MEA-I	multiple endocrine adenomatosis type I
mec	meconium
MED	median erythrocyte diameter; medial; medical; medication; medicine; minimum erythema dose; medium
MEDAC	multiple endocrine deficiency-autoimmune-candidiasis
MEE	middle ear effusion
MEF	maximum expired flow rate
MEFV	maximum expiratory flow volume
MEN (II)	multiple endocrine neoplasia (type II)
MEOS	microsomal ethanol oxidizing system
mEq	milliequivalent
M/E ratio	myeloid/erythroid ratio
META	metamyelocytes
METS	metabolic equivalents (multiples of resting oxygen uptake); metastases

MF	myocardial fibrosis; mycosis fungoides; midcavity forceps
M & F	mother and father; male and female
MFA	mid-forceps delivery
MFAT	multifocal atrial tachycardia
MFEM	maximal forced expiratory maneuver
MFH	malignant fibrous histiocytoma
MFR	mid-forceps rotation
MG	myasthenia gravis; milligram; Marcus Gunn
MGF	maternal grandfather
MGM	maternal grandmother
MGN	membranous glomerulonephritis
MGUS	monoclonal gammopathies of undetermined significance
M-GXT	multistage graded exercise test
MH	marital history; menstrual history; mental health; malignant hyperthermia
MHA	microangiopathic hemolytic anemia
MHB	maximum hospital benefit
MHC	major histocompatibility complex; mental health center
MH/MR	mental health and mental retardation
MI	myocardial infarction; mitral insufficiency; mental institution
MIA	medically indigent adult; missing in action
MIC	minimum inhibitory concentration; maternal and infant care
MICN	mobile intensive care nurse
MICU	medical intensive care unit; mobile intensive care unit
MID	multi-infarct dementia
MIDD	monoclonal immunoglobulin deposition
MIF	migration inhibitory factor
MIH	migraine with interparoxysmal headache
min	minimum; minute; minor
MIO	minimum identifiable odor
MIRP	myocardial infarction rehabilitation program
mix mon	mixed monitor
MJT	Mead Johnson tube
MKAB	may keep at bedside
ML	midline; milliliter; middle lobe
mL	milliliter
MLC	mixed lymphocyte culture; minimal lethal concentration
MLD	metachromatic leukodystrophy; minimal lethal dose
MLF	median longitudinal fasciculus
MLNS	mucocutaneous lymph node syndrome
MLR	mixed lymphocyte reaction
MM	millimeter; mucous membrane; multiple myeloma
mM	millimole
M & M	milk and molasses; morbidity and mortality

MMA	monocyte monolayer assay
MMECT	multiple monitor electroconvulsive therapy
MMEFR	maximal midexpiratory flow rate
MMF	mean maximum flow
MMFR	maximal midexpiratory flow rate
mmHg	millimeters of mercury
MMK	Marshall-Marchetti-Krantz (cystourethropexy)
MMOA	maxillary mandibular odontectomy alveolectomy
mmol	millimole
MMPI	Minnesota Multiphasic Personality Inventory
MMR	measles, mumps, rubella; midline malignant reticulosis
MMS	Mini-Mental State (examination)
MMT	manual muscle test
MMWR	*Morbidity & Mortality Weekly Report*
MN	midnight
M & N	morning and night
MNC	mononuclear leukocytes
MNG	multinodular goiter
MNR	marrow neutrophil reserve
Mn SSEPS	median nerve somatosensory evoked potentials
MNTB	medial nucleus of the trapezoid body
MO	month; medial oblique
MOA	mechanism of action
MOB	medical office building
MOD	medical officer of the day; moderate
MODY	maturity onset diabetes of youth
MOF	multiple organ failure
mono	monocyte; infectious mononucleosis
mOsm	milliosmole
mOsmol	milliosmole
MP	metacarpal phalangeal joint
MPGN	membranoproliferative glomerulonephritis
MPH	Master of Public Health
MPJ	metacarpophalangeal joint
MPL	maximum permissible level
MPR	multifetal pregnancy reduction
MPS	mucopolysaccharidosis
MPTR	motor, pain, touch reflex deficit
MQ	memory quotient
MR	mental retardation; may repeat; magnetic resonance; mitral regurgitation
MR × 1	may repeat times one
MRA	medical record administrator; magnetic resonance angiography

MRAN	medical resident admitting note
MRD	Medical Records Department
MRG	murmurs, rubs and gallops
MRI	magnetic resonance imaging
mRNA	messenger ribonucleic acid
MRS	magnetic resonance spectroscopy
MRSA	methicillin resistant *Staphylococcus aureus*
MS	multiple sclerosis; mitral stenosis; musculoskeletal; medical student; minimal support; muscle strength; mental status
M & S	microculture and sensitivity
MSAF	meconium stained amniotic fluid
MSAFP	maternal serum alpha fetoprotein
MSC	medical social consultant
MSE	Mental Status Examination
MSH	melanocyte-stimulating hormone
MSK	medullary sponge kidney
MSL	midsternal line
MSR	muscle stretch reflexes
MSS	minor surgery suite; muscular subaortic stenosis; Marital Satisfaction Scale
MST	mean survival time
MSTA®	mumps skin test antigen
MSU	midstream urine
MSUD	maple syrup urine disease
MSW	multiple stab wounds; Master of Social Work
MT	music therapy; medical technologist
MTAL	medullary thick ascending limb
MTD	Monro Tidal drainage
MTI	malignant teratoma interminate
MTM	modified Thayer-Martin medium
MTP	metatarsal phalangeal
MTU	malignant teratoma undifferentiated
MU	million units
MUDPIES	methanol, uremia, diabetic ketoacidosis, paraldehyde, idiopathic, ethylene glycol, salicylate (cause of metabolic acidosis)
MULEPAK	methanol, uremia, lactic acidosis, ethylene glycol, paraldehyde, aspirin, diabetic ketoacidosis (cause of metabolic acidosis)
MUGA	multiple gated acquisition
MUGX	multiple gated acquisition exercise
MVA	motor vehicle accident; malignant ventricular arrhythmias
MVB	mixed venous blood

MVC	maximal voluntary contraction
MVI®	parenteral multivitamins
MVO2	myocardial oxygen consumption
MVP	mitral valve prolapse
MVR	mitral valve replacement; mitral valve regurgitation
MVS	mitral valve stenosis
MVV	maximum voluntary ventilation; mixed vespid venom
MWS	Mickey-Wilson syndrome
My	myopia
myelo	myelocyte
N	normal; negative; Negro
5'-N	5'-nucleotidase
NA	nursing assistant; nurse anesthetist; not applicable
NAA	neutron activation analysis
NABS	normoactive bowel sounds
NAD	no acute distress; no apparent distress; no appreciable disease; normal axis deviation; nothing abnormal detected
NAEP	National Asthma Education Program
NAG	narrow angle glaucoma
NANB	non-A, non-B hepatitis
NANC	nonadrenergic, noncholinergic
NAS	no added salt; neonatal abstinence syndrome
NAT	no action taken
NB	newborn; note well; needle biopsy
NBM	no bowel movement; normal bowel movement; nothing by mouth
NBN	newborn nursery
NBS	normal bowel sound; no bacteria seen
NBT	nitroblue tetrazolium reduction test
NBTE	nonbacterial thrombotic endocarditis
NC	neurologic check; no complaints; not completed; nasal cannula
NCA	neurocirculatory asthenia
NC/AT	normal cephalic atraumatic
NCB	no code blue
NCD	normal childhood diseases; not considered disabling
NCF	neutrophilic chemotactic factor
NCI	National Cancer Institute
NCJ	needle catheter jejunostomy
NCL	neuronal ceroid lipofuscinosis
NCM	nailfold capillary microscopy
NCNC	normochromic, normocytic
NCPR	no cardiopulmonary resuscitation

NCS	no concentrated sweets; nerve conduction studies
NCV	nerve conduction velocity
ND	normal delivery; normal development; not done; not diagnosed; nasal deformity
NDA	new drug application
NDD	no dialysis days
NDT	neurodevelopmental treatment
NDV	Newcastle disease virus
NE	norepinephrine; not elevated; not examined
NEC	necrotizing enterocolitist elsewhere classified
NED	no evidence of disease
NEG	negative
NEMD	nonspecific esophageal motility disorder
NET	naso-endotracheal tube
neut	neutrophil
NF	Negro female; not found; neurofibromatosis
NFL	nerve fiber layer
NFTD	normal full-term delivery
NFTT	nonorganic failure to thrive
NFW	nursed fairly well
NG	nasogastric; nanogram
NGF	nerve growth factor
NGR	nasogastric replacement
NGT	nasogastric tube
NGU	nongonococcal urethritis
NH	nursing home
NHD	normal hair distribution
NHL	non-Hodgkin's lymphoma; nodular histiocytic lymphoma
NHP	nursing home placement
NCC	neonatal intensive care center
NICU	neurosurgical intensive care unit; neonatal intensive care unit
NIDD	non-insulin-dependent diabetes
NIDDM	non-insulin-dependent diabetes mellitus
NIF	negative inspiratory force
NIH	National Institutes of Health
NINVS	noninvasive neurovascular studies
NJ	nasojejunal
NK	natural killer (cells)
NKA	no known allergies
NKDA	no known drug allergies
NKHS	nonketotic hyperosmolar syndrome
NKMA	no known medication allergies
NL	normal; normal limits

NLD	necrobiosis lipoidica diabeticorum; nasolacrimal duct
NLF	nasolabial fold
NLP	nodular liquefying panniculitis; no light perception
NLT	not later than; not less than
NM	Negro male; neuromusculardular melanoma
NMD	normal muscle development
NMR	nuclear magnetic resonance
NMI	no middle initial
NMS	neuroleptic malignant syndrome
NMT	no more than
NN	neonatal; nursing notes
NND	neonatal death
NNE	neonatal necrotizing enterocolitis
NNM	Nicole-Novy-MacNeal (media)
NNO	no new orders
NNP	neonatal nurse practitioner
NNU	net nitrogen utilization
no	number
noc	night
noct	nocturnal
NOD	notify of death
NOMI	nonocclusive mesenteric infarction
NOOB	not out of bed
NOS	not otherwise specified
NOSIE	Nurse Observation Scale for Inpatient Evaluation
NP	neuropsychiatric; nasopharyngeal; newly presented; no pain; not pregnant; not present; nursed poorly; nasal prongs; nurse practitioner
NPA	near point of accommodation
NPC	near point convergences; nodal premature contractions; nonpatient contact
NPDL	nodular poorly differentiated lymphocytic
NPDR	nonproliferative diabetic retinopathy
NPH	normal pressure hydrocephalus; no previous history; neutral protamine Hagedorn (insulin)
NPO	nothing by mouth
NPR	noncardiogenic pulmonary reaction
NPT	normal pressure and temperature; nocturnal penile tumescence
NR	nonreactive
NRBS	non-rebreathing system
NRC	normal retinal correspondence
NREM	nonrapid eye movement
NREMS	nonrapid eye movement sleep

NRT	neuromuscular reeducation techniques
NS	nephrotic syndrome; nuclear sclerosis; not seen; not significant; nylon suture
NSA	normal serum albumin; no significant abnormality
NSABP	National Surgical Adjuvant Breast Project
NSC	no significant change; not service connected
NSCLC	non-small-cell lung cancer
NSD	normal spontaneous delivery; nominal standard dose
NSDA	non-steroid-dependent asthmatic
NSE	neuron-specific enolase
NSFTD	normal spontaneous full-term delivery
NSG	nursing
NSILA	nonsuppressible insulin-like activity
NSN	nephrotoxic serum nephritis
NSPVT	nonsustained polymorphic ventricular tachycardia
NSR	normal sinus rhythm; not seen regularly; nonspecific reaction; nasoseptal repair
NSSTT	nonspecific ST and T wave
NST	nutritional support team; nonstress test; not sooner than
NSU	nonspecific urethritis
NSV	nonspecific vaginitis
NSVD	normal spontaneous vaginal delivery
NT	not tested; nasotracheal; not tender
N & T	nose and throat
NTC	neurotrauma center
NTD	neural tube defects
NTE	not to exceed
NTF	normal throat flora
NTG	nontreatment group
NTMB	nontuberculous mycobacteria
NTMI	nontransmural myocardial infarction
NTP	normal temperature and pressure
NTS	nasotracheal suction; nucleus tractus solitarii
NTT	nasotracheal tube
NUD	nonulcer dyspepsia
nullip	nullipara
NV	neurovascular
N & V	nausea and vomiting
NVD	nausea, vomiting, and diarrhea; neck vein distention; no venereal disease; neurovesicle dysfunction; nonvalvular disease; neovascularization of the disc
NVE	neovascularization elsewhere
NVG	neovascular glaucoma
NVS	neurological vital signs

NWB	non-weight bearing
NWTS	National Wilms' Tumor Study
NYD	not yet diagnosed
NZ	enzyme
O	oxygen; objective finding; eye; oral; open; obvious; often; other; occlusal
1O2	singlet oxygen
O2	oxygen; both eyes
O2v	superoxide
OA	oral alimentation; occiput anterior; osteoarthritis; Overeaters Anonymous
O & A	observation and assessment
OAF	osteoclast activating factor
Ob	obstetrics
OB	occult blood
OBE-CALP	placebo capsule or tablet
Ob-Gyn	obstetrics and gynecology
OBS	organic brain syndrome
OC	oral contraceptive; obstetrical conjugate; oral care; on call; office call
OCA	oculocutaneous albinism
OCCC	open chest cardiac compression
OCCM	open chest cardiac massage
OCD	obsessive-compulsive disorder
OCG	oral cholecystogram
OCP	ova, cysts, parasites
OCT	oxytocin challenge test; optical coherence tomography
OCU	observation care unit
OD	right eye; overdose; on duty; Doctor of Optometry
OER	oxygen enhancement ratios
OFC	occipital-frontal circumference
OG	orogastric (feeding)
OGTT	oral glucose tolerance test
OH	occupational history; open heart
OHA	oral hypoglycemic agents
OHD	organic heart disease
OHF	omsk hemorrhage fever
OHG	oral hypoglycemic
OHP	oxygen under hyperbaric pressure
OHRR	open heart recovery room
OHS	open heart surgery
OI	osteogenesis imperfecta
OIF	oil-immersion field

OJ	orthoplast jacket; orange juice
OKAN	optokinetic after nystagmus
OKN	optokinetic nystagmus
OLA	occiput left anterior
OM	otitis media; every morning
OME	Office of the Medical Examiner; otitis media with effusion
OMI	old myocardial infarct
OMR	operative mortality rate
OMSC	otitis media secretory/suppurative chronic
ON	overnight; every night
ONC	over-the-needle catheter
OOB	out of bed
OOBBRP	out of bed with bathroom privileges
OOC	out of control
OOP	out on pass; out of pelvis
OOR	out of room
OOT	out of town
OP	outpatient; operation; occiput posterior; open
O & P	ova and parasites
OPB	outpatient basis
OPC	outpatient clinic
OPCA	olivopontocerebellar atrophy
OPD	outpatient department
OPG	ocular plethysmography
OPM	occult primary malignancy
OPPG	oculopneumoplethysmography
OPS	operations
OPV	oral polio vaccine
OR	operating room; oil retention
ORIF	open reduction internal fixation
ORL	otorhinolaryngology
OS	left eye; mouth; opening snap
OSA	obstructive sleep apnea
OSD	overside drainage
OSM S	osmolarity serum
OSM U	osmolarity urine
OSN	off service note
OSS	osseous
OT	old tuberculin; occupational therapy/therapist
OTC	over-the-counter
OTD	out the door
OTO	otology
OTR	Occupational Therapist, Registered
OTS	orotracheal suction

OTT	orotracheal tube
OU	both eyes
OV	office visit; ovum; ovary
OW	out of wedlock
oz	ounce
P	plan; protein; pint; pulse; peripheral; phosphorus; para
p	after
P2	pulmonic second heart sound
PA	posterior-anterior; pulmonary artery; pernicious anemia; physician assistant; presents again; psychiatric aide; professional association
P & A	percussion and auscultation
PAB	premature atrial beat
PAC	premature atrial contraction
PACH	pipers to after coming head
PACO	pivot ambulating crutchless orthosis
PaCO2	arterial carbon dioxide tension
PADP	pulmonary artery diastolic pressure
PAF	paroxysmal atrial fibrillation; platelet activating factors
PAGE	polyacrylamide gel electrophoresis
PAIVS	pulmonary atresia with intact ventricle septum
Pa Line	pulmonary artery line
PALN	para-aortic lymph node
PAN	periodic alternating nystagmus; polyarteritis nodosa
PAO2	arterial oxygen tension
PAOG	primary open angle glaucoma
PAOP	pulmonary artery occlusion pressure
PAP	pulmonary artery pressure; prostatic acid phosphatase
Pap smear	Papanicolaou smear
PA/PS	pulmonary atresia/pulmonary stenosis
PAR	postanesthetic recovery; platelet aggregate ratio
PARA	number of pregnancies
para	paraplegic
PARU	postanesthetic recovery unit
PAS	periodic acid-Schiff (reagent); peripheral anterior synechia; pulmonary artery stenosis
PasEx	passive exercise
PAT	paroxysmal atrial tachycardia; preadmission testing; percent acceleration time
Path	pathology
PAWP	pulmonary artery wedge pressure
Pb	lead
PB	powder board; paraffin bath

PBA	percutaneous bladder aspiration
PBC	point of basal convergence; primary biliary cirrhosis
PBD	percutaneous biliary drainage
PBL	peripheral blood lymphocyte
PBMC	peripheral blood mononuclear cell
PBMNC	peripheral blood mononuclear cell
PBO	placebo
PC	after meal; packed cells; professional corporation; platelet concentrate
PCA	patient care assistant/aide; patient-controlled analgesia; posterior cerebral artery; procoagulation activity; passive cutaneous anaphylaxis
PCCU	postcoronary care unit
PCG	phonocardiogram
PCH	paroxysmal cold hemoglobinuria
PCI	prophylactic cranial irradiation
PCIOL	posterior chamber intraocular lens
PCL	posterior chamber lens; posterior cruciate ligament
PCM	protein-calorie malnutrition
PCO	polycystic ovary
PCO2	carbon dioxide pressure/tension
PCOD	polycystic ovarian disease
PCP	*Pneumonocystis carinii* pneumonia; pulmonary capillary pressure
PCR	protein catabolic/caloric rate; polymerase chain reaction
PCT	porphyria cutanea
PCTA	percutaneous transluminal angioplasty
PCU	progressive care unit
PCV	packed cell volume
PCWP	pulmonary capillary wedge pressure
PD	peritoneal dialysis; postural drainage; Parkinson's disease; interpupillary distance; percutaneous drain
P/D	packs per day (cigarettes)
PDA	patent ductus arteriosus
PDE	paroxysmal dyspnea on exertion; pulsed Doppler echocardiography
PDFC	premature dead female child
PDGF	platelet-derived growth factor
PDL	poorly differentiated lymphocytic
PDL-D	poorly differentiated lymphocytic-diffuse
PDL-N	poorly differentiated lymphocytic-nodular
PDMC	premature dead male child
PDN	private duty nurse
PDR	proliferative diabetic reinopathy; *Physician's Desk Reference*

PDS	pain dysfunction syndrome
PDGXT	predischarge graded exercise test
PDT	photodynamic therapy
PDU	pulsed Doppler ultrasonography
PE	physical examination; pulmonary embolism; pressure equalization; pleural effusion
PECHO	prostatic echogram
PECO2	mixed expired carbon dioxide tension
Peds	pediatrics
PEEP	positive end-expiratory pressure
PEER	peak expiratory flow rate
PEG	pneumoencephalogram; percutaneous endoscopic gastrostomy
PEN	parenteral and enteral nutrition
PENS	percutaneous epidural nerve stimulator
PEP	protein electrophoresis; pre-ejection period; Parkinson's educational program
PER	pediatric emergency room
perf	perforation
PERL	pupils equal, reactive to light
per os	by mouth
PERR	pattern evoked retinal response
PERRLA	pupils equal, round, reactive to light and accommodation
PES	pre-excitation syndrome
PET	positron-emission tomography; pre-eclamptic toxemia; pressure equalizing tubes
PF	power factor
PFC	persistent fetal circulation
PFM	porcelain fused to metal
PFR	peak flow rate; parotid flow rate
PFT	pulmonary function test
PFU	plaque-forming unit
PG	pregnant
PGF	parenteral grandfather
PGH	pituitary growth hormones
PGL	persistent generalized lymphadenopathy
PGM	paternal grandmother
PgR	progesterone receptor
PGU	postgonococcal urethritis
pH	hydrogen ion concentration
PH	past history; poor health; public health
PHA	passive hemagglutinating; phytohemagglutinin; arterial pH; phytohemagglutinin antigen; peripheral hyperalimentation

Pharm	pharmacy
PHC	primary hepatocellular carcinoma
PHH	posthemorrhagic hydrocephalus
PHN	public health nurse; postherpetic neuralgia
PHPT	primary hyperparathyroidism
PHPV	persistent hyperplastic primary vitreous
Phx	pharynx
PI	present illness; pulmonary infarction; peripheral iridectomy
PIAT	Peabody Individual Achievement Test
PICA	posterior inferior communicating artery; posterior inferior cerebellar artery
PICU	pediatric intensive care unit
PID	pelvic inflammatory disease; prolapsed intervertebral disc
PIE	pulmonary infiltration with eosinophilia; pulmonary interstitial emphysema
PIFR	peak inspiratory flow rate
PIH	pregnancy-induced hypertension
PIOK	poikilocytosis
PIP	proximal interphalangeal joint; postinspiratory pressure
PISA	phase invariant signature algorithm
PITR	plasma iron turnover rate
PIV	peripheral intravenous
PIVD	protruded intervertebral disc
PJB	premature junctional beat
PJC	premature junctional contractions
PJS	Peutz-Jeghers syndrome
PK	penetrating keratoplasty
PKD	polycystic kidney disease
PK test	Prausnitz-Kustner transfer test
PKU	phenylketonuria
PL	plantar; place; light perception
PLAP	placental alkaline phosphatase
PLFC	premature living female child
PLH	paroxysmal localized hyperhidrosis
PLL	prolymphocytic leukemia
PLMC	premature living male child
PLN	pelvic lymph node; popliteal lymph node
PLS	primary lateral sclerosis
plts	platelets
PM	postmortem; evening; pretibial myxedema; primary motivation; presents mainly
PMA	Prinzmetal's angina; premenstrual asthma
PMB	postmenopausal bleeding; polymorphonuclear basophils
PMC	pseudomembranous colitis

PMD	private medical doctor
PME	postmenopausal estrogen
PMF	progressive massive fibrosis
PMH	past medical history
PMI	point of maximal impulse; patient medication instructions
PML	progressive multifocal leukoencephalopathy
PMN	polymorphonuclear neutrophil
PMP	pain management program; previous menstrual period
PMR	polymyalgia rheumatica; polymorphic reticulosis
PM & R	physical medicine and rehabilitation
PMS	premenstrual syndrome
PMT	premenstrual tension
PMTS	premenstrual tension syndrome
PMV	prolapse of mitral valve
PMW	pacemaker wires
PN	parenteral nutrition; progress note; percussion note
PNAS	prudent no added salt
PNB	premature nodal beat
PNC	premature nodal contraction; peripheral nerve conduction
PND	paroxysmal nocturnal dyspnea; postnasal drip
PNET-MB	primitive neuroectodermal tumors—medulloblastoma
PNF	proprioceptive neuromuscular fasciculation reaction
PNH	paroxysmal nocturnal hemoglobinuria
PNI	prognostic nutrition index; peripheral nerve injury
PNMG	persistent neonatal myasthenia gravis
PNP	Pediatric Nurse Practitioner; progressive nuclear palsy
PNS	peripheral nervous system; partial nonprogressing stroke; practical nursing student
PNT	percutaneous nephrostomy tube
PNU	protein nitrogen units
PNV	prenatal vitamins
Pnx	pneumothorax
PO	postoperative; phone order; by mouth (per os)
PO2	partial pressure of oxygen
POA	pancreatic oncofetal antigen
POAG	primary open-angle glaucoma
POC	product of conception; postoperative care
POD 1	postoperative day one
POEMS	plasma cell dyscrasia with polyneuropathy, organomegaly, endocrinopathy, monoclonal (M)-protein, skin changes
POG	Pediatric Oncology Group
POIK	poikilocytosis
POL	premature onset of labor
POLY	polymorphonuclear leukocyte

POMR	problem-oriented medical record
poplit	popliteal
PORT	postoperative respiratory therapy
POS	parosteal osteosarcoma; point of service
POSM	patient-operated selector mechanism
post	postmortem examination (autopsy)
post op	postoperative
PP	postpartum; postprandial; paradoxical pulse; pin prick; patient profile; protoporphyria; proximal phalanx; private patient; near point of accommodation
P & P	pins and plater
PPB	parts per billion
PPBG	postprandial blood glucose
PPBS	postprandial blood sugar
PPC	progressive patient care
PPD	packs per day; postpartum day; posterior polymorphous dystrophy; purified protein derivative
P & PD	percussion and postural drainage
PPD-B	purified protein derivative, Battey
PPD-S	purified protein derivative, standard
PPF	plasma protein fraction
PPG	photoplethysmography
PPH	postpartum hemorrhage
PPHN	persistent pulmonary hypertension of the newborn
PPI	patient package insert
PPL	pars planus lensectomy
PPLO	pleuro-pneumonia-like organisms
PPM	parts per million
PPN	peripheral parenteral nutrition
PPNG	penicillinase producing *Neisseria* gonorrhoeae
PPO	preferred provider organization
PPP	postpartum psychosis
PPPG	postprandial plasma glucose
PPPBL	peripheral pulses palpable both legs
PPROM	prolonged premature rupture of membranes
PPS	postpartum sterilization; pneumococcal polysaccharide (vaccine)
PPTL	postpartum tubal ligation
PPVT	Peabody Picture Vocabulary Test
PR	per rectum; pulse rate; profile; Puerto Rican; far point of accommodation
P & R	pulse and respiration; pelvic and rectal
PRA	plasma renin angiotensin
PRAT	platelet radioactive antiglobulin test

PRBC	packed red blood cells
PRCA	pure red cell aplasia
PRE	progressive/passive resistive exercise
pre-op	before surgery
prep	prepare for surgery
PRG	phleborrheogram
PRIMP	primipara (first pregnancy)
PRN	as needed
PRO	protein; peer review organization
prob	probable
PROC-TO	proctology; proctoscopic
prog	prognosis; prognathism
PROM	passive range of motion; premature rupture of membranes
ProMACE	a drug protocol combination
prov	provisional
PRP	panretinal photocoagulation
PRRE	pupils round, regular, equal
PRSs	positive rolandic spikes
PRTH-C	prothrombin time control
PRV	polycythemia rubra vera
PRVEP	pattern reversal visual evoked potentials
PRW	polymerized ragweed
PS	pulmonary stenosis; paradoxic sleep; pathologic stage; plastic surgery; serum from pregnant women; performance status
P & S	paracentesis and suction; pain and suffering
PSA	prostate-specific antigen
PS I	healthy patient with localized pathological process
PS II	patient with mild to moderate systemic disease
PS III	patient with severe systemic disease limiting activity, but not incapacitating
PS IV	patient with incapacitating systemic disease
PS V	moribund patient not expected to live
PsA	psoriatic arthritis
PSC	posterior subcapsular cataract; priimary sclerosing cholangitis
PSE	portal systemic encephalopathy
PSF	posterior spinal fusion
PSG	polysomnography
PSGN	poststreptococcal glomerulonephritis
PSH	postspinal headache
PSI	pounds per square inch
PSM	presystolic murmur
PSP	pancreatic spasmolytic peptide; progressive supranuclear palsy

PSRBOW	premature spontaneous rupture of bag of waters
PSS	progressive systemic sclerosis; physiologic saline solution
PSW	psychiatric social worker
PSVT	paroxysmal supraventricular tachycardia
PT	physical therapy/therapist; patient; prothrombin time; pine tar; posterior tibial; pint
PTA	prior to admission; plasma thromboplastin antecdent; pre-treatment anxiety; puretone average; physical therapy assistant; percutaneous transluminal angioplasty
PTB	patellar tendon bearing
PTBD-EF	percutaneous transhepatic biliary drainage—enteric feeding
PTC	plasma thromboplastin components; percutaneous transhepatic cholangiography
PTCA	percutaneous transluminal coronary angioplasty
PTD	period to discharge; permanent and total disability
PTE	proximal tibial epiphysis; pulmonary thromboembolism; pretibial edema
PTF	plasma thromboplastin factor
PTH	post transfusion hepatitis; parathyroid hormone
PTL	pre-term labor
PTMDF	pupils, tension, media, disc, fundus
pTNM	postsurgical resection—pathologic staging of cancer
PTPM	posttraumatic progressive myelopathy
PTPN	peripheral (vein) total parenteral nutrition
PTS	prior to surgery
PTSD	posttraumatic stress disorder
PTT	partial thromboplastin time
PTX	pneumothorax
PU	peptic ulcer; pregnancy urine
PUBS	percutaneous umbilical blood sampling
PUD	peptic ulcer disease
PUFA	polyunsaturated fatty acids
pul	pulmonary
PUN	plasma urea nitrogen
PUO	pyrexia of undetermined origin
PUPPP	pruritic urticarial papules and plaques of pregnancy
PUVA	psoralen-ultraviolet light
PV	polycythemia vera; polio vaccine; portal vein; pulmonary vein; per vagina
P & V	pyloroplasty and vagotomy
PVB	premature ventricular beat
PVC	premature ventricular contraction; pulmonary venous congestion

PVD	patient very disturbed; peripheral vascular disease; posterior vitreous detachment
PVE	premature ventricular extrasystole; perivenous encephalomyelitis
PVO	peripheral vascular occlusion; pulmonary venous occlusion
PVOD	pulmonary vascular obstructive disease
PVP	peripheral venous pressure
PVR	peripheral vascular resistance; postvoiding residual; proliferative vitreoretinopathy; pulse-volume recording
PVS	peritoneovenous shunt; pulmonic valve stenosis; vibration, and suction
PVT	paroxysmal ventricular tachycardia; private
PWB	partial weight bearing
PWLV	posterior wall of left ventricle
PWM	pokeweed mitogens
PWP	pulmonary wedge pressure
PWV	polistes wasp venom
Px	physical exam; prognosis; pneumothorax; practice
PXE	pseudoxanthoma elasticum
PTx	parathyroidectomy
PY	pack years
q	every
QA	quality assurance
QAM	every morning
QCA	quantitative coronary angiography
qd	every day
QEEG	quantitative electroencephalogram
q4h	every four hours
qh	every hour
qhs	every night
qid	four times daily
qn	every night
qns	quantity not sufficient
qod	every other day
qoh	every other hour
qon	every other night
qpm	every evening
QRS	principal deflection in an electrocardiogram
QS	sufficient quantity; every shift
QUART	quadrantectomy, axillary dissection, and radiotherapy
qwk	once a week
R	respiration; right; rectum; regular; rate; regular insulin

RA	rheumatoid arthritis; right atrium; right auricle; right arm; room air
RABG	room air blood gas
RAC	right atrial catheter
RAD	right axis deviation; radical
RAE	right atrial enlargement
RAEB	refractory anemia, erythroblastic
RAG	room air gas
RAI	resident assessment instrument
RAIU	radioactive iodine uptake
RALT	routine admission laboratory tests
RAM	rapid alternating movements
RAN	resident admission notes
RAO	right anterior oblique
RAP	right atrial pressure; resident assessment protocol
RAPD	relative afferent pupillary defect
RAS	renal artery stenosis
RAST	radioallergosorbent test
RAT	right anterior thigh
RA test	test for rheumatoid factor
R (AW)	airway resistance
RB	retrobulbar; right buttock
R & B	right and below
RBA	right brachial artery
RBB	right breast biopsy
RBBB	right bundle branch block
RBCD	right border cardiac dullness
RBC	red blood cell/count
RBD	right border or dullness
RBE	relative biologic effectiveness
RBF	renal blood flow
RBOW	rupture bag of water
RBP	retinol-binding protein
RBV	right brachial vein
R/C	reclining chair
RCA	right coronary artery; radionuclide cerebral angiogram; regional citrate anticoagulation
RCC	renal cell carcinoma
RCD	relative cardiac dullness
RCM	right costal margin; radiographic contrast media
RCR	replication-competent retrovirus
RCS	reticulum cell sarcoma
RCT	root canal therapy
RCV	red cell volume

RD	registered dietitian; renal disease; retinal detachment; respiratory disease
RDA	recommended daily allowance
RDPE	reticular degeneration of pigment epithelium
RDH	Registered Dental Hygienist
RDI	respiratory disturbance/distress index
RDS	respiratory distress syndrome
RDT	regular dialysis/hemodialysis treatment
RDVT	recurrent deep vein thrombosis
RDW	red cell size distribution width
RE	reticuloendothelial; rectal examination; regional enteritis; right eye; concerning
REE	resting energy expenditure
REF	renal erythropoietic factor; referred
rehab	rehabilitation
Rel	religion
REM	rapid eye movement
REMS	rapid eye movement sleep
REP	repeat; report; repair
repol	repolarization
RER	renal excretion rate
RES	reticuloendothelial system; resident; rehabilitation evaluation system
RESC	resuscitation
resp	respiratory; respiration
retic	reticulocyte
REV	revolutions; review; reverse
RF	rheumatoid factor; rheumatic fever; renal failure
RFA	right fronto-anterior; right femoral artery
RFL	right frontolateral
RFP	right frontoposterior
RFT	right frontotransverse
RG	right gluteal
RGM	right gluteus medius
Rh	Rhesus factor in blood
RH	right hyperphoria; right hand; reduced haloperidol; room humidifier
RHB	raise head of bed
RHC	respiration has ceased
RHD	rheumatic heart disease; relative hepatic dullness
RHE	recombinant human erythropoietin
RHF	right heart failure
RHL	right hemisphere lesions
R-HuEPO	recombinant human erythropoietin

RHT	right hypertropia
RIA	radioimmunoassay
RIC	right iliac crest; right internal carotid (artery)
RICE	rest and immobilization, ice, compression, elevation
RICS	right intercostal space
RICU	respiratory intensive care unit
RID	radial immunodiffusion
RIF	rigid internal fixation; right iliac fossa
RIH	right inguinal hernia
RIMA	right internal mammary anastomosis
RIND	reversible ischemic neurologic defect
RIP	radioimmunoprecipitin test; rapid infusion pump
RISA	radioactive iodinated serum albumin
RIST	radioimmunosorbent test
RK	radial keratotomy
RL	right leg; right lung; right lateral
R-L	right to left
RLE	right lower extremity
RLF	retrolental fibroplasia
RLL	right lower lobe
RLQ	right lower quadrant
RLR	right lateral rectus
RLT	right lateral thigh
RM	repetitions maximum; room; radical mastectomy; respiratory movement
R & M	routine and microscopic
RMA	right meno-anterior
RMCA	right main coronary artery
RMCL	right midclavicular line
RMD	rapid movement disorder
RME	right medilateral episiotomy
RMEE	right middle ear exploration
RMI	repetitive motion injuries
RML	right middle lobe
RMP	right mentoposterior
RMR	right medial rectus; resting metabolic rate
RMSF	Rocky Mountain spotted fever
RMT	right mentotransverse; registered music therapist
RN	registered nurse
RNA	radionuclide angiography
RND	radial neck dissection
RNEF	resting/radionuclide ejection fraction
RO	rule out; routine order
ROA	right occiput anterior

ROM	range of motion
ROP	right occiput posterior; retinopathy of prematurity
ROS	review of systems
ROSC	restoration of spontaneous circulation
RoRx	radiation therapy
ROT	right occipital transverse; remedial occupational therapy
RP	retinitis pigmentosa; retrograde pyelogram; Raynaud's phenomenon
RPA	right pulmonary artery; radial photon absorptiometry; registered physician assistant/associate
RPCF	Reiter protein complement fixation
RPD	removable partial denture
RPE	retinal pigment epithelium; rating of perceived exertion
RPF	renal plasma flow; relaxed pelvic floor
RPGN	rapidly progressive glomerulonephritis
RPH	retroperitoneal hemorrhage; registered pharmacist
RPICCE	round pupil intracapsular cataract extraction
RPLND	retroperitoneal lymphadenectomy
RPM	renal parenchymal malacoplakia
RPN	renal papillary recrosis
RPO	right posterior oblique
RPP	rate-pressure product
RPR	rapid plasma reagin; Reiter protein reagin
RPT	registered physical therapist
RQ	respiratory quotient
RR	recovery room; respiratory rate; regular respirations
R & R	rate and rhythm
RRE	round, regular, and equal
RREF	resting radionuclide ejection fraction
rRNA	ribosomal ribonucleic acid
RRND	right radical neck dissection
RRR	regular rhythm and rate
RRRN	round, regular, react normally
RS	Reiter's syndrome; Reye's syndrome; rhythm strip; right side
RSA	right sacrum anterior; right subclavian artery
RSDS	reflex-sympathetic dystrophy syndrome
RSI	repetitive stress injury
R-SICU	respiratory-surgical intensive care unit
RSO	right salpingo-oophorectomy; radiation safety officer
RSP	right sacroposterior
RSR	regular sinus rhythm; relative survival rate
RSTs	Rodney Smith tubes
RSV	respiratory syncytial virus

RSW	right-sided weakness
RT	right; radiation therapy; recreational therapy; renal transplant; running total; respiratory therapist; radiologic technician
R/t	related to
RTA	renal tubular acidosis
RTC	return to clinic; round the clock
RTL	reactive to light
rTNM	retreatment staging of cancer
RTO	return to office
RTOG	Radiation Therapy Oncology Group
rtPA	recombinant tissue-type plasminogen
RTRR	return to recovery room
RTS	real time scan
RT3U	resin triiodothyronine uptake
RTx	radiation therapy
RUA	routine urine analysis
RUE	right upper extremity
RUG	retrograde urethrogram
RUL	right upper lobe
rupt	ruptured
RUQ	right upper quadrant
RURTI	recurrent upper respiratory tract infection
RUSB	right upper sternal border
RV	right ventricle; residual volume; rectovaginal; rubella vaccine
RVD	relative vertebral density
RVE	right ventricular enlargement
RVET	right ventricular ejection time
RVG	radionuclide ventriculography
RVH	right ventricular hypertrophy; renovascular hypertension
RVL	right vastus lateralis
RVO	retinal vein occlusion; relaxed vaginal outlet
RVOT	right ventricular outflow tract
RVR	rapid ventricular response
RVSWI	right ventricular stroke work index
RV/TLC	residual volume to total lung capacity ratio
RVV	rubella vaccine virus
Rx	therapy; drug; medication; treatment; take
RXN	reaction
S	subjective findings; serum; suction; sacral; single; sister
S1	first heart sound; sacral vertebrae 1
S2	second heart sound

SA	sinoatrial; salicylic acid; sustained action; surface area; Spanish American
S/A	sugar and acetone
SAARD	slow-acting antirheumatic drugs
SAB	subarachnoid block/bleed
SAC	short arm cast
SACH	solid ankle cushion heel
SAD	sugar and acetone determination; seasonal affective disorder
SAE	signal-averaged electrocardiogram
SAF	self-articulating femoral
SAFE	stationary attachment and flexible endoskeletal (prosthesis)
Sag D	sagittal diameter
SAH	subarachnoid hemorrhage; systemic arterial hypertension
SAL 12	sequential analysis of 12 chemistry constituents
SAM	systolic anterior motion; self-administered medication
SAN	sinoatrial node
sang	sanguinous
SAPD	self-administration of psychotropic drugs
SAPHO	synovitis, acne, pustulosis, hyperostosis, osteitis
SAS	sleep apnea syndrome
SAT	subacute thyroiditis; saturation
SAVD	spontaneous assisted vaginal delivery
SB	stillbirth; stillborn; spina bifida; sternal border; Sengstaken-Blakemore (tube); sinus bradycardia; small bowel
SBE	subacute bacterial endocarditis
SBFT	small bowel follow through
SBGM	self blood glucose monitoring
SBI	systemic bacterial infection
SB-LM	Stanford Binet Intelligence Test—Form LM
SBO	small bowel obstruction
SBP	systolic blood pressure; spontaneous bacterial peritonitis
SBR	strict bed rest
SBT	serum bacterial titers
SC	subcutaneous; subclavian; sternoclavicular; sickle-cell; sulfur colloid; service connnected
SCA	subcutaneous abdominal (block)
SCB	strictly confined to bed
SCBC	small cell bronchogenic carcinoma
SCC	squamous cell carcinoma; sickle cell crisis
SCCa	squamous cell carcinoma
SCCA	semi-closed circle absorber
SCD	sudden cardiac death; sickle cell disease; subacute combined degeneration; service connected disability; spinal cord disease

SCE	sister chromatic exchange
SCI	spinal cord injury
SCID	severe combined immunodeficiency disorder
SCIV	subclavian intravenous
SCLC	small-cell lung cancer
SCLE	subcutaneous lupus erythematosis
SCLs	soft contact lenses
SCM	sternocleidomastoid; spondylitic caudal myelopathy
SCR	spondylitic caudal radiculopathy
SC/SP	supracondylar/suprapatellar prosthesis
SCT	sickel cell trait; sugar coated tablet; sentence completion test
SCUT	schizophrenia chronic undifferentiated type
SCV	subcutaneous vaginal (block)
SD	senile dementia; scleroderma; spontaneous delivery; sterile dressing; surgical drain
S & D	stomach and duodenum
SDA	steroid-dependent asthmatic; Seventh-Day Adventist
SDAT	senile dementia of Alzheimer's type
SDH	subdual hematoma
SDL	serum digoxin level
SDS	same day surgery
SDT	speech detection threshold
SE	side effect
sec	secondary
sed	sedimentation
sed rt	sedimentation rate
SEER	Surveillance, Epidemiology, and End Results (program)
seg	segment; segmented neutrophil
SEM	systolic ejection murmur; scanning electron microscopy; standard error of mean
SEMI	subendocardial myocardial infarction
SENS	sensorium
SEP	systolic ejection period; somatosensory evoked potential; separate
SER-IV	supination external rotation, type 4 fracture
SERs	somatosensory-evoked responses
SES	socioeconomic status
SF	scarlet fever; sugar free; salt free; symptom free; spinal fluid
SFA	superficial femoral artery; saturated fatty acids
SFC	spinal fluid count
SFEMG	single-fiber electromyography
SFP	spinal fluid pressure

SFPT	standard fixation preference test
SG	specific gravity; serum glucose; Swan-Ganz
SGA	small for gestational age
SGD	straight gravity drainage
SGE	significant glandular enlargement
s gl	without correction/glasses
SGOT	serum glutamic oxaloacetic transaminase
SGPT	serum glutamic pyruvic transaminase
SH	serum hepatitis; social history; shower; short; shoulder
S & H	speech and hearing
S/H	suicidal/homicidal ideation
SHA	super heater aerosol
S Hb	sickle hemoglobin screen
SHEENT	skin, head, eyes, ears, nose, throat
SHS	Student Health Service
SI	sacroiliac
SIADH	syndrome of inappropriate antidiuretic hormone secretion
S & I	suction and irrigation
SIB	self-injurious behavior
sibs	siblings
SICT	selective intracoronary thrombolysis
SICU	surgical intensive care unit
SIDS	sudden infant death syndrome
sig	let it be marked
SIJ	sacroiliac joint
SIMV	synchronized intermittent mandatory ventilation
SISI	short increment sensitivity index
SIT	sperm immobilization test; Slossen Intelligence Test
SIW	self-inflicted wound
SJS	Stevens-Johnson syndrome
SK	SmithKline®
SL	sublingual; slight
SLB	short leg brace
SLC	short leg cast
SLE	systemic lupus erythematosus; slit lamp examination
SLGXT	symptom limited graded exercise test
SLK	superior limbic keratoconjunctivitis
SLR	straight leg raising
SLRT	straight leg raising cast
SLWC	short leg walking cast
SM	systolic murmur; small
SMA	sequential multiple analyzer; simultaneous multichannel autoanalyzer; superior mesenteric artery; spinal muscular atrophy

SMC	special mouth care; somatomedin-C
SMD	senile macular degeneration
SMI	small volume infusion; sustained maximal inspiration
SMON	subacute myelopticoneuropathy
SMP	self-management program
SMR	submucosal resection; standardized mortality ratio; skeletal muscle relaxant; senior medical resident
SMS	senior medical student
SMVT	sustained monomorphic ventricular tachycardia
SN	student nurse
SNAP	sensory nerve action potential
SNCV	sensory nerve conduction velocity
SND	sinus node dysfunction
SNE	subacute necrotizing encephalomyelopathy
SNGFR	single nephron glomerular filtration rate
SNT	Suppan nail technique
S-O	salpingo-oophorectomy
SOA	swelling of ankles; supraorbital artery
SOAA	signed out against advice
SOAP	subjective, objective, assessment, and plan
SOB	shortness of breath
S & OC	signed and on chart (permission)
SOD	surgical officer of the day; superoxide dismutase
SOFAS	Social and Occupational Functioning Assessment Scale
sol	solution
SOM	serous otitis media
SOMI	sterno-occipital mandibular immobilizer
Sono	sonogram
SONP	solid organs not palpable
SOP	standard operating procedure
SOS	may be repeated once if urgently required
SOT	stream of thought
SP	suprapubic; sequential pulse; sacrum to pubis; speech pathologist
S/P	status post
SPA	albumin human; stimulation produced analgesia
SPAG	small particle aerosol generator
SPBI	serum protein bound iodine
SPBT	suprapubic bladder tap
SPE	serum protein electrolytes
spec	specimen
SPECT	single photon emission computer tomography
Spec Ed	special education
SPEP	serum protein electrophoresis

SPF	sun protective factor
sp fl	spinal fluid
sp gr	specific gravity
SPK	superficial punctate keratitis
SPMA	spinal progressive muscle atrophy
SPMSQ	Short Portable Mental Status Questionnaire
SPN	solitary pulmonary nodule
SPP	suprapubic prostatectomy
SPROM	spontaneous premature rupture of membrane
SPT	skin prick test
SP TAP	spinal tap
SPU	short procedure unit
SPVR	systemic peripheral vascular resistance
SQ	subcutaneous
Sq CCa	squamous cell carcinoma
SR	sedimentation rate; sustained release; side rails; system review; sinus rhythm
SRBC	sickle/sheep red blood cells
SRBOW	spontaneous rupture of bag of waters
SRC	scleroderma renal crisis
Sr Cr	serum creatinine
SRF	somatotropin releasing factor
SRF-A	slow releasing factor of anaphylaxis
SRIF	somatotropin-release-inhibiting factor
SRMD	stress-related mucosal damage
SR/NE	sinus rhythm, no ectopy
SRNS	steroid responsive nephrotic syndrome
SROM	spontaneous rupture of membrane
SRS-A	slow reacting substance of anaphylaxis
SRT	speech reception threshold; sedimentation rate test
SRU	side rails up
SS	saline solution; salt substitute; sickle cell; social security/service; slip sent; symmetrical strength
S & S	signs and symptoms
SSCA	single shoulder contrast arthrography
SSD	social security disability; source to skin distance
SSDI	social security disability income
SSE	saline solution/soapsuds enema; systemic side effects
SSEPs	somatosensory evoked potentials
SSM	superficial spreading melanoma
SSOP	Second Surgical Opinion Program
SSPE	subacute sclerosing panencephalitis
SSS	sick sinus syndrome; sterile saline soak
SSSS	staphylococcal scalded skin syndrome

ST	speech therapist; sinus tachycardia; split thickness
STA	superficial temporal artery
stab	polymorphonuclear leukocytes in nonmature form
staph	*Staphylococcus aureus*
stat	immediately
STB	stillborn
ST BY	standby
STD	sexually transmitted disease; skin test dose
STD TF	standard tube feeding
STET	submaximal treadmill exercise test
STF	special tube feeding
STG	short-term goals
STH	soft tissue hemorrhage; somatotrophic hormone
STJ	subtalar joint
STM	short-term memory
sTNM	surgical-evaluative staging of cancer
STNR	symmetrical tonic neck reflex
STORCH	syphilis, toxoplasmosis, other agents, rubella, cytomegalovirus, and herpes
STPD	standard temperature and pressure-dry
strep	streptococcus
STS	serologic test for syphilis
STSG	split thickness skin graft
STU	shock trauma unit
S & U	supine and upright
SU	sensory urgency; Somogyi units
SUB	Skene's urethra and Bartholin's glands
sub q	subcutaneous
SUD	sudden unexpected death
SUID	sudden unexplained infant death
SUNDS	sudden unexpected nocturnal death syndrome
SUP	supinator; superior
supp	suppository
SUR	surgery; surgical
SV	single ventricle; stock volume; sigmoid volvulus
SVC	superior vena cava
SVCO	superior vena cava obstruction
SVD	spontaneous vaginal delivery
SVE	sterile vaginal examination
SVPB	supraventricular premature beat
SVR	supraventricular rhythm; systemic vascular resistance
SVRI	systemic vascular resistance index
SVT	supraventricular tachycardia
SW	social worker

SWD	short wave diathermy
SWFI	sterile water for injection
SWI	sterile water for injection
SWOG	Southwest Oncology Group
SWS	slow wave sleep; Sturge-Weber syndrome; student ward secretary
SWT	stab wound of the throat
Sx	symptom; signs; surgery
SZ	seizure; suction; schizophrenic
T	temperature
T1/2	half-life
T1	tricuspid first sound; first thoracic vertebra
T3	triiodothyronine
4	thyroxine
T-7	free thyroxine factor
TA	therapeutic abortion; temperature axillary; tricuspid atresia
Ta	tonometry applanation
T & A	tonsillectomy and adenoidectomy
T(A)	axillary temperature
TAA	total ankle arthroplasty; thoracic aortic aneurysm; tumor-associated antigen (antibodies); transverse aortic arch
TAB	therapeutic abortion; triple antibiotic; tablet
TAD	transverse abdominal diameter
TAE	transcatheter arterial embolization
TAF	tissue angiogenesis factor
TAH	total abdominal hysterectomy; total artificial heart
TAL	tendon Achilles lengthening
TANI	total axial node irradiation
TAO	thromboangiitis obliterans
TAPVC	total anomalous pulmonary venous connection
TAPVD	total anomalous pulmonary venous drainage
TAPVR	total anamalous pulmonary venous return
TAR	thrombocytopenia with absent radius
TARA	total articular replacement arthroplasty
TAS	therapeutics activities specialist
TAT	tetanus antitoxin; till all taken; Thematic Apperception Test
TB	tuberculosis
TBA	to be admitted; to be absorbed
TBB	transbronchial biopsy
tbc	tuberculosis
TBE	tick-borne encephalitis
TBG	thyroxine-binding globulin
TBI	total body irradiation

T bili	total bilirubin
tbl	tablespoon (15 mL)
TBM	tubule basement membrane
TBNA	treated but not admitted
TBPA	thyroxine-binding prealbumin
TBR	total bed rest
TBSA	total burn surface area
tbsp	tablespoon (15 mL)
TBV	total blood volume; transluminal balloon valvuloplasty
TBW	total body water
T/C	to consider
TC	throat culture; true conjugate
T & C	type and crossmatch; turn and cough
TCA	tricuspid atresia; terminal cancer
TCABG	triple coronary artery bypass graft
TCBS agar	thiosulfate-citrate-bile salt-sucrose agar
TCCB	transitional cell carcinoma of bladder
TCDB	turn, cough, and deep breathe
T-cell	small lymphocyte
TCH	turn, cough, hyperventilate
TCID50	median tissue culture doses
TCM	transcutaneous monitor; tissue culture media
TCMH	tumor-direct cell-mediated hypersensitivity
TCT	thrombin clotting
TCVA	thromboembolic cerebral vascular accident
TD	tardive dyskinesia; travelers diarrhea; Takayasu's disease; transverse diameter; tidal volume; treatment discontinued; tetanus-diphtheria toxoid
Td	tetanus-diphtheria toxoid
TDD	thoracic duct drainage
TDE	total daily energy (requirement)
TDF	tumor dose fractionation
TDK	tardive dyskinesia
TDM	therapeutic drug monitoring
TdP	torsades de pointes
TDT	tentative discharge tomorrow
TE	tracheoesophageal; trace elements; thromboembolism
T & E	trial and error
TEA	total elbow arthroplasty; thromboendarterectomy
TEC	total eosinophil count
TEDS®	anti-embolism stockings
TEE	transesophageal echocardiography
TEF	tracheoesophageal fistula
TEG	thromboelastogram

tele	telemetry
TEM	transmission electron microscopy
TEN	toxic epidermal necrolysis
TEN®	total enteral nutrition
TENS	transcutaneous electrical nerve stimulation
tert	tertiary
TES	treatment emergent symptoms; trace element solution
TET	treadmill exercise test
TF	tetralogy of Fallot; tactile fremitus; tube feeding; to follow
TFB	trifascicular block
TFTs	thyroid function tests
TG	triglycerides
TGA	transient global amnesia; transposition of the great arteries
TGF	tissue/transforming growth factor
TGFA	triglyceride fatty acid
TGS	tincture of green soap
TGT	thromboplastin generation test
TH	total hysterectomy; thyroid hormone; thrill
THA	total hip arthroplasty; transient hemispheric attack
THC	transhepatic cholangiogram
TH-CULT	throat culture
THE	transhepatic embolization
Ther Ex	therapeutic exercise
THI	transient hypogammaglobulinemia of infancy
THR	total hip replacement
TI	tricuspid insufficiency
TIA	transient ischemic attack
tib	tibia
TIBC	total iron binding capacity
TIE	transient ischemia episode
TIG	tetanus immune globulin
TIN	tubulointerstitial nephritis
tinct	tincture
TJ	triceps jerk
TJN	twin jet nebulizer
TKA	total knee arthroplasty
TKNO	to keep needle open
TKP	thermokeratoplasty
TKO	to keep open
TKR	total knee replacement
TL	tubal ligation; team leader; trial leave
TLC	triple lumen catheter; thin layer chromatography; total lung capacity; total lymphocyte count; tender loving care

TLI	total lymphoid irradiation
TLS	tumor lysis syndrome
TLV	total lung volume
TM	tympanic membrane; travecular meshwork
TMA	transmetatarsal amputation
TMB	transient monocular blindness
TMC	transmural colitis
TMET	treadmill exercise test
TMI	threatened myocardial infarction
TMJ	temporomandibular joint
TMP	trimethoprim; thallium myocardial perfusion
TMS	trace metal solution
TMTC	too many to count
Tn	normal intraocular tension
TNF	tumor necrosis factor
TNI	total nodal irradiation
TNM	tumor node metastasis
TNTC	too numerous to count
TO	telephone order
T(O)	oral temperature
TOA	tubo-ovarian abscess; time of arrival
TOF	tetralogy of Fallot
TOGV	transposition of the great vessels
TOL	trial of labor
tomo	tomography
TOP	termination of pregnancy
TOPP	a drug combination protocol
TOPV	trivalent oral polio vaccine
TORCH	toxoplasmosis, other (syphilis, hepatitis, Zoster), rubella, cytomegalovirus, and herpes simplex
TORP	total ossicular replacement prosthesis
TOS	thoracic outlet syndrome
TP	total protein; Todd's paralysis
TPA	tissue plasminogen activator; tissue polypeptide antigen; total parenteral alimentation
TPC	total patient care
TPD	tropical pancreatic diabetes
TPE	total protective environment
TPH	thromboembolic pulmonary hypertension
TPI	treponema pallidum immobilization test
TPM	temporary pacemaker
TPN	total parenteral nutrition
TP & P	time, place, and person
TPPE	time, person, place, and event

TPPN	total peripheral parenteral nutrition
TPR	temperature, pulse and respiration; temperature; total peripheral resistance
TPT	time to peak tension
TPVR	total peripheral vascular resistance
Tr	trace; tremor; treatment; tincture
T(R)	rectal temperature
TRA	therapeutic recreation associate
trach	tracheal; tracheostomy
Trans D	transverse diameter
TRC	tanned red cells
TRD	traction retinal detachment
Tren	Trendelenberg
TRH	thyrotropin-releasing hormone
TRIG	triglycerides
tRNA	transfer ribonucleic acid
TRNG	tetracycline resistant *Neisseria* gonorrhea
TRP	tubular reabsorption of phosphate
TRT	thermoradiotherapy
T3RU	triiodothyroxine resin uptake
TS	test solution; Tourette's syndrome
TSA	total shoulder arthroplasty
TSAR®	tape surrounded Appli-rulers®
TSBB	transtracheal selective bronchial brushing
TSD	Tay-Sachs disease; target to skin distance
T set	tracheotomy set
TSF	triceps skin fold
TSH	thyroid stimulating hormone
tsp	teaspoon (5 mL)
TSP	total serum protein
TSR	total shoulder replacement
TSS	toxic shock syndrome
TST	titmus stereocuity test
T & T	touch and tone
TT	thrombin time; thymol turbidity; twitch tension; transtracheal; tilt table
TT3	total serum triiodothyronine
TT4	total thyroxine
TTA	total toe arthroplasty
TTN	transient tachypnea of the newborn
TTNB	transient tachypnea of the newborn
TTP	thrombotic thrombocytopenic purpura
TTS	through the skin
TTVP	temporary transvenous pacemaker

TTY-TDD	teletypewriter for the deaf
TU	tuberculin units
TUN	total urinary nitrogen
TUR	transurethral resection
T3UR	triiodothyronine uptake ratio
TURB	turbidity
TURBN	transurethral resection bladder tumor
TURP	transurethral resection of prostate
TURV	transurethral resection valves
TV	tidal volume; trial visit; *Trichomonas vaginalis*
TVC	triple voiding cystogram; true vocal cord
TVH	total vaginal hysterectomy
TVP	transvenous pacemaker
TW	test weight
TWD	total white and differential count
TWE	tapwater enema
TWETC	tapwater enema till clear
TWWD	tapwater wet dressing
Tx	treatment; therapy; traction; transfuse; transplant
TxA2	thromboxane A2
Tyl	tyloma
U	units; urine
U/1	1 finger breadth below umbilicus
1/U	1 finger over umbilicus
U/	at umbilicus
UA	uric acid; urinalysis; unauthorized absence; uncertain about
UAC	umbilical artery
UAE	urinary albumin excretion
UAL	umbilical artery line
UAO	upper airway obstruction
UAT	up as tolerated
UAVC	univentricular atrioventricular connection
UBF	unknown black female
UBI	ultraviolet blood irradiation
UBM	unknown black male
UC	urine culture; urethral catheter; uterine contraction; ulcerative colitis
U & C	urethral and cervical
UCD	usual childhood diseases
UCG	urinary chorionic-gonadotropins
UCHD	usual childhood diseases
UCI	urethral catheter in
UCO	urethral catheter out

UCX	urine culture
UD	urethral discharge
UDC	usual diseases of childhood
UE	upper extremity
UES	upper esophageal sphincter
UFO	unflagged order
UFR	uroflowmetry
UG	urogenital
UGDP	University Group Diabetes Program
UGH	uveitis, glaucoma, hyphema
UGI	upper gastrointestinal series
UHBI	upper hemibody irradiation
UHDDS	Uniform Hospital Discharge Data Set
UID	once daily
UIQ	upper inner quadrant
U/L	upper and lower
ULN	upper limits of normal
ULQ	upper left quadrant
UK	urokinase; unknown
UN	urinary nitrogen
UNA	urinary nitrogen appearance; urine sodium
ung	ointment
UNK	unknown
UOQ	upper outer quadrant
UPEP	urine protein electrophoresis
UPJ	ureteropelvic junction
U/P ratio	urine to plasma ratio
UPP	urethral pressure profile studies
UPT	urine pregnancy test
UR	utilization review
URI	upper respiratory infection
urol	urology
US	ultrasonography; unit secretary
USA	unit services assistant
USB	upper sternal border
USG	ultrasonography
USI	urinary stress incontinence
USN	ultrasonic nebulizer
USP	*United States Pharmacopeia*
USRDS	United States Renal Data System
UTD	up to date
ut dict	as directed
UTF	usual throat flora
UTI	urinary tract infection

UTO	upper tibial osteotomy
UTZ	ultrasound
UUN	urine urea nitrogen
UV	ultraviolet
UVA	ultraviolet A light; ureterovesical angle
UVB	ultraviolet B light
UVC	umbilical vein catheter
UVJ	ureterovesical junction
UVL	ultraviolet light
UVR	ultraviolet rays
UWF	unknown white female
UWM	unknown white male
V	vomiting; vein; vagina; five
VA	Veterans Administration; visual acuity; vacuum aspiration
VAC	ventriculoarterial connections
VAD	vascular/venous access device
vag	vagina
VAG HYST	vaginal hysterectomy
VAH	Veterans Administration Hospital
VAMC	Veterans Administration Medical Center
VAPA	a drug combination protocol
VAR	variant
VAS	vascular; visual analogue scale
VASC	Visual-Auditory Screen Test for Children
VAS RAD	vascular radiology
VB	VanBuren (catheter)
VBAC	vaginal birth after cesarean
VBI	vertebrobasilar insufficiency
VBS	vertebral-basilar system
VC	vital capacity; vena cava; vocal cords; color vision; vomiting center
VCG	vectorcardiography
VCT	venous clotting time
VCU	voiding cystourethrogram
VCUG	vesicoureterogram; voiding cystourethrogram
VD	venereal disease; volume of distribution; voided
VDA	visual discriminatory acuity; venous digital angiogram
VDG	venereal disease—gonorrhea
VDH	valvular disease of the heart
VDRL	Venereal Disease Research Laboratory (test for syphilis)
VDRR	vitamin D-resistant rickets
VDS	venereal disease—syphilis
VDT	video display terminal

VE	vaginal examination; vertex; volume of expired gas
VEB	ventricular ectopic beat
VEE	Venezuelan equine encephalitis
vent	ventricular; ventral
VEP	visual evoked potential
VER	visual evoked response; ventricular escape rhythm
VF	ventricular fibrillation; vision field; vocal fremitus
V fib	ventricular fibrillation
VFP	vitreous fluorophotometry
VG	vein graft; ventricular gallop; very good
VH	vaginal hysterectomy; viral hepatitis; vitreous hemorrhage; Veterans Hospital
VI	volume index; six
vib	vibration
VID	videodensitometry
VIG	vaccinia immune globulin
VIP	voluntary interruption of pregnancy; vasoactive intestinal peptide
VISC	vitreous infusion suction cutter
VIT	vitamin; vital; venom immunotherapy
vit cap	vital capacity
VKC	vernal keratoconjunctivitis
VLBW	very low birth weight
VLDL	very low density lipoprotein
VLH	ventrolateral nucleus of the hypothalamus
VMH	ventromedial hypothalamus
VNA	Visiting Nurses Association
VO	verbal order
VOCTOR	void on call to operating room
VOD	vision right eye; venocclusive disease
VOL	voluntary
VOR	vestibular ocular reflex
VOS	vision left eye
VOU	vision both eyes
VP	venous pressure; variegate porphyria; ventriculoperitoneal; ventricular-peritoneal
V & P	ventilation and perfusion; vagotomy and pyloroplasty
VPB	ventricular premature beat
VPC	ventricular premature contractions
VPDs	ventricular premature depolarizations
VPL	ventro-posterolateral
V/Q	ventilation/perfusion (scan)
VR	ventricular rhythm; verbal reprimand
VRA	visual reinforcement audiometry

VS	vital signs; versus
VSD	venous stasis retinopathy
VSS	vital signs stable
VT	ventricular tachycardia; tidal volume
v tach	ventricular tachycardia
VTE	venous thromboembolism
VTX	vertex
VV	varicose veins
V & V	vulva and vagina
V/V	volume to volume ratio
VVFR	vesicovaginal fistula repair
VVOR	visual-vestibulo-ocular-reflex
VW	vessel wall
VWM	ventricular wall motion
VZ	varicella zoster
VZIG	varicella zoster immune globulin
VZV	varicella zoster virus
w	white; with; widowed
WA	while awake; when awake
WAIS	Wechsler Adult Intelligence Scale
WAIS-R	Wechsler Adult Intelligence Scale—Revised
WAP	wandering atrial pacemaker
WAS	Wiskott-Aldrich syndrome
WASS	Wasserman test
WB	whole blood; weight bearing
WBAT	weight bearing as tolerated
WBC	white blood cell/count
WBH	whole-body hyperthermia
WBN	wellborn nursery
WC	wheelchair; white count; ward clerk; whooping cough
W/D	warm and dry; withdrawal
W–D	wet to dry
WDHA	watery diarrhea; hypokalemia, and achlorhydria
WDL	well-differentiated lymphocyte
WDLL	well-differentiated lymphocytic lymphoma
WDWN-BF	well-developed, well-nourished black female
WDWN-BM	well-developed, well-nourished black male
WDWN-WF	well-developed, well-nourished white female
WDWN-WM	well-developed, well-nourished white male
WE	weekend
WEE	western equine encephalitis
WEP	weekend pass
WF	white female

WFI	water for injection
WFL	within functional limits
WFR	wheel-and-flare reaction
WHO	World Health Organization
WHV	woodchuck hepatitis virus
WHVP	wedged hepatic venous pressure
WIA	wounded in action
WIC	women, infants, and children
WID	widow; widower
WISC	Wechsler Intelligence Scale for Children
WLS	wet lung syndrome
WLT	waterload test
WKS	Wernicke-Korsakoff syndrome
WM	white male
WMA	wall motion abnormality
WN	well-nourished
WND	wound
WNL	within normal limits
W/O	without
WO	written order; weeks old
WP	whirlpool
WPFM	Wright peak flow meter
WPPSI	Wechsler Preschool Primary Scale of Intelligence
WPW	Wolff-Parkinson-White
WR	Wasserman reaction; wrist
WS	ward secretary; watt seconds
wt	weight
WWAC	walk with aid of cane
W/U	workup
W/V	weight-to-volume ratio
W/W	weight-to-weight ratio
X	cross-match; start of anesthesia; except; times, ten; break
X3	orientation as to person, place, and time
X & D	examination and diagnosis
XM	cross-match
X-mat	cross-match
XMM	xeromammography
XRT	radiotherapy
XS-LIM	exceeds limits of procedure
XT	exotropia
XX	normal female sex chromosome type
XY	normal male sex chromosome type

YACP	young adult chronic patient
YAG	yttrium aluminum garnert (laser)
YF	yellow fever
YJV	yellow jacket venom
YLC	youngest living child
YO	years old
YORA	younger-onset rheumatoid arthritis
YSC	yolk sac carcinoma
ZEEP	zero end-expiratory pressure
ZES	Zollinger-Ellison syndrome
Z-ESR	zeta erythrocyte sedimentation rate
ZIFT	zygote intrafallopian transfer
ZIG	zoster serum immune globulin
ZIP	zoster immune plasma
ZIZ	zoster serum immune globulin
ZMC	zygomatic
Zn	zinc

Terms Used in Prescription Writing

Term	Meaning	Abbreviation
acidum	an acid	*acid, ac.*
ad	to, up to	*ad*
adde, addatur	add, let be added	*add.*
ad libitum	as much as desired	*ad lib.*
admove, admoveatur	apply, let be applied	*admov.*
ad partes dolentes	to the painful parts	*ad part. dolent.*
agita, agitetur	shake, stir	*agit.*
albus, -a, -um	white	*alb.*
aluminum	aluminum	*al.*
ampulla	an ampul	*ampul.*
ana	of each	*aa*
ante	before	*a.*
ante cibos	before meals	*a.c., ac*
ante cibum	before food	*a.c., ac*
aqua	water	*aq.*
aqua bulliens	boiling water	*aq. bull.*
aqua destillata	distilled water	*aq. dest.*
balneum	bath	*baln.*
balneum vaporis	steam bath	*baln. vap., b.v.*
bene	well	*bene*
bis in die	twice a day	*b.i.d., BID*
bromidum	a bromide	*brom.*
calcium	calcium	*calc., Ca*
capsula, capsulae	capsule, capsules	*cap., caps.*
carbons	carbonate	*carb.*
cataplasma	a cataplasm, poultice	*catapl.*
charta, chartae	paper(s), powder(s)	*chart.*
charta cerata	waxed paper	*chart. cerat.*
chartula	(small) paper, powder	*chart.*
chioridum	chloride	*chlorid.*
cochleare amplum	tablespoonful	*coch. ampl/.*

Term	Meaning	Abbreviation
cochleare magnum	tablespoonful	*coch. mag.*
cochleare parvum	teaspoonful	*coch. parv.*
collodium	collodion	*collod.*
collunarium	nasal douche	*collun.*
collyrium	eye lotion, eyewash	*collyr.*
compositus, -a, -um	compound	*comp., co.*
congius	gallon	*cong., C.*
cum	with	*c*
cum aqua	with water	*cum aq.*
cum cibos	with meals, food	*cc*
da, detur, dentur	give, let be given	*d., det.*
dentur tales doses	give of such doses	*d.t.d. DTD*
diebus alternis	on alternate days	*dieb. alt., QOD*
dilutus, -a, -um	dilute	*dil.*
dimidius, -a, -um	one half	*dim.*
dividatur in partes aequales	let be divided into equal parts	*div. in par. aeq.*
dosis	dose	*dos.*
durante	while pain lasts	*dur. dol.*
elixir	an elixir	*elix., el.*
emplastrum	a plaster	*emp.*
emulsum	emulsion	*emuls.*
et	and	*et*
ex aqua	in water	*ex aq.*
ex modo praescripto	in the manner prescribed	*e.m.p.*
extractum	an extract	*ext.*
fac, fiat, fiant	make	*ft.*
ferrum	iron	*ferr.*
fiant	let them be made	*ft.*
fiat	let it be made	*ft.*
fiat lege artis	let be made according to the law of the art	*f.l.a.*
filtra	filter	*filt.*
gargarisma	a gargle	*garg.*
gelatum	a gel, jelly	*gel.*
glyceritum	a glycerite	*glycer.*
glycerogelatinum	glycerogelatin	*glycerogel.*
granum, grana	a grain, grains	*gr.*
gutta, guttae	drop, drops	*gt., gtt.*
guttatim	drop by drop	*guttat.*
hora decubitus	at bed hour, at bedtime	*hor. decub., h.d.*
hora somni	before sleep	*h.s., HS*

Term	Meaning	Abbreviation
hydrargyrum	mercury	*hydrarg.*
in	in, into, within	*in*
in aqua	in water	*in aq.*
in die	in a day	*in d.*
infusum	an infusion	*inf.*
inhalatio	inhalation	*inhal.*
in vitro	in glass	*in vit.*
iodidum	an iodide	*iodid.*
kalium	potassium	*K*
lavatio	a wash	*lavat.*
leviter	lightly	*lev., levit.*
linimentum	a linament	*lin.*
liquor	a liquor, solution	*liq.*
lotio	a lotion	*lot.*
magma	a magma, milk	*mag.*
magnesium	magnesium	*Mg*
magnus, -a, -um	large	*mag.*
mane primo	first thing in the morning	*man. prim.*
misce	you mix	*M.*
mistura	a mixture	*mist.*
mitte tales	send such	*mitt. tal.*
modo dictu	as directed	*m. dict.*
modo praescripto	in the manner prescribed	*mod. praes., m.p.*
mollis	soft	*moll.*
moro dicto	in the manner directed	*mor. dict.*
mucliago	a mucilage	*mucil.*
natrium	sodium	*Na*
nebula	a spray	*nebul.*
nihil album	zinc oxide	*nihil alb.*
nocte	at night	*noct.*
nocte maneque	night and morning	*noct. maneq.*
non repetatur	do not repeat	*non rep.*
octarius	a pint	*O., oct.*
oculo dextro	in the right eye	*ocul. dext., o.d., O.D.*
oculo sinistro	in the left eye	*ocul. sinist., o.s., O.S.*
oculo utro	each eye	*ocul. utro, o.u., O.U.*
odontalgicum	toothache drops	*odont.*
oleum	an oil	*ol.*
omni hora	every hour	*omn. hor., qh*

Term	Meaning	Abbreviation
omni mane vel nocte	every morning or night	*omn. man. vel noct.*
omni quarta hora	every four hours	*omn. 4 hr., q4h*
omnis	all, every	*omn.*
omni secunda hora	every two hours	*omn. 2 hr, q2h*
omni tertia hora	every three hours	*omn. tert. hor., q3h*
optimus, -a, -um	the best	*opt.*
partes aequales	equal parts	*p.e., part. aeq.*
parvus, -a, -um	small	*parv.*
pasta	a paste	*pat.*
pastillus	lozenge, pastille	*pastil.*
per diem	per day	*per diem*
per os	by mouth	*per os, PO*
phosphas	a phosphatate	*phos.*
pilula, pilulae	a pill, pills	*pil.*
placebo	I please	*placebo*
ponderosus	heavy	*pond.*
post cibum, post cibos	after food, after meals	*p.c., PC*
praecipitatus	precipitated	*ppt.*
pro dose	for a dose	*pro dos.*
pro ratione aetatis	according to age	*pro rat. aet.*
pro recto	rectally	*pro rect.*
pro re nata	as occasion arises	*p.r.n., PRN*
pro urethra	urethral	*pro ureth*
pro usu externo	for external use	*pro us. ext.*
pro vagina	vaginal	*pro vagin.*
pulvis, pulveres	a powder, powders	*pulv.*
quantum libet/ placet/vis	as much as you wish	*q.l., q.p., q.v.*
quantum sufficit	as much as suffices	*q.s., QS*
quaque die	every day	*q.d., QD*
quaque hora	every hour	*qq. hor., qh*
quater in die	four times a day	*q.i.d.*
recipe	take thou	*Rx.*
ruber, rubra, rubrum	red	*rub.*
sal	salt	*sal*
saturatus, -a, -um	saturated	*sat.*
secundum artem	according to art	*s.a.*
semel	once	*semel*
semi, semis	one half	*ss, sem.*
semihora	half hour	*semih.*
sesqui	one and one half	*sesq.*
signa, signetur	write, let it be written	*sig., S.*

Term	Meaning	Abbreviation
simul	at the same time	*sumul*
sine	without	*s., w/o*
sine aqua	without water	*sine aq.*
si opus sit	if there is need	*si op. sit, s.o.s.*
sodium	sodium	*sod., Na*
solutio	a solution	*sol.*
solutio saturata	a saturated solution	*sol. sat.*
spiritus	a spirit	*sp.*
spiritus vini rectifi-catus	alcohol	*sp. vin. rect., s.v.r.*
spiritus vini tenuis	proof spirit, diluted alcohol	*sp. vin. ten., s.v.t.*
statim	immediately	*stat., STAT*
sume, sumendus	take, to be taken	*sum.*
suppositoria	suppositories	*suppos.*
suppositoria rectalia	rectal suppositories	*suppos. rect., RS*
suppositorium	a suppository	*suppos.*
syrupus	a syrup	*syr.*
tabletta	tablet	*tab.*
tales doses	such doses	*tal. dos.*
talis, tales, talia	such	*tal.*
ter	three times, thrice	*t.*
ter in die	three times a day	*t.i.d., TID*
tinctura	a tincture	*tr., tinct.*
trituratio	a trituration	*trit.*
trochiscus, trochisci	a troche, troches	*troch.*
uncia	ounce	*oz.*
unguentum	an ointment	*ungt.*
ut dictum	as told, as directed	*ut dict.*
vaccinum	a vaccine	*vac.*
vel	vel	*or*
vinum	a wine	*vin.*
viridis	green	*vir.*

TABLES AND STANDARDS

This section is designed to put a number of needed information points into one place. The Conversion Factors segment provides the formulas and data needed to quickly calculate milliequivalents and a list of weights and measures. The Anthropometric segment provides creatine clearance formulas, ideal body weight and surface area nomograms. The Laboratory Indices provide typical reference ranges for most common clinical laboratory tests. This segment is followed by a list of tests that is organized first by body system and then by type of test. The clinical laboratory segments are particularly helpful when confronted with a patient who knows what was tested but not necessarily for what. The normal values are also helpful but care needs to be exercised when applying them to individual patients since reference ranges can vary widely depending on where the test was done.

Finally, a quick checklist to help in evaluating the clinical literature is included as is the Indian Health Service patient counseling algorithm.

Conversion Calculations

TEMPERATURE

Fahrenheit to Celsius (°F−32) × 5/9 = °C
Celsius to Fahrenheit (°C × 9/5) + 32 = °F
Celsius to Kelvin °C + 273 = K

WEIGHTS AND MEASURES

Metric Weight Equivalents

1 kilogram (kg)	=	1000 grams
1 gram (g)	=	1000 milligrams
1 milligram (mg)	=	0.001 gram
1 microgram (mcg, μg)	=	0.001 milligram
1 nanogram (ng)	=	0.001 microgram
1 picogram (pg)	=	0.001 nanogram
1 femtogram (fg)	=	0.001 picogram

Metric Volume Equivalents

1 liter (L)	=	1000 milliliters
1 deciliter (dL)	=	100 milliliters
1 milliliter (mL)	=	0.001 liter
1 microliter (μL)	=	0.001 milliliter
1 nanoliter (nL)	=	0.001 microliter
1 picoliter (pL)	=	0.001 nanoliter
1 femtoliter (fL)	=	0.001 picoliter

Apothecary Weight Equivalents

1 scruple (℈)	=	20 grains (gr)
60 grains (gr)	=	1 dram (ʒ)
8 drams (ʒ)	=	1 ounce (℥)
1 ounce (℥)	=	480 grains
12 ounces (℥)	=	1 pound (lb)

Apothecary Volume Equivalents

60 minims (m)	=	1 fluidram (fl ʒ)
8 fluidrams (fl ʒ)	=	1 fluid ounce (fl ʒ)
1 fluid ounce (fl ʒ)	=	480 minims
16 fluid ounces (fl ʒ)	=	1 pint (pt)

Avoirdupois Equivalents

1 ounce (oz)	=	437.5 grans
16 ounces (oz)	=	1 pound (lb)

Weight/Volume Equivalents

1 mg/dL	=	10 μg/mL
1 mg/dL	=	1 mg%
1 ppm	=	1 mg / L

Conversion Equivalents

1 gram (g)	=	15.43 grains
1 grain (gr)	=	64.8 milligrams
1 ounce (ʒ)	=	31.1 grams
1 ounce (oz)	=	28.35 grams
1 pound (lb)	=	453.6 grams
1 kilogram (kg)	=	2.2 pounds
1 milliliter (mL)	=	16.23 minims
1 minim (m)	=	0.06 milliliter
1 fluid ounce (fl oz)	=	29.57 mL
1 pint (pt)	=	473.2 mL
0.1 mg	=	1/600 gr
0.12 mg	=	1/500 gr
0.15 mg	=	1/400 gr
0.2 mg	=	1/300 gr
0.3 mg	=	1/200 gr
0.4 mg	=	1/150 gr
0.5 mg	=	1/120 gr
0.6 mg	=	1/100 gr
0.8 mg	=	1/80 gr
1.0 mg	=	1/65 gr

MICROMOLECULES

SI units (*le Système International d'Unités*) are used to express clinical laboratory and serum drug concentrations. The SI system uses moles (mol) to designate the amount of a substance instead of using units of mass such as micrograms. A molar solution contains one mole (grams of the substance divided by molecular weight) of the solute in one liter of solution. Below is the formula used to covert units of mass to moles (mg/mL to mmol/L or ng/mL to nmol/L, etc.)

Micromoles per Liter (mmol/L)

$$\mu mol/L = \frac{\text{Drug Concentration } (\mu g/mL) \times 1000}{\text{Molecular weight (g/mol)}}$$

MILLIEQUIVALENTS

A milliequivalent is the gram weight of a substance that will combine with or replace one milligram (one millimole) of hydrogen. A milliequivalent is 1/1000 of an equivalent weight.

Milliequivalents per Liter (mEq/L)

$$mEq/L = \frac{\text{Weight of salt} \times \text{Valence of ion} \times 1000}{\text{Molecular weight of salt}}$$

$$\text{Weight of salt (g)} = \frac{mEq/L \times \text{Molecular Weight of salt}}{\text{Valence of ion} \times 1000}$$

Valences and Atomic Weights of Selected Ions.

Substance	Electrolyte	Valence	Molecular Weight
Calcium	Ca^{2+}	2	40
Chloride	Cl^-	1	35.5
Magnesium	Mg^{2+}	2	24
Phosphate	HPO_4^{2-} (80%)	1.8	96
(ph = 7.4)	$H_2PO_4^-$ (20%)	1.8	96
Potassium	K^+	1	39
Sodium	Na^+	1	23
Sulfate	SO_4^{2-}	2	96

Approximate Milliequivalents and Weights of Selected Ions.

Salt	mEq/g Salt	Mg Salt/mEq
Calcium Carbonate [$CaCO_3$]	20	50
Calcium Chloride [$CaCl_2-2H_2O$]	14	73
Calcium Gluconate (Ca gluconate$_2-1H_2O$)	4	224
Calcium Lactate (Ca lactate$-5H_2O$)	6	154
Magnesium sulfate ($MgSO_4$)	16	60
Magnesium sulfate ($MgSO_4-7H_2O$)	8	123
Potassium acetate (K acetate)	10	98
Potassium chloride (KCl)	13	75
Potassium citrate K_3 citrate$-1H_2O$)	9	108
Potassium iodide (KI)	6	166
Sodium bicarbonate ($NaHCO_3$)	12	84
Sodium chloride (NaCl)	17	58
Sodium citrate (Na_3 citrate$-2H_2O$)	10	98
Sodium iodide (NaI)	7	150
Sodium lactate (Na lactate)	9	112

ANION GAP

The anion gap is the concentration of plasma anions that is normally not measured by plasma electrolyte assays. It is useful in the evaluation of acid-base disorders. The anion gap is greater with increased plasma concentrations of endogenous (e.g., phosphate, sulfate, lactate, ketoacids) or exogenous (e.g., salicylate, penicillin, ethylene glycol, ethanol, methanol) compounds. The formulas for calculating the anion gap are as follow:

$$(1) \text{ Anion Gap} = (Na^+ + K^+) - (Cl^- + HCO_3^-)$$

or

$$(2) \text{ Anion Gap} = Na^+ - (Cl^- + HCO_3^-)$$

where

the anticipated normal value for 1 is 11–20 mmol/L
the anticipated normal value is 7–16 mmol/L (Note that there are variances at the upper and lower limits of the normal range. Ranges may vary from laboratory to laboratory.)

Anthropometrics

CREATININE CLEARANCE FORMULAS

Formulas for Evaluating Creatinine Clearance in Patients with Stable Renal Function

Adults (Age 18 Years and Older) [1]

$$Cl_{cr} \text{ (Males)} = \frac{(140 - Age) \times (Weight)}{Cl_s \times 72}$$

$$Cl_{cr} \text{ (Females)} = 0.85 \times (male\ Cl_{cr})$$

where

Cl_{cr} = creatinine clearance in mL/min
Cl_s = serum creatinine in mg/dL
Age in years.
Weight in kilograms.
(Some studies suggest that the prediction accuracy of this formula for women is better *without* the correction factor of 0.85)

Children (Age 1–18 Years) [2]

$$Cl_{cr} = \frac{0.48 \times (Height) \times (BSA)}{Cr_s \times 1.73}$$

where

BSA = body surface area in m^2
Cl_{cr} = creatinine clearance in mL/min
Cl_s = serum creatinine in mg/dL
Height is in centimeters.

Creatinine Clearance from a Measured Urine Collection

$$\text{Formula: } Cl_{cr} \text{ (mL/min)} = \frac{U \times V^*}{P \times t}$$

where

U = concentration of creatinine in specimen (in same units as P)

V = volume of urine (mL)

P = concentration of creatinine in serum at the midpoint of the urine collection period (same units as U)

t = time of the urine collection period in minutes

IDEAL BODY WEIGHT

Ideal body weight (IBW) is the weight expected for person of normal weight for a given height. The IBW formulas below, as well as many life-insurance tables, can be used to estimate IBW. Most dosing methods described in the literature make use of IBW as a method in dosing obese patients.

Adults (18 Years and Older) [3]

IBW (Males) = 50 + (2.3 × Height in inches over 5 feet)

IBW (Females) = 45.5 + (2.3 × Height in inches over 5 feet)

where ideal body weight is in kilograms

Children (1–18 Years) [2]
Children Under 5 Feet Tall

$$IBW = \frac{(\text{Height}^2 \times 1.65)}{1000}$$

where ideal body weight is in kilograms and height is in centimeters

Children 5 Feet or Taller in Height

IBW (Males) = 39 + (2.27 × Height in inches over 5 feet)

IBW (Females) = 42.2 + (2.27 × Height in inches over 5 feet)

where ideal body weight is in kilograms

---

*The product of $U \times V$ equals the production of creatinine during the collection period and should equal 20–25 mg/kg/day ideal body weight in males and 15–20 mg/kg/day ideal body weight in females. If the value is less than this value, insufficient urine collection may have occurred and Cl_{cr} will be underestimated.)

BODY SURFACE AREA OF ADULTS AND CHILDREN—NOMOGRAMS

Calculating Body Surface Area in Infants and Adults

To determine body surface area for infants and adults, lay a straightedge on the corresponding height and weight points for the child and read the intersecting point on the surface area scale.

Nomogram for Determining Body Surface Area from Height and Weight (Infants) [4]

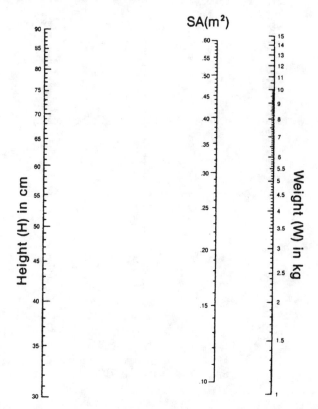

$$SA = W^{0.5378} \times H^{0.3964} \times 0.024265$$

SA(m^2)
Height (H) in centimeters
Weight (W) in kilograms

Nomogram for Determining Body Surface Area from Height and Weight (Adults) [5]

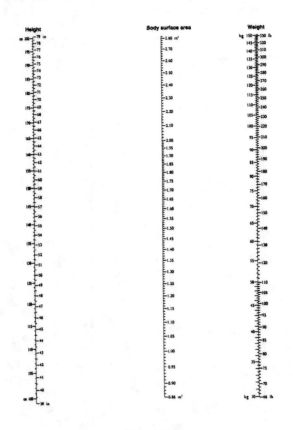

$$SA = W^{0.425} \times H^{0.725} \times 71.84$$

SA(m^2)
Height (H) in centimeters
Weight (W) in kilograms

REFERENCES

1. Cockcroft DW, Gault MH. Prediction of creatinine clearance from serum creatinine. *Nephron*, 1976; 16:31–41.

2. Traub SL, Johnson CE. Comparison of methods of estimating creatinine clearance in children. *Am J Hosp Pharm*, 1980; 37:195–201.

3. Devine BJ, Gentamicin therapy. *Drug Intell Clin Pharm*. 1974; 8:650–5.

4. From Haycock GB et al. Geometric method for measuring body surface area: a height-weight formula validated in infants, children, and adults. *J. Pediatr*, 1978; 93:62–6.

5. DuBois and DuBois. *Arch Intern Med*, 1916; 17:863.

Laboratory Indices

BLOOD, SERUM, PLASMA CHEMISTRY; URINE, RENAL FUNCTION TESTS; HEMATOLOGY

The following table includes typical reference ranges for clinical laboratory tests in common use. Reference ranges for laboratory tests may vary widely among testing facilities, often as a result of methodologic differences. It is therefore always advisable to obtain reference ranges from the laboratory performing the analyses. Laboratory test results should never be accepted without correct identification of the units of measurement, because most tests can be reported in several systems of measurement. The table presents both conventional and international (usually the same as *Système International*, or SI) units.

The following abbreviations are used to identify the specimen:

(P)—Plasma
(S)—Serum
(U)—Urine
(WB)—Whole Blood
(WB, art)—Whole Blood, Arterial

This section was reprinted from *1999 Handbook of Clinical Drug Data*, 9th edition, P. O. Anderson et al., © 1999, Appleton & Lange. Reproduced with permission of The McGraw-Hill Companies.

Blood, Serum, Plasma Chemistry.

Test/Specimen	Age Group or Other Factor	Reference Range	
		Conventional	International Units
Acid Phosphatase (S)		0.11–0.60 units/L	0.11–0.60 units/L
Alanine Aminotransferase (S) (ALT, SGPT)		units/L	units/L
	Adult	8–20	8–20
	>60 yr, M	7–24	7–24
	>60 yr, F	7–16	7–16
Alkaline Phosphatase (S)		units/L	units/L
	Child	20–150	20–150
	Adult	20–70	20–70
	>60 yr	30–75	30–75
Ammonia Nitrogen (S,P)	Adult	15–45 µg/dL	11–32 µmol/L
Amylase (S)		units/L	units/L
	Adult	25–125	25–125
	>70 yr	20–160	20–160
Anion Gap ($Na^+ - [Cl^- + HCO_3^-])(P)$		7–16 mEq/L	7–16 mmol/L
Aspartate Aminotransferase (S) (AST, SGOT)		units/L	units/L
	Adult	8–20	8–20
	>60 yr, M	11–26	11–26
	>60 yr, F	10–20	10–20
Bicarbonate (S)		mEq/L	mmol/L
	Arterial	21–28	21–28
	Venous	22–29	22–29
(WB, art)	Adult	18–23	18–23

Blood, Serum, Plasma Chemistry (continued).

Test/Specimen	Age Group or Other Factor	Reference Range	
		Conventional	International Units
Bilirubin (S)		*mg/dL*	*mmol/L*
Total	Child, Adult	0.2–10	3.4–17.1
Conjugated (direct)	Child, Adult	0–0.2	0–3.4
Calcium (S)		*mg/dL*	*µmol/L*
Ionized	Adult	4.48–4.92	1.12–1.23
Total	Child	8.8–10.8	2.20–2.70
	Adult	8.4–10.2	2.10–2.55
Carbon Dioxide, Partial Pressure (WB, art) (pCO$_2$)		*mm Hg*	*kPa*
	Adult, M	35–48	4.66–6.38
	Adult, F	32–45	4.26–5.99
Chloride (S,P)		98–107 mEq/L	98–107 mmol/L
Cholesterol, Total (S,P)		*mg/dL*	*mmol/L*
	Child	120–200	3.11–5.18
	Adolescent	120–210	3.11–5.44
	Adult	140–310	3.63–8.03
	Desired, Adult	140–220	3.63–5.70
Cortisol (S,P)		*µg/dL*	*nmol/L*
	08:00 hr	5–23	138–635
	16:00 hr	3–15	83–414
	20:00 hr	≤50% of 08:00 hr	≤50% of 08:00 hr
Creatine Kinase (CK)(S)		*units/L*	*units/L*
	Adult, M	38–174	38–174
	Adult, F	26–140	26–140

Blood, Serum, Plasma Chemistry (continued).

Test/Specimen	Age Group or Other Factor	Conventional		International Units	
		Normal	Diabetic	Normal	Diabetic
Creatinine (S,P)		*mg/dL*		*µmol/L*	
	Child	0.3–0.7		27–62	
	Adolescent	0.5–1.0		44–88	
	Adult, M	0.7–1.3		62–115	
	Adult, F	0.6–1.1		53–97	
(γ)-Glutamyltransferase (S) (GGT)		*units/L*		*units/L*	
	Adult, M	9–50		9–50	
	Adult, F	8–40		8–40	
Glucose, 2-hr Postprandial (S)		<120 mg/dL		<6.7 mmol/L	
Glucose Tolerance Test (S) (Oral)		*mg/dL*		*mmol/L*	
	Fasting	70–105	>140	3.9–5.8	>7.8
	60 min	120–170	≥200	6.7–9.4	≥11.1
	90 min	100–140	≥200	5.6–7.8	≥11.1
	120 min	70–120	≥140	3.9–6.7	≥7.8
HDL-Cholesterol (S,P)		*mg/dL*		*mmol/L*	
	15–19 yr, M	30–65		0.78–1.68	
	15–19 yr, F	30–70		0.78–1.81	
	20–29 yr, M	30–70		0.78–1.81	
	20–29 yr, F	30–75		0.78–1.94	
	30–39 yr, M	30–70		0.78–1.81	
	30–39 yr, F	30–80		0.78–2.07	
	>40 yr, M	30–70		0.78–1.81	
	>40 yr, F	30–85		0.78–2.20	

Values for Blacks 10 mg/dL higher.

Blood, Serum, Plasma Chemistry (continued).

Test/Specimen	Age Group or Other Factor	Reference Range Conventional	International Units
Iron (S)		*µg/dL*	*mmol/L*
	Child	50–120	8.95–21.48
	Adult, M	65–170	11.64–30.43
	Adult, F	50–170	8.95–30.43
Iron Binding Capacity, Total (S) (TIBC)		250–450 µg/dL	44.75–80.55 µmol/L
Isocitrate Dehydrogenase (S)		1.2–7.0 units/L	1.2–7.0 units/L
Lactate Dehydrogenase (S)		*units/L*	*units/L*
	Child	60–170	60–170
	Adult	100–190	100–190
	>60 yr	110–210	110–210
Isozymes (S)		*% of Total*	*Fraction of Total*
	Fraction 1	14–26	0.14–0.26
	Fraction 2	29–39	0.29–0.39
	Fraction 3	20–26	0.20–0.26
	Fraction 4	8–16	0.08–0.16
	Fraction 5	6–16	0.06–0.16
Lead (WB)		*µg/dL*	*µmol/L*
	Child	<15	<0.72
	Adult	<30	<1.45
Lipase (S)		*units/L*	*units/L*
	Adult	10–150	10–150
	>60 yr	18–180	18–180

Blood, Serum, Plasma Chemistry (continued).

Test/Specimen	Age Group or Other Factor	Reference Range	
		Conventional	International Units
β-Lipoprotein (LDL)(S)		28–53% of total lipoproteins	0.28–0.53
Magnesium (S)		*mEq/L*	*mmol/L*
	6–12 yr	1.7–2.1	0.70–0.86
	12–20 yr	1.7–2.2	0.70–0.91
	Adult	1.6–2.6	0.66–1.07
Osmolality (S)		*mOsmol/kg*	*mOsmol/kg*
	Child, Adult	275–295	275–295
	>60 yr	280–301	280–301
Osmolal Gap		≤10	≤10
Measured Osmolality—Calculated Osmolality			
Calculated Osmolality = 2(Na⁺) + (Glucose/18) + (BUN/2.8)			
Oxygen, Partial Pressure (WB, art) (pO₂) (Decreases with age and attitude)		83–108 mm Hg	11.04–14.36 kPa
pH (WB, art)		7.35–7.45	7.35–7.45
Phosphorus, Inorganic (S)		*mg/dL*	*mmol/L*
	Child	4.5–5.5	1.45–1.78
	Adult	2.7–4.5	0.87–1.45
	>60 yr, M	2.3–3.7	0.74–1.20
	>60 yr, F	2.8–4.1	0.90–1.32
Potassium (S,P)		*mEq/L*	*mmol/L*
	Child	3.4–4.7	3.4–4.7
	Adult	3.5–5.1	3.5–5.1

Blood, Serum, Plasma Chemistry (continued).

Test/Specimen	Age Group or Other Factor	Reference Range	
		Conventional	International Units
Protein, Total (S)	Adult	*g/dL*	*g/L*
	Ambulatory	6.4–8.3	64–83
	Recumbent	6.0–7.8	60–78
Albumin	>60 yr	lower by 0.2	lower by 2
	Adult	3.5–5.0	35–50
	>60 yr	3.7–4.7	37–47
Globulins	Adult	2.3–3.5	23–35
Prealbumin	Adult	10–40 mg/dL	100–400 mg/L
Sodium (S,P)		*mEq/L*	*mmol/L*
	Child	138–145	138–145
	Adult	136–146	136–146
Thyroid Stimulating Hormone (S,P) (TSH)		*μunits/mL*	*munits/L*
	Child	4.5 ± 3.6	4.5 ± 3.6
	Adult	<10	<10
	>60 yr, M	2–7.3	2–7.3
	>60 yr, F	2–16.8	2–16.8
Thyroxine, Total (S) (T₄)		*μg/dL*	*nmol/L*
	5–10 yr	6.4–13.3	83–172
	Adult	5–12	65–155
	>60 yr, M	5–10	65–129
	>60 yr, F	5.5–10.5	71–135
	4–9 mo pregnant	6.1–17.6	79–227

Blood, Serum, Plasma Chemistry (continued).

Test/Specimen	Age Group or Other Factor	Reference Range			
		Conventional		International Units	
Transferrin (S)		*mg/dL*		*g/L*	
	Adult	220–400		2.20–4.00	
	>60 yr	180–380		1.80–3.80	
Triglycerides (S)		*mg/dL*		*mmol/L*	
		M	F	M	F
	12–15 yr	36–138	41–138	0.41–1.56	0.46–1.56
	16–19 yr	40–163	40–128	0.45–1.84	0.45–1.45
	20–29 yr	44–185	40–128	0.50–2.09	0.45–1.45
	30–39 yr	49–284	38–160	0.55–3.21	0.43–1.81
	40–49 yr	56–298	44–186	0.63–3.37	0.50–2.10
	50–59 yr	62–288	55–247	0.70–3.25	0.62–2.79
	Desired, Adult	40–160	35–135	0.45–1.81	0.40–1.53
Triiodothyronine Resin Uptake (S) (T_3RU)		*% of Total*		*Fraction of Total*	
	Adult	24–34		0.24–0.34	
	>60 yr, M	24–32		0.24–0.32	
	>60 yr, F	22–32		0.22–0.32	
Triiodothyronine, Total (S) (T_3)		*ng/dL*		*nmol/L*	
	10–15 yr	80–210		1.23–3.23	
	Adult	120–195		1.85–3.00	
	>60 yr, M	105–175		1.62–2.69	
	>60 yr, F	108–205		1.66–3.16	

Blood, Serum, Plasma Chemistry (continued).

| | | Reference Range | |
Test/Specimen	Age Group or Other Factor	Conventional	International Units
Urea Nitrogen (S) (BUN)		*mg/dL*	*mmol/L urea*
	Child	5–18	0.8–3.0
	Adult	7–18	1.2–3.0
	>60 yr	8–21	1.3–3.5
Uric Acid (S) (Uricase Method)		*mg/dL*	*mmol/L*
	Child	2.0–5.5	0.12–0.32
	Adult, M	3.5–7.2	0.21–0.42
	Adult, F	2.6–6.0	0.15–0.35

Urine, Renal Function Tests.

| | | Reference Range | |
Test/Specimen	Age Group or Other Factor	Conventional	International Units
Catecholamines, 24-hr (U)		<110 µg	<650 nmol
Creatinine, 24-hr (U)		*mg/kg*	*µmol/kg*
	Child	8–22	71–195
	Adolescent	8–30	71–265
	Adult, M	14–26	124–230
	Adult, F	11–20	97–177
	Decreases with age to 10 mg/kg/day at age 90		

Urine, Renal Function Tests (continued).

Test/Specimen	Age Group or Other Factor	Reference Range	
		Conventional	International Units
Creatinine Clearance (S, P, and U)		$mL/min/1.73\ m^2$	$mL/sec/m^2$
	<40 yr, M	97–137	0.93–1.32
	<40 yr, F	88–128	0.85–1.23
		Decreases with age <40 yr.	

Inulin Clearance (S and U)

		$mL/min/1.73\ m^2$		$mL/sec/m^2$	
		M	F	M	F
	20–29 yr	90–174	84–156	0.87–1.68	0.81–1.50
	30–39 yr	88–168	82–150	0.85–1.62	0.79–1.44
	40–49 yr	78–162	82–146	0.75–1.56	0.79–1.41
	50–59 yr	68–152	66–142	0.65–1.46	0.63–1.37
	60–69 yr	57–137	58–130	0.55–1.32	0.56–1.25
	70–79 yr	42–122	45–121	0.40–1.17	0.43–1.17
	80–89 yr	39–105	39–105	0.38–1.01	0.38–1.01

Test/Specimen	Age Group or Other Factor	Conventional	International Units
pH (U)		4.5–8	4.5–8
Protein, Total (U)		1–14 mg/dL	10–140 mg/L
	At Rest	50–80 mg/day	50–80 mg/day
Specific Gravity, Random (U)		1.002–1.030	1.002–1.030
Uric Acid, 24-hr (U)		250–750 mg	1.48–4.43 mmol

Hematology.

Test/Specimen	Age Group or Other Factor	Reference Range	
		Conventional	International Units
Bleeding Time		3–9 min	180–540 sec
Erythrocyte Count (WB)	M	4.6–6.2 ×10^6/µL	4.6–6.2 ×10^{12}/L
	F	4.2–5.4	4.2–5.4
Erythrocyte Indices (WB)			
Mean Corpuscular Volume		80–96 µm³	80–96 fL
Mean Corpuscular Hemoglobin		27–31 pg	27–31 pg
Erythrocyte Sedimentation Rate (WB)		mm/hr	mm/hr
	M	1–13	1–13
	F	1–20	1–20
Fibrinogen (P)		200–400 mg/dL	2.00–4.00 g/L
Hematocrit (WB)		% Packed RBC Volume	Volume Fraction
	6–12 yr	35–45	0.35–0.45
	12–18 yr, M	37–49	0.37–0.49
	12–18 yr, F	36–46	0.36–0.46
	18–49 yr, M	41–53	0.41–0.53
	18–49 yr, F	36–46	0.36–0.46
Hemoglobin (WB)		g/dL	mmol/L
	6–12 yr	11.5–15.5	1.78–2.40
	12–18 yr, M	13.0–16.0	2.02–2.48
	12–18 yr, F	12.0–16.0	1.86–2.48
	18–49 yr, M	13.5–17.5	2.09–2.71
	18–49 yr, F	12.0–16.0	1.86–2.48
Hemoglobin A$_{1c}$ (WB)		5.3–7.5% of total Hb	0.053–0.075

Hematology (continued).

Test/Specimen	Age Group or Other Factor	Reference Range	
		Conventional	**International Units**
Leukocyte Count (WB)		$4.5\text{–}11 \times 10^3/\mu L$	$4.5\text{–}11 \times 10^9/L$
	Segs	31–71%	31–71%
	Bands	0–12%	0–12%
	Lymphocytes	15–50%	15–50%
	Monocytes	0–12%	0–12%
	Eosinophils	0–5%	0–5%
	Basophils	0–2%	0–2%
Absolute Neutrophil Count (ANC)			
ANC = (% Segs % Bands) × Leukocyte Count			
Partial Thromboplastin Time, Activated (WB) (aPTT)		25–37 sec	25–37 sec
Platelets (WB)		$150\text{–}440 \times 10^3/\mu L$	$0.15\text{–}0.44 \times 10^{12}/L$
Prothrombin Time (WB)		Less than 2 sec deviation from control	
Reticulocytes (WB)		0.5–1.5% of erythrocytes	0.005–0.015

REFERENCES

1. Burtis CA, Ashwood ER, eds. *Tietz textbook of clinical chemistry,* 2nd ed. Philadelphia: WB Saunders; 1994.

2. Henry JB, ed. *Clinical diagnosis and management by laboratory methods,* 18th ed. Philadelphia: WB Saunders; 1991.

3. Preventing lead poisoning in young children: a statement by the Centers for Disease Control, 4th Rev. ed. Atlanta: Centers for Disease Control; 1991.

4. Système International (SI) units conversion table for common laboratory tests. *Ann Pharmacother* 1995; 29:100–7.

5. Tietz NW, ed. *Clinical guide to laboratory tests,* 2nd ed. Philadelphia: WB Saunders; 1990.

6. Wallach J. *Interpretation of diagnostic tests: a synopsis of laboratory medicine,* 5th ed. Boston: Little, Brown; 1996.

List of Tests by Body System

CANCER STUDIES

Acid phosphatase
Bence Jones protein
Bone scan
CA 27.29 and CA 15-3 tumor
    markers
CA 19-9 tumor marker
CA-125 tumor marker
Carcinoembryonic antigen
Estrogen-receptor assay
Gallium scan
Lymphangiography
Mammography
Octreotide scan
Oncoscinct scan
Papanicolaou smear
Progesterone receptor assay
Prostate-specific antigen
Sputum cytology

CARDIOVASCULAR SYSTEM

Adenosine stress test

Aldosterone assay, blood
Antimyocardial antibodies
Antistreptolysin O titer
Apolipoproteins
Arteriography
Aspartate aminotransferase
Atrial natriuretic factor
Cardiac catheterization
Cardiac exercise stress testing
Cardiac nuclear scanning
Carotid duplex scanning
Catecholamines
Chest x-ray
Cholesterol
Computed tomography of
    chest
Creatine phosphokinase
Cryoglobulin
Digital subtraction angiography
Dipyridamole-thallium scan
Dobutamine stress test
Doppler studies
Echocardiography
Electrocardiography
Electrophysiologic study
Fibrinogen

Tests in this list are grouped by the following: cancer studies; cardiovascular, endocrine, gastrointestinal, hematologic, hepatobiliary, and immunologic systems; miscellaneous studies; and nervous, pulmonary, reproductive, skeletal, and urologic systems.

This section was reprinted from *Mosby's Diagnostic and Laboratory Test Reference*, 5th edition, Pagana and Pagana, © 2001, Mosby, Inc.

Holter monitoring
Homocysteine
Isonitrile scan
Lactic dehydrogenase
Lipoproteins
MUGA scan
Myoglobin
Pericardiocentesis
Plethysmography
   arterial
   venous
Positron-emission tomography
Renin assay
   plasma
   renal vein
Tilt-table testing
Transesophageal echocardiography
Transthoracic echocardiography
Triglycerides
Troponins
Vanillylmandelic acid
Venography of lower extremities

ENDOCRINE SYSTEM

Adrenal angiography
Adrenal venography
Adrenocorticotropic hormone
   stimulation test
Aldosterone assay, blood
Androstenedione
Antidiuretic hormone
Antithyroglobulin antibody
Antithyroid microsomal antibody
Blood glucose
Calcitonin
Calcium
Catecholamines
Chromosome karyotype
Computed tomography of adrenals
Cortisol
   blood
   urine
C-peptide

Dexamethasone suppression test
Estriol excretion
Follicle-stimulating hormone
Free thyroxine
Gastrin
Glucagon
Glucose
   blood
   postprandial
   urine
Glucose tolerance test
Glycosylated hemoglobin
Growth hormone
   stimulation test
17-Hydroxycorticosteroids
Insulin antibody
Insulin assay
Ketones
17-Ketosteroids
Long-acting thyroid stimulator
Luteinizing hormone assay
Metyrapone
Osmolality, blood
Parathyroid hormone
Phosphorus
Postprandial glucose
Prolactin levels
Renin assay
   plasma
   renal vein
Somatomedin C
Testosterone
Thyroid scanning
Thyroid-stimulating hormone
Thyroid ultrasound
   stimulation test
Thyrotropin-releasing hormone test
Thyrotine-binding globulin
Thyroxine, free
Thyroxine, total
Thyroxine index, free
Triiodothyronine
Urine glucose
Vanillylmandelic acid

GASTROINTESTINAL SYSTEM

Abdominal ultrasound
Barium enema
Barium swallow
Carcinoembryonic antigen
Clostridial toxin assay
Colonoscopy
Computed tomography of abdomen
Computed tomography portogram
Esophageal function studies
Esophagogastroduodenoscopy
Fecal fat
Gastrin
Gastroesophageal reflux scan
Gastrointestinal bleeding scan
Helicobactor pylori antibodies
5-Hydroxyindoleacetic acid
Lactose tolerance test
Laparoscopy
Meckel's diverticulum nuclear scan
Obstruction series
Paracentesis
Prealbumin
Protein, blood
Schilling test
Sialography
Sigmoidoscopy
Small bowel follow-through
Stool culture
Stool for occult blood testing
Transrectal ultrasonography
Upper gastrointestinal x-ray study
Urea nitrogen blood test
Videofluoroscopy
D-Xylose absorption test

HEMATOLOGIC SYSTEM

Activated clotting time
Antithrombin III
Basophils
Bleeding time
Blood smear
Blood typing
Bone marrow biopsy
Clot retraction test
Coagulating factors concentration
Complete blood count differential count
Coomb's test
  direct
  indirect
D-Dimer test
Delta-aminolevulinic acid
2,3-Diphosphoglycerate
Disseminated intravascular coagulation screening
Eosinophils
Euglobulin lysis time
Ferritin
Fibrin degradation products
Fibrinogen
Folic acid
Glucose-6-phosphate dehydrogenase
Ham's test
Haptoglobin
Hematocrit
Hemoglobin electrophoresis
Iron level and total iron-binding capacity
Lymphocytes
Monocytes
Neutrophils
Partial thromboplastin time, activated
Plasminogen
Platelet aggregation
Platelet antibody detection tests
Platelet count
Platelet volume, mean
Porphyrins and porphobilinogens
Prothrombin time
Red blood cell count
Red blood cell indices
Red blood cell survival study

Red blood cells and casts, urine
Reticulocyte count
Sickle cell test
Uroporphyrinogen-I-synthase
Vitamin B$_{12}$
White blood cell count and
    differential count

HEPATOBILIARY SYSTEM

Abdominal ultrasound
Alanine aminotransferase
Aldolase
Alkaline phosphatase
Alpha-fetoprotein
Ammonia level
Amylase
   blood
   urine
Aspartate aminotransferase
Bilirubin blood
CA 19-9 tumor marker
Cholesterol
Computed tomography of abdomen
Endoscopic retrograde
   cholangiopancreatography
Epstein-Barr virus
Fecal fat
Gallbladder scanning
Gallium scan
Gamma-glutamyl
   transpeptidase
Hepatitis virus studies
Lactic dehydrogenase
Leucine aminopeptidase
Lipase
Liver biopsy
Liver and pancreatobiliary system
   ultrasonography
Liver/spleen scanning
5'-Nucleotidase
Obstruction series
Percutaneous transhepatic
   cholangiography

Protein, blood
Secretin-pancreozymin
Sweat electrolytes test

IMMUNOLOGIC SYSTEM

Agglutinins, febrile/cold
AIDS serology
Aldolase
Allergy blood testing
Allergy skin testing
Anticardiolipin antibodies
Anticentromere antibody
Antideoxyribonuclease-B titer
Anti-DNA antibody
Anti-extractable nuclear antigens
Antiglomerular basement membrane
   antibody
Antimitochondrial antibody
Antimyocardial antibodies
Antineutrophil cytoplasmic
   antibody
Antinuclear antibody
Antiscleroderma antibody
Anti-smooth muscle antibody test
Anti-SS-A and anti-SS-B
   antibody
CD4/CD8 for HIV
Complement assay
Cryoglobulin
Cutaneous immunofluorescence
   biopsy
Epstein-Barr virus
HIV oral testing
HIV urine testing
HLA-B27 antigen
Human T-cell lymphotropic virus
Immunoglobulin electrophoresis
Lyme disease test
Mononucleosis spot test
Parvovirus B-19 antibody
Protein electrophoresis
Rabies-neutralizing antibody test
Rheumatoid factor

MISCELLANEOUS TESTS

Blood culture and sensitivity
Blood glucose
Carbon dioxide content
Carboxyhemoglobin
Chloride, blood
Cholinesterase
C-Reactive protein
Erythrocyte sedimentation rate
Ethanol
Magnesium
Positron emission tomography
Potassium
  blood
  urine
Protein, blood
Sialography
Sleep studies
Sodium
  blood
  urine
Therapeutic drug monitoring
Throat culture and sensitivity
Toxicology screening
Urine culture and sensitivity
Urine glucose
White blood cell scan
Wound culture and sensitivity

NERVOUS SYSTEM

Acetylcholine receptor-binding
    antibody
Amyloid beta protein precursor,
    soluble
Apolipoprotein E4
Caloric study
Cerebral angiography
Cerebrospinal fluid examination
Computed tomography of brain
C-reactive protein
Digital subtraction angiography
Electroencephalography

Electromyography
Electroneurography
Electronystagmography
Evoked-potential studies
Hexosaminidase
Lumbar puncture
Magnetic resonance angiography
Magnetic resonance imaging
Magnetic resonance spectroscopy
Myelography
Positron emission tomography
Skull x-ray
Spinal x-rays
Tau protein

PULMONARY SYSTEM

Acid-fast bacilli
Alpha$_1$-antitrypsin
Angiotensin-converting enzyme
Blood gases
Bronchoscopy
Carbon dioxide content
Carboxyhemoglobin
Chest x-ray
Computed tomography of
    chest
Legionnaires' disease antibody
Lung biopsy
Lung scan
Mediastinoscopy
Nose culture
Oximetry
Pleural biopsy
Pulmonary angiography
Pulmonary function tests
Sleep studies
Sputum culture and sensitivity
Sputum cytology
Strept screen
Thoracentesis and pleural fluid
    analysis
Thoracoscopy
Throat culture

Tuberculin test
Tuberculosis culture
Urine pH

RENAL/UROLOGIC SYSTEM

Acid phosphatase
Aldosterone assay
Anion gap
Antidiurectic hormone
Antistreptolysin O titer
Bilirubin, urine
Captopril renal scan
Carbon dioxide content
Catecholamines
Chloride, blood
Computed tomography of
    kidney
Creatinine, blood
Creatinine clearance
Crystals
Cystography
Cystometry
Cystoscopy
Epithelial casts
Fatty casts
Granular casts
Hyaline casts
Intravenous pyelogram
Ketones
Kidney sonogram
Kidney, ureter, and bladder x-ray
    study
Lactic acid
Leukocyte esterase
Nitrites
Osmolality
    blood
    urine
Pelvic floor sphincter
    electromyography
Percent free PSA
Potassium
    blood
    urine
Prostate sonogram
Prostate-specific antigen
PSA velocity
Protein, urine
Renal angiography
Renal biopsy
Renal scanning
Renin assay
    plasma
    renal vein
Retrograde pyelography
Scrotal scan
Scrotal ultrasound
Sodium
    blood
    urine
Testicular sonogram
Urea nitrogen blood test
Urethral pressure profile
Uric acid
Urinalysis
Urine appearance and color
Urine culture and sensitivity
Urine flow studies
Urine odor
Urine pH
Urine specific gravity
Vanillylmandelic acid
Waxy casts
White blood cells and casts

REPRODUCTIVE SYSTEM

Alpha-fetoprotein
Amniocentesis
Antispermatozoal antibody
Breast cancer genetic screening
Breast scintography
Breast sonogram
CA 27.29 and CA 15-3 tumor
    markers
CA-125 tumor marker

Chlamydia
Chorionic villus sampling
Colposcopy
Cytomegalovirus
Endometrial biopsy
Estriol excretion
Fetal biophysical profile
Fetal contraction stress test
Fetal nonstress test
Fetal scalp blood pH
Fetoscopy
Follicle-stimulating hormone
Gonorrhea culture
Herpes genitalis
Hysterosalpingography
Hysteroscopy
IUD localization
Lamellar body count
Laparoscopy
Luteinizing hormone assay
Mammography
Obstetric ultrasonography
Papanicolaou smear
Phenylketonuria test
Pregnancy tests
Pregnanediol
Progesterone assay
Prolactin

Rubella antibody test
Semen analysis
Sexually transmitted disease cultures
Sims-Huhner test
Syphilis detection test
TORCH test
Toxoplasmosis antibody titer

SKELETAL SYSTEM

Aldolase
Alkaline phosphatase
Arthrocentesis with synovial fluid
    analysis
Arthrography
Arthroscopy
Bone densitometry
Bone scan
Bone x-ray
Electromyography
HLA-B27 antigen
Lactate dehydrogenase
Magnetic resonance imaging
Myoglobin
N-telopeptide
Rheumatoid factor
Spinal x-rays
Uric acid

List of Tests by Type

BLOOD TESTS

Acetylcholine receptor antibody
Acid phosphatase
Activated clotting time (ACT)
Adrenocorticotropic hormone stimulation test
Agglutinins, febrile/cold
AIDS serology
Alanine aminotransferase
Aldolase
Aldosterone assay
Alkaline phosphatase
Allergy blood testing
Alpha$_1$-antitrypsin
Alpha-fetoprotein
Ammonia level
Amylase
Androstenedione
Angiotensin-converting enzyme
Anion gap
Anticardiolipin antibodies
Anticentromere antibody test
Antideoxyribonuclease-B titer
Antidiuretic hormone
Anti-DNA antibody

Anti-extractable nuclear antigens antibody
Antiglomerular basement membrane antibody
Antimitochondrial antibody
Antimyocardial antibodies
Antineutrophil cytoplasmic antibody
Antinuclear antibody test
Antiscleroderma antibody
Anti-smooth muscle antibody
Antispermatozoal antibody
Anti-SS-A and anti-SS-B antibody
Antistreptolysin O titer
Antithrombin III
Antithyroglobulin antibody
Antithyroid microsomal antibody
Apolipoproteins
Aspartate aminotransferase
Atrial natriuretic factor
Basophils
Bilirubin
Bleeding time
Blood culture and sensitivity
Blood gases
Blood smear

Tests in this list are grouped by the following types: blood, electrodiagnostic, endoscopy, fluid analysis, manometric, microscopic examination, nuclear scan, other studies, sputum, stool, ultrasound, urine, and x-ray.

This section was reprinted from *Mosby's Diagnostic and Laboratory Test Reference*, 5th edition, Pagana and Pagana, © 2001, Mosby, Inc.

Lyme disease test
Lymphocytes
Lymphocyte immunophenotyping
Magnesium
Metyrapone
Monocytes
Mononucleosis spot test
Myoglobin
Neutrophils
N-telopeptide
5'-Nucleotidase
Osmolality
Parathyroid hormone
Partial thromboplastin time,
    activated
Parvovirus B-19 antibody
Percent free PSA
Phenylketonuria test
Phosphorus
Plasminogen
Platelet aggregation
Platelet antibody detection tests
Platelet count
Platelet volume, mean
Potassium
Prealbumin
Pregnancy tests
Progesterone assay
Prolactin level
Prostate-specific antigen
Protein
Prothrombin time
PSA velocity
Rabies-neutralizing antibody test
Red blood cell count
Red blood cell indices
Renin assay
    plasma
    renal vein
Reticulocyte count
Rheumatoid factor
Rubella antibody test
Sexually transmitted diseases
Sickle cell test

Sodium
Somatomedin C
Syphilis detection test
Testosterone
Therapeutic drug monitoring
Thyroid-binding globulin
Thyroid-stimulating hormone
    stimulation test
Thyrotropin-releasing hormone test
Thyroxine, free
Thyroxine, total
Thyroxine index, free
Toxicology screening
Toxoplasmosis antibody titer
Triglycerides
Triiodothyronine
Troponins
Urea nitrogen blood test
Uric acid
Uroporphyrinogen-I-synthase
Vitamin B_{12}
White blood cell count and
    differential count
D-Xylose absorption test

ELECTRODIAGNOSTIC TESTS

Caloric study
Cardiac exercise stress testing
Contraction stress (fetal)
Electrocardiography
Electroencephalography
Electromyography
Electroneurography
Electronystagmography
Electrophysiologic study
Evoked potential studies
Holter monitoring
Nonstress (fetal)
Pelvic floor sphincter
    electromyography
Signal-averaged electrocardiography
Sleep studies

ENDOSCOPY

Arthroscopy
Bronchoscopy
Colonoscopy
Colposcopy
Cystoscopy
Endoscopic retrograde
    cholangiopancreatography
Esophagogastroduodenoscopy
Fetoscopy
Gastroscopy
Hysteroscopy
Laparoscopy
Mediastinoscopy
Sigmoidoscopy
Thoracoscopy
Transesophageal echocardiography

FLUID ANALYSIS

Amniocentesis
Amyloid beta protein precursor,
    soluble
Antispermatozoal antibody
Arthrocentesis with synovial fluid
    analysis
HIV oral testing
Lumbar puncture and cerebrospinal
    fluid examination
Paracentesis
Pericardiocentesis
Secretin-pancreozymin
Semen analysis
Sims-Huhner test
Sweat electrolytes test
Tau protein
Thoracentesis and pleural fluid
    analysis

MANOMETRIC TESTS

Cystometry
Esophageal function studies

Plethysmography
    arterial
    venous
Urethral pressure profile

MICROSCOPIC EXAMINATIONS

Antiglomerular basement membrane
    antibodies
Bone marrow biopsy
Chlamydia
Cutaneous immunofluorescence
    biopsy
Endometrial biopsy
Estrogen receptor assay
Gonorrhea culture
Helicobacter pylori antibodies
Herpes genitalis
Liver biopsy
Lung biopsy
Nose culture
Papanicolaou smear
Pleural biopsy
Progesterone receptor assay
Renal biopsy
Sexually transmitted disease
    cultures
Strept screen
Throat culture
Tuberculosis culture
Urine culture
Wound culture and sensitivity

NUCLEAR SCANS

Bone scan
Breast scintography
Cardiac nuclear scanning
Gallbladder scanning
Gallium scan
Gastroesophageal reflux scan
Gastrointestinal bleeding scan
Isonitrile scan

Liver/spleen scanning
Lung scan
Meckel's diverticulum nuclear scan
MUGA scan
Octreotide scan
Oncoscint scan
Positron emission tomography
Red blood cell survival study
Renal scanning
Scrotal scan
Thallium scan
Thyroid scanning
White blood cell scan

OTHER STUDIES

Allergy skin testing
Chorionic villus sampling
Colposcopy
Fetal nonstress test
Magnetic resonance angiography
Magnetic resonance imaging
Magnetic resonance spectroscopy
Oximetry
Pulmonary function tests
Tilt-table testing
TORCH test
Tuberculin test
Urine flow studies

SPUTUM TESTS

Acid-fast bacilli
Culture and sensitivity
Cytology

STOOL TESTS

Clostridial toxin assay
Culture
Fecal fat
Occult blood testing
Ova and parasites

ULTRASOUND TESTS

Abdominal ultrasound
Breast sonogram
Carotid duplex scanning
Doppler studies
Echocardiography
Fetal biophysical profile
IUD localization
Kidney sonogram
Liver and pancreatobiliary system
    ultrasonography
Obstetric ultrasonography
Prostate/rectal sonogram
Scrotal ultrasound
Testicular ultrasound
Thyroid ultrasound
Transesophageal echocardiography
Transrectal ultrasonography

URINE TESTS

Aldosterone
Amylase
Appearance and color
Bence Jones protein
Cortisol
Creatinine clearance
Crystals
Culture and sensitivity
Delta-aminolevulinic acid
Dexamethasone suppression
    test
Epithelial casts
Estriol excretion
Ethanol
Fatty casts
Flow studies
Glucose
Glucose tolerance test
Granular casts
HIV urine testing
Hyaline casts
17-Hydroxycorticosteroids

5-Hydroxyindoleacetic acid
Ketones
17-Ketosteroids
Leucine aminopeptidase
Leukocyte esterase
Metyrapone
N-telopeptide
Nitrites
Odor
Osmolality
pH
Phenylketonuria test
Porphyrins and
    porphobilinogens
Potassium
Prealbumin
Pregnancy
Pregnanediol
Protein
Red blood cells and casts
Schilling test
Sodium
Specific gravity
Toxicology screening
Uric acid
Urinalysis
Vanillylmandelic acid and
    catecholamines
Waxy casts
White blood cells and casts
D-Xylose absorption test

X-RAY EXAMINATIONS

Adrenal angiography
Adrenal venography
Arteriography
Arthrography

Barium enema
Barium swallow
Bone densitometry
Bone x-ray
Cardiac catheterization
Cerebral angiography
Chest X-ray
Computed tomography
    of abdomen
    of adrenals
    of brain
    of chest
    of kidney
Computed tomography portogram
Cystography
Digital subtraction angiography
Hysterosalpingography
Intravenous pyelogram
Kidney, ureter, and bladder
    x-ray study
Lymphangiography
Magnetic resonance imaging
Mammography
Myelography
Obstruction series
Percutaneous transhepatic
    cholangiography
Positron emission tomography
Pulmonary angiography
Renal angiography
Retrograde pyelography
Sialography
Skull x-rays
Small bowel follow-through
Spinal x-rays
Upper gastrointestinal x-ray study
Venography of lower extremities
Videofluoroscopy

Patient Counseling Principles

INDIAN HEALTH SERVICE INTERACTIVE PATIENT COUNSELING TECHNIQUE EVALUATION FORM

A. Setting the Stage	Yes	No	N/A
1. Did the pharmacist identify the patient?			
2. Did the pharmacist identify him/herself and the purpose of the counseling?			
3. Were the physical and patient barriers identified and dealt with?			
B. Consultation Process			
1. Were the open-ended "Prime" or "Show & Tell" questions used appropriately to direct the dialogue to cover the three major areas of understanding?			
a. What did the doctor tell you the medication was for? (What do you take this for?)			
b. How did the doctor tell you to take the medication? (How do you take it?)			
c. Were other open-ended questions used to break up "How" discussion? e.g., "What does three times a day mean to you?"			
d. What did the doctor tell you to expect? (What kind of problems are you having?)			
2. Was dialogue for each Prime Question completed before moving onto the next one?			
3. Did the pharmacist talk continuously for more than 60 seconds at a time?			
4. Was the patient asked to demonstrate wherever possible?			

C. Closure	Yes	No	N/A
1. Was the patient asked to verify overall understanding (Final Verification)? e.g., "Just to make sure I didn't leave anything out, please go over how you are going to use the medicine."			
2. Was an appropriate closure used? e.g., "Is there anything else I can do for you?"			
Pharmacist Name: Date:			

Principles of Literature Evaluation

OVERVIEW

1. What is the journal's reputation? Are the clinical studies refereed?
2. Is the title of abstract misleading? Does the author's bias show?
3. Are the researcher's qualified to undertake this study?
4. Is the location of the study adequate or appropriate?
5. Is the article referenced with key up-to-date articles?

INTRODUCTION

6. Is there a brief review of previous work and background on why the study was done?
7. Is the hypothesis or objectives of the trial clearly stated?

METHODOLOGY

8. Was the study design appropriate for the hypothesis? Ethical?
9. Was subject selection and exclusion criteria clearly detailed? Was subject selection adequate for extrapolation to the appropriate population?
10. Was the number of subjects enrolled adequate?
11. Was the subject sample described sufficiently (age range, sex, severity of disease) to make sure groups were comparable? Were group differences subjected to statistical analysis?
12. Were appropriate controls used?
13. Was allocation to treatment groups truly random?
14. Were doses, schedules, and duration of drug treatment adequate and comparable?
15. Were washouts used? Were they of sufficient duration?
16. Was concurrent therapy allowed? Controlled?
17. Was the study blinded? Was it truly blinded?
18. Were observers identified? Were they qualified? Were they blinded?
19. Were the test measures used indicative of therapeutic efficacy?

20. Did the test measurements use subjective or objective assessment?
21. What is the test measurement's sensitivity, specificity and reliability? Could a more reliable test measure have been used?
22. How long were subjects followed? Was it long enough?

RESULTS

23. Were the results clearly, accurately and adquately presented?
24. Were the results presented?
25. Were dropouts adequately accounted for?
26. Was an appropriate statistical method used?

DISCUSSION AND CONCLUSIONS

27. Does a statistically significant difference necessarily imply clinical significance?
28. Were valid conclusions based upon the results presented?
29. Were valid conclusions based upon the hypotheses of the study?
30. Does the discussion place the results of this study into the perspective of previous clinical trials comparing and contrasting results? Does the discussion honestly outline the clinical trial's shortcomings?

ASSOCIATIONS AND CONTACTS

Professional associations are an important part of pharmacy. State and national associations represent the profession in a number of venues. The addresses and other contact information are provided for the national and state associations. Contact information for the state boards of pharmacy is also provided. Contact information and addresses on Canadian national associations as well as regulatory and voluntary organizations are included.

National Pharmacy Associations

AACP   American Association of Colleges of Pharmacy
1426 Prince Street, Alexandria, VA 22314-2841
Tel: 703/739-2330, Fax: 703/836-8982, http://www.aacp.org

AAPS   American Association of Pharmaceutical Scientists
1650 King Street, Alexandria, VA 22314
Tel: 703/243-2800, Fax: 703/243-9650, http://www.aaps.org

ACA   American College of Apothecaries
P.O. Box 341266, Memphis, TN 38184
Tel: 901/383-8119, Fax: 901/383-8882, http://www.acainfo.org

ACCP   American College of Clinical Pharmacy
3101 Broadway, Suite 650, Kansas City, MO 64111
Tel: 816/531-2177, Fax: 816/531-4990, http://www.accp.com

ACPE   American Council of Pharmaceutical Education
311 West Superior Street, Suite 512, Chicago, IL 60610-3537
Tel: 312/664-3575, Fax: 312/664-4652, http://www.acpe-accredit.org

AFPC   Association of Faculties of Pharmacy of Canada
2609 Eastview, Saskatoon, Saskatchewan, Canada S7J 3G7
Tel: 306/374-6327

AFPE   American Foundation for Pharmaceutical Education
One Church Street, Suite 202, Rockville, MD 20850
Tel: 301/738-2160, Fax: 301/738-2161, http://www.afpenet.org

AIHP   American Institute for the History of Pharmacy
425 North Charter Street, Madison, WI 53706-1515
Tel: 608/262-5378, Fax: 608/262-3397, http://www.aihp.org

AMCP   Academy of Managed Care Pharmacy
100 North Pitt Street, Suite 400, Alexandria, VA 22314
Tel: 703/683-8416, Fax: 703/683-8417, http://www.amcp.org

ANMP   Association of Natural Medicine Pharmacists
P.O. Box 150727, San Rafael, CA 94915-0727
Tel: 415/453-3534, Fax: 415/453-4963, http://www.anmp.org

APhA   American Pharmaceutical Association
2215 Constitution Avenue, NW, Washington, DC 20037-2985
Tel: 202/628-4410, Fax: 202/429-6300, http://www.apha.org

ASAP American Society of Automation in Pharmacy
492 Norristown Road, Suite 160, Blue Bell, PA 19422
Tel: 610/825-7783, Fax: 610/825-7641, http://www.asapnet.org

ASCP American Society of Consultant Pharmacists
1321 Duke Street, Alexandria, VA 22314
Tel: 703/739-1300, Fax: 703/739-1321, http://www.ascp.com

ASHP American Society of Health-System Pharmacists
7272 Wisconsin Avenue, Bethesda, MD 20814
Tel: 301/657-3000, Fax: 301/664-8877, http://www.ashp.org

ASPL American Society of Pharmacy Law
13017 Wisteria Drive, #336, Germantown, MD 20874
Tel: 301/916-6968, Fax: 301/916-6961, http://www.aspl.org

BPS Board of Pharmaceutical Specialties
2215 Constitution Avenue, NW, Washington, DC 20037-2985
Tel: 202/429-7591, Fax: 202/429-6304, http://www.bpsweb.org

CCAPP Canadian Council for Accreditation of Pharmacy Programs
Thorvaldson Building, Room 123, 110 Science Place,
Saskatoon, Saskatchewan, Canada S7J 5C9
Tel: 306/966-6388, Fax: 306/966-6377

CPhA Canadian Pharmacists Association
1785 Alta Vista Drive, Ottawa, Ontario, Canada K1G 3Y6
Tel: 613/523-7877, Fax: 613/523-0445, http://www.cdnpharm.ca

FIP International Federation of Pharmacy
P.O. Box 84200, 2508 Hague, Netherlands
Tel: 31/70-302-1970, Fax: 31/70-302-1999, http/www.fip.nl

NABP National Association of Boards of Pharmacy
700 Busse Highway, Park Ridge, IL 60068-2402
Tel: 847/698-6227, Fax: 847/698-0124, http://www.nabp.net

NACDS National Association of Chain Drug Stores
P.O. Box 1417-D49, Alexandria, VA 22313-1480
Tel: 703/549-3001, Fax: 703/836-4869, http://www.nacds.org

NAPRA National Association of Pharmacy Regulatory Authorities
http://www.napra.org

NCPA National Community Pharmacists Association
205 Daingerfield Road, Alexandria, VA 22314
Tel: 703/683-8200, Fax: 703/683-3619, http://www.ncpanet.org

NCPIE National Council on Patient Information and Education
4915 Saint Elmo Avenue, Suite 505, Bethesda, MD 20814-6053
Tel: 301/656-8565, www.talkaboutrx.org

NPhA National Pharmaceutical Association
107 Kilmayne Drive, Suite C, Cary, NC 27511
Tel: 800/944-6742, Fax: 919/469-5870, http://www.npha.net

PCMA   Pharmaceutical Care Management Association
        2300 Ninth Street, Suite 210, Arlington, VA 22204
        Tel: 703/920-8480, Fax: 703/920-8491, http://www.pcmanet.org
USP   United States Pharmacopeial Convention, Inc.
        12601 Twinbrook Parkway, Rockville, MD 20852
        Tel: 301/881-0666, Fax: 301/816-8299, http://www.usp.org
USPHS   U.S. Public Health Service
        5600 Fishers Lane, Room 9A-05, Rockville, MD 20857
        Tel: 301/827-5846, Fax: 301/443-3847

State Pharmacy Associations

Alabama Pharmacy Association
  1211 Carmichael Way, Montgomery, AL 36106-3672
  Tel: 334/271-5423, Fax: 334/271-5423, http://www.aparx.org
Alaska Pharmaceutical Association
  Box 101185, Anchorage, AK 99510
  Tel: 907/563-8880, Fax: 907/563-7880
  http://www.alaska.net/~akphrmcy
Arizona Pharmacy Association
  1845 E. Southern Avenue, Tempe, AZ 85282-5831
  Tel: 480/838-3385, Fax: 480/838-3557, http://www.azpharmacy.org
Arkansas Pharmacists Association
  417 South Victory, Little Rock, AR 72201
  Tel: 501/372-5250, Fax: 501/372-0546, http://www.arpharmacists.org
California Pharmacists Association
  1112 "I" Street, Suite 300, Sacramento, CA 95814
  Tel: 916/444-7811, Fax: 916/444-7929, http://www.cpha.com
Colorado Pharmacists Association
  5150 East Yale Circle, Suite 304, Denver, CO 80222
  Tel: 303/756-3069, Fax: 303/756-3649
  http://www.coloradopharmacy.org/CphA.htm
Connecticut Pharmacists Association
  35 Cold Spring Road, Suite 125, Rocky Hill, CT 06067
  Tel: 860/563-4619, Fax: 860/257-8241, http://www.ctpharmacists.org
Delaware Pharmacists Society
  P.O. Box 454, Smyrna, DE 19977
  Tel: 800/782-3716, Fax: 302/659-3089
  http://www.depharmacy.org/Index.htm
Florida Pharmacy Association
  610 North Adams Street, Tallahassee, FL 32301
  Tel: 850/222-2400, Fax: 850/561-6758, http://www.pharmview.com
Georgia Pharmacy Association
  20 Lenox Pointe, NE, Atlanta, GA 30327
  Tel: 404/231-5074, Fax: 404/237-8435, http://www.gpha.org

Hawaii Pharmacists Association
  2448 East Manoa Drive, Honolulu, HI 96807
  Tel: 808/739-1230, Fax: 808/235-5189
  http://www.helix.com/helix/assoc/assn_pharm/hpha/hpha.htm
Idaho State Pharmacy Association
  P.O. Box 140117, Boise, ID 83714
  Tel: 208/424-1107, Fax: 208/424-1102, http://www.idahopharmacy.org
Illinois Pharmacists Association
  204 West Cook, Springfield, IL 62704
  Tel: 217/522-7300, Fax: 217/522-7349, http://www.ipha.org
Indiana Pharmacists Association
  729 N. Pennsylvania Street, Indianapolis, IN 46204-1171
  Tel: 317/634-4968, Fax: 317/632-1219
  http://www.indianapharmacists.org
Iowa Pharmacy Association
  8515 Douglas Avenue, Suite 16, Des Moines, IA 50322
  Tel: 515/270-0713, Fax: 515/270-2979, http://www.iarx.org
Kansas Pharmacists Association
  1020 SW Fairlawn Road, Topeka, KS 66604
  Tel: 785/228-2327, Fax: 785/228-9147, http://www.kansaspharmacy.org
Kentucky Pharmacists Association
  1228 U.S. 127 South, Frankfort, KY 40601-4330
  Tel: 502/227-2303, Fax: 502/227-2258, http://www.kphanet.org
Louisiana Pharmacists Association
  P.O. Box 14446, Baton Rouge, LA 70898
  Tel: 225/926-2666, Fax: 225/926-1020
Maine Pharmacy Association
  P.O. Box 346, Brewer, ME 04412
  Tel: 207/989-6190, Fax: 207/989-6743,
  http://www.mainepharmacyassoc.com
Maryland Pharmacists Association
  650 W. Lombard Street, Baltimore, MD 21201
  Tel: 410/727-0746, Fax: 410/727-2253
  http://www.users.erols.com/mpha
Massachusetts Pharmacists Association
  681 Main Street, Suite 3-32, Waltham, MA 02451-0621
  Tel: 781/736-0101, Fax: 781/736-0080
  http://www.channel1.com/users/mpha
Michigan Pharmacists Association
  815 N. Washington Avenue, Lansing, MI 48906-5198
  Tel: 517/484-1466, Fax: 517/484-4893, http://www.mipharm.com
Minnesota Pharmacists Association
  1935 W. County Road, B2#450, Roseville, MN 55113
  Tel: 651/697-1771, Fax: 651/697-1776, http://www.mpha.org

Mississippi Pharmacists Association
  341 Edgewood Terrace Drive, Jackson, MS 39211
  Tel: 601/981-0416, Fax: 601/981-0451
Missouri Pharmacy Association
  211 E. Capitol Avenue, Jefferson City, MO 65101
  Tel: 573/636-7522, Fax: 573/636-7485, http://www.morx.com
Montana State Pharmaceutical Association
  P.O. Box 4718, Helena, MT 59604
  Tel: 406/449-3843, Fax: 406/443-1592, http://www.rxmt.com
Nebraska Pharmacists Association
  6221 South 58th Street, Suite A, Lincoln, NE 68516-3687
  Tel: 402/420-1500, Fax: 402/420-1406, http://www.npa.creighton.edu
Nevada Pharmacy Alliance
  100 N. Green Valley Parkway, Henderson, NV 89014
  Tel: 702/732-4610, Fax: 702/990-6018, http://www.nvphall.org
New Hampshire Pharmacists Association
  2 Eagle Square, Suite 400, Concord, NH 03301-4956
  Tel: 603/229-0292, Fax: 603/224-7769
  http://www.state.nh.us/pharmacy/nhpa.htm
New Jersey Pharmacists Association
  3 Marlen Drive, #B, Robbinsville, NJ 08691-1604
  Tel: 609/584-9063, Fax: 609/586-8186
New Mexico Pharmaceutical Association
  4800 Zuni Southeast, Albuquerque, NM 87108
  Tel: 505/265-8729, Fax: 505/255-8476
  http://www.nm-pharmacy.com
Pharmacists Society of the State of New York
  210 Washington Avenue Ext., Albany, NY 12203
  Tel: 518/869-6595, Fax: 518/464-0618, http://www.pssny.org
North Carolina Association of Pharmacists
  109 Church Street, Chapel Hill, NC 27516
  Tel: 919/967-2237, Fax: 919/968-9430,
  http://www.ncpharmacists.org
North Dakota Pharmaceutical Association
  1906 East Broadway Avenue, Bismark, ND 58501
  Tel: 701/258-4968, Fax: 701/258-9312
  http://www.nodakpharmacy.com
Ohio Pharmacists Association
  6037 Frantz Road, Suite 106, Dublin, OH 43017
  Tel: 614/798-0037, Fax: 614/798-0978,
  http://www.ohiopharmacists.org
Oklahoma Pharmacists Association
  P.O. Box 18731, Oklahoma City, OK 73154
  Tel: 405/528-3338, Fax: 405/528-1417, http://www.opha.com

Oregon State Pharmacists Association
  1460 State Street, Salem, OR 97301
  Tel: 503/585-4887, Fax: 503/378-9067
  http://www.oregonpharmacists.com
Pennsylvania Pharmacists Association
  508 North 3rd Street, Harrisburg, PA 17101-1199
  Tel: 717/234-6151, http://www.papharmacists.com
Colegio de Farmeceuticos de Puerto Rico
  P.O. Box 360206, San Juan, PR 00936-4087
  Tel: 787/753-7167, Fax: 787/759-9793, http://www.cfpr.org
Rhode Island Pharmacists Association
  500 Prospect Street, Pawtucket, RI 02860
  Tel: 401/725-4141, Fax: 401/725-9960, http://www.ripharm.com
South Carolina Pharmacy Association
  1405 Calhoun Street, Columbia, SC 29201
  Tel: 803/254-1065, Fax: 803/254-9379
  http://www.scpharmacyasssociation.org
South Dakota Pharmacists Association
  P.O. Box 518, Pierre, SD 57501
  Tel: 605/224-2338, Fax: 605/224-1280, http://www.sdpha.org
Tennessee Pharmacists Association
  226 Capitol Boulevard, Suite 810, Nashville, TN 37219-1893
  Tel: 615/256-3023, Fax: 615/255-3528, http://www.tnpharm.org
Texas Pharmacy Association
  P.O. Box 14709, Austin, TX 78761
  Tel: 512/836-8350, Fax: 512/836-0308
  http://www.txpharmacy.com
Utah Pharmaceutical Association
  1805 South Columbia Lane, Orem, UT 84058
  Tel: 801/762-0452, Fax: 801/762-0454, http://www.upha.com
Vermont Pharmacists Association
  P.O. Box 790, Richmond, VT 05477-0790
  Tel: 802/434-3001, Fax: 802/434-4803
Virginia Pharmacists Association
  5501 Patterson Ave., Suite 200, Richmond, VA 23226
  Tel: 800/527-8742, Fax: 804/285-4227
  http://www.pharmacy.su.edu/vpha/homepage.htm
Washington State Pharmacists Association
  1501 Taylor Avenue SW, Renton, WA 98055-3139
  Tel: 425/228-7171, Fax: 425/277-3897
  http://www.pharmcare.org
West Virginia Pharmacists Association
  2003 Quarrier Street, Charleston, WV 25311-2212
  Tel: 304/344-5302, Fax: 304/344-5316

Pharmacy Society of Wisconsin
  701 Heartland Tr., Madison, WI 53717
  Tel: 608/827-9200, Fax: 608/827-9292, http://www.pswi.org
Wyoming Pharmacists Association
  P.O. Box 541, Powell, WY 82435
  Tel: 307/754-4284, Fax: 307/754-4284, http://www.wpha.net
District of Columbia Pharmaceutical Association
  6406 Georgia Avenue SW, Suite 202, Washington, DC 20012-2953
  Tel: 202/829-1515, Fax: 202/829-1514

State Boards
of Pharmacy

Alabama Board of Pharmacy
  1 Perimeter Park South, Suite 425 South, Birmingham, AL 35243
  Tel: 205/967-0130, Fax: 205/967-1009, http://www.albop.com
Alaska Board of Pharmacy
  P.O. Box 110806, 333 Willoughby Avenue, Juneau, AK 99811
  Tel: 907/465-2589, Fax: 907/465-2974
  http://www.dced.state.ak.us/occ/ppha.htm
Arizona State Board of Pharmacy
  4425 West Olive Avenue, Suite 140, Glendale, AZ 85302
  Tel: 623/463-2727, Fax: 623/934-0583
  http://www.pharmacy.state.az.us
Arkansas State Board of Pharmacy
  101 E. Capitol, Suite 218, Little Rock, AR 72201
  Tel: 501/682-0191, Fax: 501/682-0195, http://www.state.ar.us/asbp
California Board of Pharmacy
  400 R. Street, Suite 4070, Sacramento, CA 95814
  Tel: 916/445-5014, Fax: 916/327-6308
  http://www.pharmacy.ca.gov
Colorado State Board of Pharmacy
  1560 Broadway, Suite 1310, Denver, CO 80202-5146
  Tel: 303/894-7750, Fax: 303/894-7764
  http://www.dora.state.co.us/pharmacy
Connecticut Commission of Pharmacy
  State Office Building, 165 Capitol Avenue, Room 147, Hartford, CT 06106
  Tel: 860/713-6065, Fax: 860/713-7242
  http://www.ctdrugcontrol.com/rxcommission.htm
Delaware State Board of Pharmacy
  P.O. Box 637, Dover, DE 19901
  Tel: 302/739-4798, Fax: 302/739-3071
Florida Board of Pharmacy
  4052 Bald Cypress Way, Bin #C04, Tallahassee, FL 32399-3254
  Tel: 850/245-4292, Fax: 850/413-6982
  http://www.doh.state.fl.us/mqa/pharmacy/pshome.htm

Georgia State Board of Pharmacy
  237 Coliseum Drive, Macon, GA 31217-3858
  Tel: 438/207-1686, Fax: 438/207-1699
  http://www.sos.state.ga.us/ebd-pharmacy
Hawaii State Board of Pharmacy
  P.O. Box 3469, Honolulu, HI 96801
  Tel: 808/586-2698, Fax: 808/586-2689
Idaho Board of Pharmacy
  3380 American Terrace, Suite 320, P.O. Box 83720, Boise, ID 83720-0067
  Tel: 208/334-2356, Fax: 208/334-3536, http://www.state.id.us/bop
Illinois Department of Professional Regulation
  320 W. Washington, 3rd Floor, Springfield, IL 62786
  Tel: 217/785-0800, Fax: 217/782-7645, http://www.dpr.state.il.us
Indiana Board of Pharmacy
  402 W. Washington Street, Room 041, Indianapolis, IN 46204-2739
  Tel: 317/232-1140, Fax: 317/232-4236, http://www.ai.org/hbp/isbp
Iowa Board of Pharmacy Examiners
  400 S.W. Eighth Street, Suite F, Des Moine, IA 50309-4688
  Tel: 515/281-5944, Fax: 515/281-4609, http://www.state.ia.us/ibpe
Kansas State Board of Pharmacy
  900 Jackson, Room 513, Topeka, KS 66612
  Tel: 785/296-4056, Fax: 785/296-8420
  http://www.ink.org/public/pharmacy
Kentucky Board of Pharmacy
  1024 Capitol Center Drive, Suite 210, Frankfort, KY 40601-8204
  Tel: 502/573-1580, Fax: 502/573-1582, http://www.kyboardrx.org
Louisiana Board of Pharmacy
  5615 Corporate Boulevard, Suite 8E, Baton Rouge, LA, 70808-2537
  Tel: 225/925-6496, Fax: 225/925-6499, http://www.labp.com
Maine Board of Pharmacy
  35 State House Station, Augusta, ME 04333
  Tel: 207/624-8603, Fax: 207/624-8637
  http://www.state.me.us/pfr/olr
Maryland Board of Pharmacy
  4201 Patterson Avenue, Baltimore, MD 21215-2299
  Tel: 410/764-4755, Fax: 410/358-6207
Massachusetts Board of Registration in Pharmacy
  239 Causeway Street, Boston, MA 02113
  Tel: 617/727-9953, Fax: 617/727-2197
  http://www.state.ma.us/reg/boards/ph
Michigan Board of Pharmacy
  611 W. Ottawa, First Floor, P.O. Box 30670, Lansing, MI 48909-8170
  Tel: 517/373-9102, Fax: 517/373-2179
  http://www.cis.state.mi.us:8020/public/lic_reg$.startup

Minnesota Board of Pharmacy
   2829 University Avenue SE, Suite 530, Minneapolis, MN 55414-3251
   Tel: 612/617-2201, Fax: 612/617-2212
   http://www.phcybrd.state.mn.us
Mississippi Board of Pharmacy
   P.O. Box 24507, Jackson, MS 39225-4507
   Tel: 601/354-6750, Fax: 601/354-6071, http://www.mbp.state.ms.us
Missouri Board of Pharmacy
   P.O. Box 625, 3605 Missouri Blvd., Jefferson City, MO 65102
   Tel: 573/751-0091, Fax: 573/526-3464
   http://www.ecodev.state.mo.us/pr/pharmacy
Montana Board of Pharmacy
   P.O. Box 200513, 111 North Jackson, Helena, MT 59620-0513
   Tel: 406/841-2356, Fax: 406/841-2343
   http://www.com.state.mt.us/License/POL/pol_boards/pha_board/board_page.htm
Nebraska Board of Examiners in Pharmacy
   P.O. Box 94986, 301 Centennial Mall South, Lincoln NE 68509
   Tel: 402/471-2115, Fax: 402/471-0555, http://www.hhs.state.ne.us
Nevada State Board of Pharmacy
   555 Double Eagle Court, Suite 1100, Reno, NV 89511-8991
   Tel: 775/850-1440, Fax: 775/850-1444
   http://www.state.nv.us/pharmacy
State of New Hampshire Board of Pharmacy
   57 Regional Drive, Concord, NH 03301-8518
   Tel: 603/271-2350, Fax: 603/271-2856, http://www.state.nh.us/pharmacy
New Jersey Board of Pharmacy
   P.O. Box 45013, 124 Halsey Street, Newark, NJ 07101
   Tel: 973/504-6450, Fax: 973/648-3355
   http://www.state.nj.us/lps/ca/brief/pharm.htm
New Mexico Board of Pharmacy
   1650 University Boulevard NE, Suite 400B, Albuquerque, NM 87102
   Tel: 505/841-9102, Fax: 505/841-9113
   http://www.state.nm.us/pharmacy
New York Board of Pharmacy
   Cultural Education Center, Room 3035, Madison Avenue,
   Albany, NY 12230
   Tel: 518/474-3817, ext. 130, Fax: 518/473-6995
   http://www.op.nysed.gov.pharm.htm
North Carolina Board of Pharmacy
   P.O. Box 459, Carrboro Plaza, Carrboro, NC 27510-0459
   Tel: 919/942-4454, Fax: 919/967-5757, http://www.ncbop.org
North Dakota State Board of Pharmacy
   P.O. Box 1354, 405 E. Broadway, 3rd Floor, Bismarck, ND 58502-1354
   Tel: 701/328-9535, Fax: 701/258-9312

Ohio State Board of Pharmacy
   77 S. High Street, 17th Floor, Room 1702, Columbus, OH 43215-6126
   Tel: 614/466-4143, Fax: 614/752-4836
   http://www.state.oh.us/pharmacy
Oklahoma State Board of Pharmacy
   4545 Lincoln Boulevard, Suite 112, Oklahoma City, OK 73105-3488
   Tel: 405/521-3815, Fax: 405/521-3758
   http://www.state.ok.us/~pharmacy
Oregon Board of Pharmacy
   800 NE Oregon Street #9, State Office Building Room 425
   Portland, OR 97232
   Tel: 503/731-4032, Fax: 503/731-4067
   http://www.pharmacy.state.or.us
Pennsylvania State Board of Pharmacy
   124 Pine Street, P.O. Box 2649, Harrisburg, PA 17105-2649
   Tel: 717/783-7156, Fax: 717/787-7769
   http://www.dos.state.pa.us/bpoa/phabd/mainpage.htm
Puerto Rico Board of Pharmacy
   800 Avenida Robert T. Todd, Office #201, Stop 18, Santurce, PR 00908
   Tel: 787/725-8161, Fax: 787/725-7903
Rhode Island Board of Pharmacy
   3 Capitol Hill, Room 205, Providence, RI 02908
   Tel: 401/277-2837, Fax: 401/277-2499
South Carolina Board of Pharmacy
   1026 Sumter Street, Room 209, P.O. Box 11927
   Columbia, SC 29211-1927
   Tel: 803/896-4700, Fax: 803/734-1552
   http://www.llr.state.sc.us/POL/Pharmacy
South Dakota Board of Pharmacy
   4305 South Louise Avenue, Suite 104, Sioux Falls, SD 57106
   Tel: 605/362-2737, Fax: 605/362-2738
   http://www.state.sd.us/dcr/pharmacy
Tennessee Board of Pharmacy
   500 James Robertson Parkway, 2nd Floor, Davey Crockett Tower
   Nashville, TN 37243
   Tel: 615/741-2718, Fax: 615/741-2722
   http://www.state.tn.us/commerce/pharmacy
Texas State Board of Pharmacy
   333 Guadalupe, Tower 3, Suite 600, Box 21, Austin, TX 78701-3942
   Tel: 512/305-8000, Fax: 512/305-8082
   http://www.tsbp.state.tx.us
Utah Board of Pharmacy
   160 E. 300 South, P.O. Box 146741, Salt Lake City, UT 84114-6741
   Tel: 801/530-6767, Fax: 801/530-6511

Vermont Board of Pharmacy
   26 Terrace Street, Drawer 09, Montpelier, VT 05609-1106
   Tel: 802/828-2875, Fax: 802/828-2465
   http://www.vtprofessionals.org/pharmacists
Virginia Board of Pharmacy
   6606 W. Broad Street, Suite 400, Richmond, VA 23230-1717
   Tel: 804/662-9911, Fax: 804/662-9313
   http://www.dhp.state.va.us/pharmacy
Washington State Board of Pharmacy
   P.O. Box 47863, Olympia, WA 98504-7863
   Tel: 360/236-4825, Fax: 360/586-4359, http://www.doh.wa.gov/pharmacy
West Virginia Board of Pharmacy
   232 Capitol Street, Charleston, WV 25301
   Tel: 304/558-0558, Fax: 304/558-0572
Wisconsin Pharmacy Examining Board
   1400 E. Washington, P.O. Box 8935, Madison, WI 53708
   Tel: 608/266-2812, Fax: 608/261-7083,
   http://www.state.wi.us/agencies/drl
Wyoming State Board of Pharmacy
   1720 S. Poplar Street, Suite 4, Casper, WY 82601
   Tel: 307/234-0294, Fax: 307/234-7226
   http://www.pharmacyboard.state.wy.us
District of Columbia Board of Pharmacy
   825 North Capitol Street, N.E., Room 2224, Washington, DC 20002
   Tel: 202/442-9200, Fax: 202/442-9431

Canadian Provincial Voluntary Organizations

Pharmacy Association of Alberta
  10130–112th Street, 7th Floor, Edmonton, Alberta, T5K 2K4
  Tel: 780/990-0326, Fax: 780/990-0328
  http://www.altapharm.org
Alberta College of Pharmacists
  10130–112th Street, 7th Floor, Edmonton, Alberta, T5K 2K4
  Tel: 780/990-0321, Fax: 780/990-0328
  http://www.altapharm.org
British Columbia Pharmacy Association
  150–3751 Shell Road, Richmond, British Columbia, V6X 2W2
  Tel: 604/279-2053, Fax: 604/279-2065
College of Pharmacists of British Columbia
  200–1765 West 8th Avenue, Vancouver, British Columbia, V6J 1V8
  Tel: 604/733-2440, Fax: 604/733-2493
  http://www.collpharmbc.org
Manitoba Society of Pharmacists
  22–90 Garry Street, Winnipeg, Manitoba, R3C 4H1
  Tel: 204/956-6680, Fax: 204/956-6686, http://www.msp.mb.ca
New Brunswick Pharmacists' Association Inc.
  410–212 Queen Street, Fredericton, New Brunswick, E3B 1A8
  Tel: 506/459-6008, Fax: 506/453-0736
Pharmacy Association of Nova Scotia
  P.O. Box 3214 (S), 1526 Dresden Row, Halifax, Nova Scotia, B3J 3H5
  Tel: 902/422-9583, Fax: 902/422-2619, http://www.pans.ns.ca
Ontario Pharmacist Association
  301–23 Lesmill Road, Don Mills, Ontario, M3B 3P6
  Tel: 416/441-0788, Fax: 416/441-0791, http://www.opatoday.com
Prince Edward Island Pharmaceutical Association
  P.O. Box 1404, Summerside, Prince Edward Island, C1N 4K2
  Tel: 902/854-3127, Fax: 902/854-3127

Association québécoise des pharmaciens propriétaires
    4378, avenue Pierre-de-Coubertin, Montréal, Québec, H1V 1A6
    Tel: 514/254-0676 or 800/361-7765, Fax: 514/254-1288
Representative Board of Saskatchewan Pharmacists
    700–4010 Pasqua Street, Regina, Saskatchewan, S4S 7B9
    Tel: 306/359-7277, Fax: 306/584-9695

Canadian Provincial Regulatory Authorities

Alberta College of Pharmacists
  10130–112th Street, 7th Floor, Edmonton, Alberta, T5K 2K4
  Tel: 780/990-0321, Fax: 780/990-0328
  http://www.altapharm.org
College of Pharmacists of British Columbia
  200–1765 West 8th Avenue, Vancouver, British Columbia, V6J 1V8
  Tel: 604/733-2440, Fax: 604/733-2493, http://www.collpharmbc.org
Manitoba Pharmaceutical Association
  187 St. Mary's Road, Winnipeg, Manitoba, R2H 1J2
  Tel: 204/233-1411, Fax: 204/237-3468
New Brunswick Pharmaceutical Society
  Burbank Complex, 101–30 Gordon Street, Moncton,
  New Brunswick, E1C 1L8
  Tel: 506/857-8957, Fax: 506/857-8838
Newfoundland Pharmaceutical Association
  Apothecary Hall, 488 Water Street, St. John's, Newfoundland, A1E 1B3
  Tel: 709/753-5877, Fax: 709/753-8615
Northwest Territories Regulatory Authority
  P.O. Box 1320, Yellowknife, Northwest Territories, X1A 2L9
  Tel: 867/920-8058, Fax: 867/873-0484
Nova Scotia Pharmaceutical Society
  P.O. Box 3363 (S), 1526 Dresden Row, Halifax, Nova Scotia, B3J 3J1
  Tel: 902/422-8528, Fax: 902/422-2619
Ontario College of Pharmacists
  483 Huron Street, Toronto, Ontario, M5R 2R4
  Tel: 416/962-4861, Fax: 416/962-1619
  http://www.ocpharma.com
Prince Edward Island Pharmacy Board
  P.O. Box 89, Crapaud, Prince Edward Island, C0A 1J0
  Tel: 902/658-2780, Fax: 902/658-2198

Ordre des pharmaciens du Québec
266, rue Notre-Dame Ouest, Bureau 301, Montréal, Québec, H2Y 1T6
Tel: 800/363-0324 or 514/284-9588, Fax: 514/284-3420
http://www.opq.org
Saskatchewan Pharmaceutical Association
700–4010 Pasqua Street, Regina, Saskatchewan, S4S 7B9
Tel: 306/584-2292, Fax: 306/584-9695
Yukon Regulatory Authority
P.O. Box 2703, Whitehorse, Yukon, Y1A 2C6
Tel: 867/667-5111, Fax: 867/667-3609

Canadian National Pharmacy Associations

Canadian Association of Pharmacy Students and Interns
  14 Kingsbridge Road, St. John's, Newfoundland, A1C 3K3
  Tel: 709/754-2739, Fax: 709/737-7044
Canadian College of Clinical Pharmacy
  275 Armand Frappier Boulevard, Laval, Québec, H7V 4A7
  Tel: 450/978-7870, Fax: 450/978-7946
Canadian Council on Continuing Education in Pharmacy
  3861 Athol Street, Regina, Saskatchewan, S4S 3J2
  Tel: 306/584 5703, Fax: 306/584-5703
Canadian Pharmacists Association
  1785 Alta Vista Drive, Ottawa, Ontario, K1G 3Y6
  Tel: 800/917-9489 (inside Canada) or 613/523-7877 (outside Canada)
  Fax: 613/523-0445, http://www.cdnpharm.ca
Canadian Society of Consultant Pharmacists
  243 Consumers Road, Toronto, Ontario, M2J 4W8
  Tel: 416/490-2865, Fax: 416/493-1581, http://www.ascp.com
Canadian Society of Hospital Pharmacists
  350–1145 Hunt Club Road, Ottawa, Ontario, K1V 0Y3
  Tel: 613/736-9733, Fax: 613/736-5660, http://www.cshp.ca
National Association of Pharmacy Regulatory Authorities
  1005–116 Albert Street, Ottawa, Ontario, K1P 5G3
  Tel: 613/569-9658, Fax: 613/569-9659, http://napra.org
Pharmacy Examining Board of Canada
  603–123 Edward Street, Toronto, Ontario, M5G 1E2
  Tel: 416/979-2431, Fax: 416/599-9244

BOTANICAL NOMENCLATURE

The typical dictionary definition of *herb* includes the fact that it is a plant that does not develop persistent, above-ground woody tissue and that it is used for both medical reasons and for flavoring foods. Professor Varro Tyler, a world-famous pharmacy educator, takes this definition a step further and presents it in a fashion truly relevant to pharmacy: "crude drugs of vegetable origin utilized for the treatment of disease states, often of a chronic nature, or to attain or maintain a condition of improved health."[1]

In 1900, over 50% of the medicines in the *United States Pharmacopoeia* were still botanical products. These "weeds and seeds" were usually bought in bulk or intermediate form and then compounded to meet the requirements set down in the physician's prescription. In order to be a successful apothecary, one had to know the names, both common and official, of these botanical medicines.

Thanks to the modern herbal movement, many botanical products are again gaining popularity. This time it is the consumer who is making decisions about which herbs, and in which dosage forms, they will use. Many of these consumers are seeking information on the proper use and expected consequences of herbal use, and will turn to the pharmacist for this information.

This Section provides a list of the common and official names of the most popular herbs used for health purposes.

---

[1]Tyler, Varro E. *Herbs of Choice: The Therapeutic Use of Phytomedicinals,* Haworth Press, Binghamton, NY, 1994.

Herbal Taxonomy

PRIMARY COMMON NAME SORT

Primary Common Name	Latin Name	Common Names
Agrimony	*Agrimonia eupatoria*	Church steeples, cocklebur
Alfalfa	*Medicago sativa*	Buffalo grass
Aloe	*Aloe vera*	
Angelica	*Angelica archangelica*	Wild celery
Arnica	*Arnica montana*	Mountain tabacco, wolfsbane
Artichoke	*Cynara scolymus*	
Ashwaganda	*Withania somnifera*	Indian ginseng, winter cherry
Asparagus	*Asparagus officinalis*	
Astragalus	*Astragalus membranaceus*	Milk vetch, yellow leader
Balm	*Melissa officinalis*	Bee balm, lemon balm
Barberry	*Berberis vulgaris*	Sowberry
Basil	*Ocimum basilicum*	St. Josephwort
Bearberry	*Arctostaphylos uva ursi*	Upland cranberry
Bilberry	*Vaccinium myrtillus*	Bog bilberry
Black Cohosh	*Cimicifuga racemosa*	Black snakeroot, squaw root, bugbane
Blessed Thistle	*Centaurea benedictus*	Holy ghost herb, holy thistle
Bloodroot	*Sanguinaria canadensis*	Redroot, sanguinara
Blue Cohosh	*Caulophyllum thalictroides*	Blue ginseng, papoose root
Boldo	*Peumus boldus*	Boldea
Borage	*Borago officinalis*	Bee plant, ox's tongue, starflower

Primary Common Name	Latin Name	Common Names
Broom	*Cytisus scoparius*	Banal, hogweed
Burdock	*Articum lappa*	Beggar's buttons, burr
Butcher's Broom	*Ruscus aculeatus*	Box holly
Calendula	*Calendula officinalis*	Goldblood, pot marigold
Cardamom	*Elettaria cardamomum*	
Cascara Sagrada	*Rhamnus purshiana*	Buckthorn, sacred bark
Castor	*Ricinus communis*	
Cat's-Claw	*Uncaria tomentosa*	Life-giving vine of Peru
Cayenne	*Capsicum annuum*	
Celery	*Apium graveolens*	Marsh parsley
Chamomile	*Matricaria recutita*	
Chaparral	*Larrea tridentate*	Creosote bush, greasewood
Chickweed	*Stellaria media*	Mouse-ear, starweed
Cinnamon	*Cinnamonum verum*	
Comfrey	*Symphytum officinale*	Blackwort, slippery root
Coriander	*Coriandrum sativum*	Chinese parsley, cilantro
Cranberry	*Vaccinium macrocarpon*	
Damiana	*Turnera diffusa*	Old woman's broom
Dandelion	*Taraxacum officinale*	Wild endive
Devil's Claw	*Harpagophytum procumbens*	Grapple plant, wood spider
Dong-quai	*Angelica sinensis*	
Echinacea	*Echinacea*	American coneflower, black susan
Elder	*Sambucus canadensis*	Elderberry
Eleuthero	*Eleutherococcus senticosus*	
Ephedra	*Ephedra sinica*	Cao mahaung
Eucalyptus	*Eucalyptus globules*	Blue gum, fever tree
Evening Primrose	*Oenothera biennis*	King's cure-all
Eyebright	*Euphrasia officinalis*	Augentrot, eufrasia
Fennel	*Foeniculum vulgare*	Carosella, finocchio
Fenugreek	*Trigonella foenum graecum*	Bird's foot, trigonella
Feverfew	*Tanacetum parthenium*	Altamisa, midsummer daisy, wild chamomile
Flax	*Linum usitatissimum*	Flaxseed, linseed

Primary Common Name	Latin Name	Common Names
Fo-ti	*Polygonum multiflorum*	Climbing knotweed, knotweed
Foxglove	*Digitalis purpurea*	Fairy cap, fairy finger
Garcinia	*Garginia cambogia*	
Garlic	*Allium sativum*	Camphor of the poor, stinking rose
Gentian	*Gentiana lutea*	Bitterroot, gall weed
Ginger	*Zinigiber officinale*	Gan jiang
Ginkgo	*Ginko biloba*	Kew tree, maidenhair tree
Ginseng	*Panax ginseng*	
Goldenseal	*Hydrastis canadensis*	Indian paint, yellowroot
Gotu Kota	*Centella asiatica*	Indian pennywort, marsh penny, sheep rot
Grapeseed	*Vitis vinifera*	
Hawthorn	*Crataegus* spp.	May blossom, mayflower
Hops	*Humulus lupulus*	
Horehound	*Marrubium vulgare*	
Horse Chestnut	*Aesculus hippocastanum*	Aesculus
Horseradish	*Armoracia rusticana*	
Horsetail	*Equisetum arvense*	Bottle brush, scouring rush
Hyssop	*Hyssopus officinalis*	
Iceland Moss	*Cetraria islandica*	Consumption moss
Ipecac	*Cephaelis ipecacuanha*	
Jojoba	*Simmondsia chinensis*	Deernut oil, goatnut oil
Juniper	*Juniperus communis*	Geneva, giniver
Kava-kava	*Piper methysticum*	Intoxicating pepper
Kudzu	*Pueraria montana*	Ge gen, Japanese arrowroot
Lemon Balm	*Melissa officinalis*	
Lemon Grass	*Cymbopogon citratus*	
Licorice	*Glycyrrhiza glabra*	Gan cao
Lobelia	*Lobelia inflata*	Indian tobacco, pukeweed
Marshmallow	*Althaea officinalis*	Kitme, mallards
Mayapple	*Podophyllum peltati*	American mandrake

Primary Common Name	Latin Name	Common Names
Meadowsweet	*Filipendula ulmaria*	Bridewort, queen-of-the meadow
Milk Thistle	*Silybum marianum*	Marian, Our Lady's thistle
Motherwort	*Leonurus cardiaca*	Heartwort, lion's tail
Mullein	*Varbascum densiflorum*	Aaron's rod, flannel plant, shepherd's staff
Myrrh	*Commiphora myrrhea*	Ma yao
Neem	*Azadirachta indica*	Margosa
Nopal	*Opuntia ficus-indica*	
Oatstraw	*Avena sativa*	
Olive	*Olea europaea*	
Onion	*Allium cepa*	
Oregano	*Origanum heracleoticum*	Wild sage
Parsley	*Petroselinum crispum*	
Passionflower	*Passiflora incarnata*	Apricot vine, maypop, water lemon
Pau d'arco	*Tabebuia impetiginosa*	Ipe roxo
Peppermint	*Mentha x piperita*	
Plantain	*Plantago major*	
Pokeweed	*Phytolacca americana*	Cancer root, pigeon berry
Poppy	*Papaver somniferum*	Opium poppy
Prickly Ash	*Zanthoxylum americanum*	Angelica tree, toothache tree
Psyllium	*Plantago ovata*	Fleawort seed
Pumpkin	*Cucurbita pepo*	
Pygeum	*Prunus africana*	
Red Clover	*Trifolium pratense*	Cow clover, trefoil
Reishi	*Ganoderma lucidum*	Holy mushroom
Rhubarb	*Rheum officinale*	
Rose hips	*Rosa canina*	Heps, hipberries
Rosemary	*Rosmarinus officinalis*	Mi die xiang, old man
Sage	*Salvia officinalis*	
Sarsaparilla	*Smilax* spp.	
Sassafras	*Sassafras albidum*	Ague tree, saloop
Saw Palmetto	*Serenoa repens*	Cabbage palm, serenoa
Schisandra	*Schisandra chinensis*	Five-flavor seed
Senega	*Polygala senega*	Rattlesnake root, milkwort

Primary Common Name	Latin Name	Common Names
Senna	*Senna alexandrina*	
Shepard's Purse	*Capsella bursa pastoris*	Lady's purse, shovelweed
Skullcap	*Scutellaria lateriflora*	
Slippery Elm	*Ulmus rubra*	Moose elm
Squill	*Urginea maritime*	Sea onion
St. John's Wort	*Hypericum perforatum*	Goat weed, rosin rose
Stinging Nettle	*Urtica dioica*	
Tea Tree	*Melaleuca alternifolia*	Cajeput
Thyme	*Thymus vulgaris*	
Tumeric	*Curcuma domestica*	Indian saffron, curcuma
Valerian	*Valeriana officinalis*	Garden heliotrope
Vitex	*Vitex agnus castus*	Chasteberry, hemp tree
White Oak	*Quercus alba*	
Wild Yam	*Dioscorea villosa*	Colic root
Willow	*Salix* spp.	
Witch Hazel	*Hamamelis virginiana*	Tobacco wood, winter bloom
Yellow Dock	*Rumex crispus*	Rumex
Yohimbe	*Pausinystalia yohimbe*	
Yucca	*Yucca schidigera*	Adam's needle, dagger plant, Joshua tree

Herbal Nomenclature

LATIN NAME SORT

Latin Name	Primary Common Name	Common Names
Aesculus hippocastanum	Horse chestnut	Aesculus
Agrimonia eupatoria	Agrimony	Church steeples, cocklebur
Allium cepa	Onion	
Allium sativum	Garlic	Camphor of the poor, stinking rose
Aloe vera	Aloe	
Althaea officinalis	Marshmallow	Kitme, mallards
Angelica archangelica	Angelica	Wild celery
Angelica sinensis	Dong-quai	
Apium graveolens	Celery	Marsh parsley
Arctostaphylos uva ursi	Bearberry	Upland cranberry
Armoracia rusticana	Horseradish	
Arnica montana	Arnica	Mountain tabacco, wolfsbane
Articum lappa	Burdock	Beggar's buttons, burr
Asparagus officinalis	Asparagus	
Astragalus membranaceus	Astragalus	Milk vetch, yellow leader
Avena sativa	Oatstraw	
Azadirachta indica	Neem	Margosa
Berberis vulgaris	Barberry	Sowberry
Borago officinalis	Borage	Bee plant, ox's tongue, starflower
Calendula officinalis	Calendula	Goldblood, pot marigold
Capsella bursa pastoris	Shepard's Purse	Lady's purse, shovelweed

Latin Name	Primary Common Name	Common Names
Capsicum annuum	Cayenne	
Caulophyllum thalictroides	Blue Cohosh	Blue ginseng, papoose root
Centaurea benedictus	Blessed Thistle	Holy ghost herb, holy thistle
Centella asiatica	Gotu Kola	Indian pennywort, marsh penny, sheep rot
Cephaelis ipecacuanha	Ipecac	
Centraria islandica	Iceland moss	Consumption moss
Cimicifuga racemosa	Black Cohosh	Black snakeroot, squaw root, bugbane
Cinnamomum verum	Cinnamon	
Commiphora myrrhea	Myrrh	Ma yao
Coriandrum sativum	Coriander	Chinese parsley, cilantro
Crataegus spp.	Hawthorn	May blossom, mayflower
Cucurbita pepo	Pumpkin	
Curcuma domestica	Tumeric	Indian saffron, curcuma
Cymbopogon citratus	Lemon Grass	
Cynara scolymus	Artichoke	
Cytisus scoparius	Broom	Banal, hogweed
Digitalis purpurea	Foxglove	Fairy cap, fairy finger
Dioscorea villosa	Wild Yam	Colic root
Echinacea	Echinacea	American coneflower, black susan
Elettaria cardamomum	Cardamom	
Eleutherococcus senticosus	Eleuthero	
Ephedra sinica	Ephedra	Cao mahaung
Equisetum arvense	Horsetail	Bottle brush, scouring rush
Eucalyptus globules	Eucalyptus	Blue gum, fever tree
Euphrasia officinalis	Eyebright	Augentrot, eufrasia
Filipendula ulmaria	Meadowsweet	Bridewort, queen-of-the medow
Foeniculum vulgare	Fennel	Carosella, finocchio
Ganoderma lucidum	Reishi	Holy mushroom
Garcinia cambogia	Garcinia	
Geniana lutea	Gentian	Bitterroot, gall weed

Latin Name	Primary Common Name	Common Names
Ginko biloba	Ginkgo	Kew tree, maidenhair tree
Glycyrrhiza glabra	Licorice	Gan cao
Hamamelis virginiana	Witch Hazel	Tobacco wood, winter bloom
Harpagophytum procumbens	Devil's Claw	Grapple plant, wood spider
Humulus lupulus	Hops	
Hydrastis canadensis	Goldenseal	Indian paint, yellowroot
Hypericum perforatum	St. John's Wort	Goat weed, rosin rose
Hyssopus officinalis	Hyssop	
Juniperus communis	Juniper	Geneva, giniver
Larrea tridentate	Chaparral	Creosote bush, greasewood
Leonurus cardiaca	Motherwort	Heartwort, lion's tail
Linum usitatissimum	Flax	Flaxseed, linseed
Lobelia inflata	Lobelia	Indian tobacco, pukeweed
Marrubium vulgare	Horehound	
Matricaria recutita	Chamomile	
Medicago sativa	Alfalfa	Buffalo grass
Melaleuca alternifolia	Tea Tree	Cajeput
Melissa officinalis	Balm	Bee balm, lemon balm
Melissa officinalis	Lemon Balm	
Mentha x piperita	Peppermint	
Ocimum basilicum	Basil	St. Josephwort
Oenothera biennis	Evening Primrose	King's cure-all
Olea europaea	Olive	
Opuntia fiscus-indica	Nopal	
Origanum heracleoticum	Oregano	Wild sage
Panax ginseng	Ginseng	
Papaver somniferum	Poppy	Opium poppy
Passiflora incarnata	Passionflower	Apricot vine, maypop, water lemon
Pausinystalia yohimbe	Yohimbe	
Petroselinum crispum	Parsley	
Peumus boldus	Boldo	Boldea
Phytolacca americana	Pokeweed	Cancer root, pigeon berry
Piper methysticum	Kava-kava	Intoxicating pepper

Latin Name	Primary Common Name	Common Names
Plantago major	Plantain	
Plantago ovata	Psyllium	Fleawort seed
Podophyllum peltati	Mayapple	American mandrake
Polygala senega	Senega	Rattlesnake root, milkwort
Polygonum multiflorum	Fo-ti	Climbing knotweed, knotweed
Prunus africana	Pygeum	
Pueraria montana	Kudzu	Ge gen, Japanese arrowroot
Quercus alba	White Oak	
Rhamnus purshiana	Cascara Sagrada	Buckthorn, sacred bark
Rheum officinale	Rhubarb	
Ricinus communis	Castor	
Rosa canina	Rose hips	Heps, hipberries
Rosmarinus officinalis	Rosemary	Mi die xiang, old man
Rumex crispus	Yellow Dock	Rumex
Ruscus aculeatus	Butcher's Broom	Box holly
Salix spp.	Willow	
Salvia officinalis	Sage	
Sambucus canadensis	Elder	Elderberry
Sanguinaria canadensis	Bloodroot	Redroot, sanguinara
Sassafras albidum	Sassafras	Ague tree, saloop
Schisandra chinensis	Schisandra	Five-flavor seed
Scutellaria lateriflora	Skullcap	
Senna alexandrina	Senna	
Serenoa repens	Saw Palmetto	Cabbage palm, serenoa
Silybum marianum	Milk Thistle	Marian, Our Lady's thistle
Simmondsia chinensis	Jojoba	Deernut oil, goatnut oil
Smilax spp.	Sarsaparilla	
Stellaria media	Chickweed	Mouse-ear, starweed
Symphytum officinale	Comfrey	Blackwort, slippery root
Tabebuia impetiginosa	Pau d'arco	Ipe roxo
Tanacetum parthenium	Feverfew	Altamisa, midsummer daisy, wild chamomile
Taraxacum officinale	Dandelion	Wild endive
Thymus vulgaris	Thyme	
Trifolium pratense	Red Clover	Cow clover, trefoil

Latin Name	Primary Common Name	Common Names
Trigonella foenum graecum	Fenugreek	Bird's foot, tirgonella
Turnera diffusa	Damiana	Old woman's broom
Ulmus rubra	Slippery Elm	Moose elm
Uncaria tomentosa	Cat's-Claw	Life-giving vine of Peru
Urginea maritime	Squill	Sea onion
Urtica dioica	Stinging Nettle	
Vaccinium macrocarpon	Cranberry	
Vaccinium myrtillus	Bilberry	Bog bilberry
Valeriana officinalis	Valerian	Garden heliotrope
Varbascum densiflorum	Mullein	Aaron's rod, flannel plant, shepherd's staff
Vitex angus castus	Vitex	Chasteberry, hemp tree
Vitis vinifera	Grapeseed	
Withania somnifera	Ashwaganda	Indian ginseng, winter cherry
Yucca schidigera	Yucca	Adam's needle, dagger plant, Joshua tree
Zanthoxylum americanum	Prickly Ash	Angelica tree, tooth-ache tree
Zinigiber officinale	Ginger	Gan jiang

PHARMACY'S PRINCIPLES

No matter which definition of profession is used, a common attribute is the requirement that the profession must fulfill a societal need. This is because it is society that determines which activities constitute a profession; an occupation cannot unilaterally declare itself to be a profession. In the case of the profession of pharmacy, this means that not only must the pharmacist be well trained and knowledgeable but that the pharmacist must apply that knowledge for the good of the patient.

One of the attributes of a profession is the existence of a code of ethics or set of standards. Such a code communicates to the public what practitioners of the profession will or will not do. Pharmacists have developed a Code of Ethics that has changed to meet the changing expectations of the public that it serves.

The Pharmacist's Code of Ethics stresses that the individual pharmacist has an obligation to the individual patient, which is to help the patient obtain the best results possible from his or her medications. All other considerations and points of ethical expectations address how this optimum outcome is to be achieved.

The Principles of Practice for Pharmaceutical Care focus attention on the patient. It is not important what pharmacists call their practice; what is important is that all activities be judged by the criteria of what good is delivered to and for the patient. For, without the patient, there is no reason to believe that pharmacy or its practitioners meet the societal needs of a profession.

Code of Ethics for Pharmacists[2]

PREAMBLE

Pharmacists are health professionals who assist individuals in making the best use of medications. This Code, prepared and supported by pharmacists, is intended to state publicly the principles that form the fundamental basis of the roles and responsibilities of pharmacists. These principles, based on moral obligations and virtues, are established to guide pharmacists in relationships with patients, health professionals, and society.

I. A pharmacist respects the covenantal relationship between the patient and pharmacist.

Considering the patient-pharmacist relationship as a covenant means that a pharmacist has moral obligations in response to the gift of trust received from society. In return for this gift, a pharmacist promises to help individuals achieve optimum benefit from their medications, to be committed to their welfare, and to maintain their trust.

II. A pharmacist promotes the good of every patient in a caring, compassionate, and confidential manner.

A pharmacist places concern for the well-being of the patient at the center of professional practice. In doing so, a pharmacist considers needs stated by the patient as well as those defined by health science. A pharmacist is dedicated to protecting the dignity of the patient. With a caring attitude and a compassionate spirit, a pharmacist focuses on serving the patient in a private and confidential manner.

---

[2]Adopted by the membership of the American Pharmaceutical Association October 27, 1994.

III. A pharmacist respects the autonomy and dignity of each patient.

A pharmacist promotes the right of self-determination and recognizes individual self-worth by encouraging patients to participate in decisions about their health. A pharmacist communicates with patients in terms that are understandable. In all cases, a pharmacist respects personal and cultural differences among patients.

IV. A pharmacist acts with honesty and integrity in professional relationships.

A pharmacist has a duty to tell the truth and to act with conviction of conscience. A pharmacist avoids discriminatory practices, behavior or work conditions that impair professional judgment, and actions that compromise dedication to the best interests of patients.

V. A pharmacist maintains professional competence.

A pharmacist has a duty to maintain knowledge and abilities as new medications, devices, and technologies become available and as health information advances.

VI. A pharmacist respects the values and abilities of colleagues and other health professionals.

When appropriate, a pharmacist asks for the consultation of colleagues or other health professionals or refers the patient. A pharmacist acknowledges that colleagues and other health professionals may differ in the beliefs and values they apply to the care of the patient.

VII. A pharmacist serves individual, community, and societal needs.

The primary obligation of a pharmacist is to individual patients. However, the obligations of a pharmacist may at times extend beyond the individual to the community and society. In these situations, the pharmacist recognizes the responsibilities that accompany these obligations and acts accordingly.

VIII. A pharmacist seeks justice in the distribution of health resources.

When health resources are allocated, a pharmacist is fair and equitable, balancing the needs of patients and society.

Principles of Practice for Pharmaceutical Care[3]

PREAMBLE

Pharmaceutical Care is a patient-centered, outcomes-oriented pharmacy practice that requires the pharmacist to work in concert with the patient and the patient's other healthcare providers to promote health, to prevent disease, and to assess, monitor, initiate, and modify medication use to assure that drug therapy regimens are safe and effective. The goal of Pharmaceutical Care is to optimize the patient's health-related quality of life, and achieve positive clinical outcomes, within realistic economic expenditures. To achieve this goal, the following must be accomplished:

A. A professional relationship must be established and maintained.

Interaction between the pharmacist and the patient must occur to assure that a relationship based upon caring, trust, open communication, cooperation, and mutual decision making is established and maintained. In this relationship, the pharmacist holds the patient's welfare paramount, maintains an appropriate attitude of caring for the patient's welfare, and uses all his/her professional knowledge and skills on the patient's behalf. In exchange, the patient agrees to supply personal information and preferences, and participate in the therapeutic plan. The pharmacist develops mechanisms to assure the patient has access to pharmaceutical care at all times.

B. Patient-specific medical information must be collected, organized, recorded, and maintained.

Pharmacists must collect and/or generate subjective and objective infor-

---

[3]Prepared by the APhA Pharmaceutical Care Guidelines Advisory Committee, approved by the APhA Board of Trustees, August 1995.

mation regarding the patient's general health and activity status, past medical history, medication history, social history, diet and exercise history, history of present illness, and economic situation (financial and insured status). Sources of information may include, but are not limited to, the patient, medical charts and reports, pharmacist-conducted health/physical assessment, the patient's family or caregiver, insurer, and other healthcare providers including physicians, nurses, mid-level practitioners and other pharmacists. Since this information will form the basis for decisions regarding the development and subsequent modification of the drug therapy plan, it must be timely, accurate, and complete, and it must be organized and recorded to assure that it is readily retrievable and updated as necessary and appropriate. Patient information must be maintained in a confidential manner.

C. Patient-specific medical information must be evaluated and a drug therapy plan developed mutually with the patient.

Based upon a thorough understanding of the patient and his/her condition or disease and its treatment, the pharmacist must, with the patient and with the patient's other healthcare providers as necessary, develop an outcomes-oriented drug therapy plan. The plan may have various components which address each of the patient's diseases or conditions. In designing the plan, the pharmacist must carefully consider the psycho-social aspects of the disease as well as the potential relationship between the cost and/or complexity of therapy and patient adherence. As one of the patient's advocates, the pharmacist assures the coordination of drug therapy with the patient's other healthcare providers and the patient. In addition, the patient must be apprised of (1) various pros and cons (i.e., cost, side effects, different monitoring aspects, etc.) of the options relative to drug therapy and (2) instances where one option may be more beneficial based on the pharmacist's professional judgment. The essential elements of the plan, including the patient's responsibilities, must be carefully and completely explained to the patient. Information should be provided to the patient at a level the patient will understand. The drug therapy plan must be documented in the patient's pharmacy record and communicated to the patient's other healthcare providers as necessary.

D. The pharmacist assures that the patient has all supplies, information and knowledge necessary to carry out the drug therapy plan.

The pharmacist providing Pharmaceutical Care must assume ultimate responsibility for assuring that his/her patient has been able to obtain, and is appropriately using, any drugs and related products or equipment called for in the drug therapy plan. The pharmacist must also assure that the patient has a thorough understanding of the disease and the therapy/medications prescribed in the plan.

E. The pharmacist reviews, monitors, and modifies the therapeutic plan as necessary and appropriate, in concert with the patient and healthcare team.

The pharmacist is responsible for monitoring the patient's progress in achieving the specific outcomes according to strategy developed in the drug therapy plan. The pharmacist coordinates changes in the plan with the patient and the patient's other healthcare providers as necessary and appropriate in order to maintain or enhance the safety and/or effectiveness of drug therapy and to help minimize overall healthcare costs. Patient progress is accurately documented in the pharmacy record and communicated to the patient and to the patient's other healthcare providers as appropriate. The pharmacist shares information with other healthcare providers as the setting for care changes, thus helping assure continuity of care as the patient moves between the community setting, the institutional setting, and the long-term care setting.

PRACTICE PRINCIPLES

1. Data Collection

1.1 The pharmacist conducts an initial interview with the patient for the purposes of establishing a professional working relationship and initiating the patient's pharmacy record. In some situations (e.g., pediatrics, geriatrics, critical care, language barriers) the opportunity to develop a professional relationship with and collect information directly from the patient may not exist. Under these circumstances, the pharmacist should work directly with the patient's parent, guardian, and/or principal caregiver.

1.2 The interview is organized, professional, and meets the patient's need for confidentiality and privacy. Adequate time is devoted to assure that questions and answers can be fully developed without either party feeling uncomfortable or hurried. The interview is used to systematically collect patient-specific subjective information and to initiate a pharmacy record which includes information and data regarding the patient's general health and activity status, past medical history, medication history, social history (including economic situation), family history, and history of present illness. The record should also include information regarding the patient's thoughts or feelings and perceptions of his/her condition or disease.

1.3 The pharmacist uses health/physical assessment techniques (blood-pressure monitoring, etc.) appropriately and as necessary to acquire necessary patient-specific objective information.

1.4 The pharmacist uses appropriate secondary sources to supplement the information obtained through the initial patient interview and health/physical assessment. Sources may include, but are not limited to, the patient's medical record or medical reports, the patient's family, and the patient's other healthcare providers.

1.5 The pharmacist creates a pharmacy record for the patient and accurately records the information collected. The pharmacist assures that the patient's record is appropriately organized, kept current, and accurately reflects all pharmacist-patient encounters. The confidentiality of the information in the record is carefully guarded and appropriate systems are in place to assure security. Patient-identifiable information contained in the record is provided to others only upon the authorization of the patient or as required by law.

2. Information Evaluation

2.1 The pharmacist evaluates the subjective and objective information collected from the patient and other sources, then forms conclusions regarding: (1) opportunities to improve and/or assure the safety, effectiveness, and/or economy of current or planned drug therapy; (2) opportunities to minimize current or potential future drug or health-related problems; and (3) the timing of any necessary future pharmacist consultation.

2.2 The pharmacist records the conclusions of the evaluation in the medical and/or pharmacy record.

2.3 The pharmacist discusses the conclusions with the patient, as necessary and appropriate, and assures an appropriate understanding of the nature of the condition or illness and what might be expected with respect to its management.

3. Formulating a Plan

3.1 The pharmacist, in concert with other healthcare providers, identifies, evaluates and then chooses the most appropriate action(s) to: (1) improve and/or assure the safety, effectiveness, and/or cost-effectiveness of current or planned drug therapy; and/or, (2) minimize current or potential future health-related problems.

3.2 The pharmacist formulates plans to effect the desired outcome. The plans may include, but are not limited to, work with the patient as well as with other health providers to develop a patient-specific drug therapy protocol or to modify prescribed drug therapy, develop and/or implement drug therapy monitoring mechanisms, recommend nutritional or dietary modifications, add non-prescription medications or non-drug treatments, refer the patient to an appropriate source of care, or institute an existing drug therapy protocol.

3.3 For each problem identified, the pharmacist actively considers the patient's needs and determines the desirable and mutually agreed upon outcome and incorporates these into the plan. The plan may include specific disease state and drug therapy endpoints and monitoring endpoints.

3.4 The pharmacist reviews the plan and desirable outcomes with the patient and with the patient's other healthcare provider(s) as appropriate.

3.5 The pharmacist documents the plan and desirable outcomes in the patient's medical and/or pharmacy record.

4. Implementing the Plan

4.1 The pharmacist and the patient take the steps necessary to implement the plan. These steps may include, but are not limited to, contacting other health providers to clarify or modify prescriptions, initiating drug therapy, educating the patient and/or caregiver(s), coordinating the acquisition of medications and/or related supplies, which might include helping the patient overcome financial barriers or lifestyle barriers that might otherwise interfere with the therapy plan, or coordinating appointments with other healthcare providers to whom the patient is being referred.

4.2 The pharmacist works with the patient to maximize patient understanding and involvement in the therapy plan, assures that arrangements for drug therapy monitoring (e.g., laboratory evaluation, blood pressure monitoring, home blood glucose testing, etc.) are made and understood by the patient, and that the patient receives and knows how to properly use all necessary medications and related equipment. Explanations are tailored to the patient's level of comprehension and teaching and adherence aids are employed as indicated.

4.3 The pharmacist assures that appropriate mechanisms are in place to ensure that the proper medications, equipment, and supplies are received by the patient in a timely fashion.

4.4 The pharmacist documents in the medical and/or pharmacy record the steps taken to implement the plan including the appropriate baseline monitoring parameters, and any barriers which will need to be overcome.

4.5 The pharmacist communicates the elements of the plan to the patient and/or the patient's other healthcare provider(s). The pharmacist shares information with other healthcare providers as the setting for care changes, in order to help maintain continuity of care as the patient moves between the ambulatory, inpatient or long-term care environment.

5. Monitoring and Modifying the Plan/Assuring Positive Outcomes

5.1 The pharmacist regularly reviews subjective and objective monitoring parameters in order to determine if satisfactory progress is being made toward achieving desired outcomes as outlined in the drug therapy plan.

5.2 The pharmacist and patient determine if the original plan should continue to be followed or if modifications are needed. If changes are necessary, the pharmacist works with the patient/caregiver and his/her other healthcare providers to modify and implement the revised plan as described in "Formulating the Plan" and "Implementing the Plans" above.

5.3 The pharmacist reviews ongoing progress in achieving desired outcomes with the patient and provides a report to the patient's other healthcare providers as appropriate. As progress towards outcomes is achieved, the pharmacist should provide positive reinforcement.

5.4 A mechanism is established for follow-up with patients. The pharmacist uses appropriate professional judgment in determining the need to notify the patient's other healthcare providers of the patient's level of adherence with the plan.

5.5 The pharmacist updates the patient's medical and/or pharmacy record with information concerning patient progress, noting the subjective and objective information which has been considered, his/her assessment of the patient's current progress, the patient's assessment of his/her current progress, and any modifications that are being made to the plan. Communications with other healthcare providers should also be noted.

APPENDIX[4]

Pharmaceutical care is a process of drug therapy management that requires a change in the orientation of traditional professional attitudes and re-engineering of the traditional pharmacy environment. Certain elements of structure must be in place to provide quality pharmaceutical care. Some of these elements are: (1) knowledge, skill, and function of personnel, (2) systems for data collection, documentation, and transfer of information, (3) efficient work flow processes, (4) references, resources and equipment, (5) communication skills, and (6) commitment to quality improvement and assessment procedures.

---

[4]From *Pharmaceutical Care, Principles of Practice*, American Pharmaceutical Association, 2001.

Knowledge, Skill, and Function of Personnel

The implementation of pharmaceutical care is supported by knowledge and skills in the area of patient assessment, clinical information, communication, adult teaching and learning principles and psychosocial aspects of care. To use these skills, responsibilities must be reassessed, and assigned to appropriate personnel, including pharmacists, technicians, automation, and technology. A mechanism of certifying and credentialling will support the implementation of pharmaceutical care.

Systems for Data Collection and Documentation

The implementation of pharmaceutical care is supported by data collection and documentation systems that accommodate patient care communications (e.g., patient contact notes, medical/medication history), interprofessional communications (e.g., physician communication, pharmacist to pharmacist communication), quality assurance (e.g., patient outcomes assessment, patient care protocols), and research (e.g., data for pharmacoepidemiology, etc.). Documentation systems are vital for reimbursement considerations.

Efficient Work Flow Processes

The implementation of pharmaceutical care is supported by incorporating patient care into the activities of the pharmacist and other personnel.

References, Resources, and Equipment

The implementation of pharmaceutical care is supported by tools that facilitate patient care, including equipment to assess medication therapy adherence and effectiveness, clinical resource materials, and patient education materials. Tools may include computer software support, drug utilization evaluation (DUE) programs, disease management protocols, etc.

Communication Skills

The implementation of pharmaceutical care is supported by patient-centered communication. Within this communication, the patient plays a key role in the overall management of the therapy plan.

Quality Assessment/Improvement Programs

The implementation and practice of pharmaceutical care is supported and improved by measuring, assessing, and improving pharmaceutical care activities utilizing the conceptual framework of continuous quality improvement.

This document will not cover each and every situation; that was not the intent of the Advisory Committee. This is a dynamic document and is intended to be revised as the profession adapts to its new role. It is hoped that pharmacists will use these principles, adapting them to their own situation and environments, to establish and implement pharmaceutical care.

Note: Although "drug therapy" typically refers to intended, beneficial effects of pharmacologic drugs, in this document, "drug therapy" refers to the intended, beneficial use of drugs—whether diagnostic or therapeutic—and thus includes diagnostic radiopharmaceuticals, X-ray contrast media, etc. in addition to pharmacologic drugs. Similarly, "drug therapy plan" includes the outcomes oriented plan for diagnostic drug use in addition to pharmacologic drug use.

GLOSSARY OF MANAGED CARE TERMS

Managed care has brought a whole new vocabulary into health care. Important concepts and definitions are more likely to be derived from the insurance or business communities than from health care. Understanding the terms of this payer community is increasingly important as third party programs become the dominant payer for prescription and nonprescription medicines.

Glossary of Managed Care Terms

access   a patient's ability to obtain medical care. The ease of access is determined by components such as the availability of medical services and their acceptability to the patient, the location of health care facilities, transportation, hours of operation and affordability of care.

accountable health plans (AHPs)   (see organized delivery systems) under various Managed Competition Acts introduced in Congress during 1994, providers and insurance companies would be encouraged (through tax incentives) to form AHPs, similar to HMOs, PPOs, and other group practices. Accountable health plans would compete on the basis of quality and cost, and would offer insurance and health care as a single product. They would be responsible for the total health of members and reporting of medical outcomes in accordance with federal and state guidelines.

accrete   a term used by Medicare to describe the process of adding new enrollees to a health plan.

accreditation   accreditation programs grant an official authorization or approval to an organization determined by a set of industry-derived standards.

actively-at-work   a requirement of many insurers' policies stipulating that if a given employee is not actively at work on the day the policy goes into effect, medical coverage will not be provided until that employee returns to work.

activities of daily living (ADLs)   activities performed as part of a person's daily routine of self-care, such as bathing, dressing, toileting, transferring, continence and eating.

actual acquisition cost   the pharmacist's net payment made to purchase a drug product, after taking into account such items as purchasing allowances, discounts, rebates and the like.

actual charge   the amount a physician or other provider actually bills a patient for a particular medical service, procedure or supply in a specific instance. The actual charge may differ from the usual, customary, prevailing and/or reasonable charge.

This section is reprinted from *NPC Pocket Glossary of Managed Care Terms,* National Pharmaceutical Counsel Inc.

actuarial table   a chart or system for determining insurance rates and eligibility created by using probability and statistics.

actuary   a person trained in the insurance field who determines policy rates and reserves dividends as well as conducts various other statistical studies.

acute care   care for a person with a single episode of short-term illness or with an exacerbation of a chronic condition.

additional drug benefit list   a list of pharmaceutical products approved by a health plan and employer for dispensing in larger quantities than the standards covered under a benefit package in order to facilitate long-term patient use. The list is subject to periodic review and modification by the health plan. Also called *drug maintenance list*.

adjudication   processing a claim through a series of edits in order to determine proper payment.

adjusted average per capita cost (AAPCC)   the estimated average cost of Medicare benefits for an individual in a county, based on the following factors: age, sex, institutional status, Medicaid, disability and end stage renal disease status. HCFA uses the AAPCCs to make monthly payments to risk and cost contractors.

adjusted community rating (ACR)   insurance premium based on community rating adjusted for group specific demographics and the group's prior experience. Also known as *prospective rating* and *factor rating*.

administrative costs   the costs incurred by a carrier such as an insurance company or HMO, for services such as claims processing, billing and enrollment, and overhead costs. Administrative costs can be expressed as a percentage of premiums or on a per member per month basis. Additional costs that are often expressed as administrative include those related to utilization review, insurance marketing, medical underwriting, agents' commissions, premium collection, claims processing, insurer profit, quality assurance activities, medical libraries and risk management.

adjusted expenses per admission   average expense to the hospital in providing care for one inpatient day. Adjusted expenses are derived by subtracting outpatient expenses from total expenses. In patient expense is divided by total admissions.

adjusted expenses per inpatient day   expenses incurred for inpatient care only, and derived by dividing total expenses by adjusted inpatient days.

adjusted inpatient days   an aggregate figure reflecting the number of days of inpatient care, plus an estimate of the volume of outpatient services, expressed in units equivalent to an inpatient day in terms of level of effort.

administrative services only (ASO)   an insurance arrangement requiring the employer to be at risk for the cost of health care services provided, while a separate company delivers administrative services. This is a common arrangement when an employer sponsors a self-funded health care program.

admissions/1000   the number of hospital admissions per 1000 health plan members. The formula for this measure is: (# of admissions/member months) × 1000 members × # of months. It can also be used to express the number of hospital admissions per 1000 members of any other given population. Example: 998 admissions/1000 elderly in a given state.

admits   the number of admissions to a hospital or inpatient facility during a reporting period (excludes newborns).

admissions   number of patients, excluding newborns, accepted for inpatient service during a reporting period.

Advanced Practice Nurse (APN)   an umbrella term which describes a registered nurse (RN) who has met advanced educational and clinical practice requirements beyond the two to four years of basic nursing education required of all RNs.

adverse selection   a term used to describe a situation in which a carrier disproportionally enrolls a population which is prone to higher than average utilization of benefits, thereby driving up costs and increasing financial risk.

affiliated provider   a health care provider of facility that is subcontracted by a primary provider in order to gain additional services for its members.

aftercare   services following hospitalization or rehabilitation, individualized for each patient's needs. Aftercare gradually phases the patient out of treatment while providing follow-up attention to prevent relapse.

age/sex factor   a measurement used in underwriting which represents the age and sex risk of medical costs of one population relative to another. A group with an age/sex factor of 1.00 is average. An age/sex factor above 1.00 indicates a higher than average demographic risk of expected medical claims. An age/sex factor below 1.00 indicates a lower than average demographic risk of expected medical claims.

Agency for Health Care Policy and Research (AHCPR)   a federal agency under Health and Human Services (HHS) whose purpose is to enhance the quality and effectiveness of health care by funding health care services research, conducting health technology assessments and outcomes studies, and developing and disseminating clinical practice guidelines.

allied health personnel   specially trained and licensed (when necessary) health workers other than physicians, dentists, optometrists, chiropractors, podiatrists, and nurses. The term is sometimes used synonymously with paramedical personnel, all health workers who perform tasks which must otherwise be performed by a physician, or health workers who do not usually engage in independent practice.

allowable charge   the maximum fee that a third party will reimburse a provider for a given service. An allowable charge may not be the same amount as either a reasonable or customary charge.

allowable costs   charges for services rendered or supplies furnished by a health provider which qualify for an insurance reimbursement.

all-payer system   1. a plan which would impose uniform prices on medical services for all payers, 2. a reimbursement set up where all insurers reimburse providers using the same accounting system.

alternative care   medical care received in lieu of inpatient hospitalization. Sometimes referred to as care available in lieu of accepted medical practices.

alternative delivery systems (ADS)   a catch-all phrase used to describe all forms of health care delivery other than traditional fee-for-service and indemnity health care. Just about all managed care organizations are called "alternative delivery systems."

alternative-detailing   a procedure utilized to contact providers in order to discuss treatment alternatives. Most often used in order to direct compliance with a formulary of medical protocol.

ambulatory care   health care services that do not require hospitalization of a patient, such as those delivered at a physician's office, clinic, medical center, or outpatient facility.

ambulatory setting   an institutional health setting in which organized health services are provided on an outpatient basis, such as a surgery center, clinic, or other outpatient facility.

ambulatory surgical facility   a freestanding or hospital-based health care center that performs surgical services not requiring overnight confinement.

ambulatory utilization review   the review of care provided in ambulatory settings.

American Association of Preferred Providers Organizations (AAPPO)   reorganized as the Association of Managed health care Organizations (AMHO).

American Association of Health Plans (AAHP)   IPA/HMO trade association

American Medical Assoc. (AMA)   prominent organization of physicians. Establishes physicians' standards of practice and accredits medical schools. Publishes the *Journal of American Medical Association* (JAMA) and the *American Medical News*. Active lobbyist organization for physicians.

American Medical Care and Review Association (AMCRA)   merged with GHAA to form the American Association of Health Plans (AAHP).

American Society of Health-Systems Pharmacists (ASHP)   trade group for pharmacists in hospitals and other health systems.

American Hospital Association (AHA)   organization of hospitals designed to promote high-quality hospital care. Conducts an annual survey of membership listing composite statistical profiles of all registered hospitals.

ancillary charge   1. the fee associated with additional service performed prior to and/or secondary to a significant procedure. 2. also referred to as hospital "extras" or misc. hospital charges. They are supplementary to a hospital's daily room and board charge. They include such items as charges for drugs, medicines and dressings, lab services, X-ray examinations, and use of the operating room.

ancillary services   hospital services other than room, board, and professional services. They may include X-ray, laboratory, or anesthesia.

any willing provider   a requirement that a health insurance plan or a health maintenance organization (HMO) must sign a contract for the delivery of health care services with any provider in the area that would like to provide such services to the plan's or HMO's enrollees.

appeal   1. a formal request by a covered person or provider for reconsideration of a decision, such as a utilization review recommendation, a benefit payment or an administrative action. 2. appropriateness of care. 3. a term used in connection with review of care to indicate whether the measures taken and the delivery setting were proper under the circumstances, and whether it would have been proper to have taken other measures or have delivered the care in another setting under the same circumstances.

approved health care facility or program   a facility or program that is licensed, certified, or otherwise authorized pursuant to the laws of the state to provide health care and which is approved by a health plan to provide the care described in a contract.

assignee   the person to whom the rights to a health insurance policy are assigned, either in part or in whole, by the original policyholder.

assignment of benefits   a method under which a claimant requests that his/her benefits under a claim be paid to some designated person or institution, usually a physician or hospital.

Association of Managed Healthcare Organizations (AMHO)   national trade association for open model managed care organizations.

at-risk   accepting prepayment as full coverage for a predetermined health care benefit having to assume the financial liability for any loss which occurs when premiums paid are less than the cost of services provided.

average cost per claim   the average dollar amount of administrative and/or medical services rendered for the unit of measure within each expenditure category. The calculation is: $ amount/# of units.

average length of stay   the average number of days in a hospital for each admission

average manufacturer price (AMP)   the average price paid by wholesalers for products distributed to the retail class of trade.

average wholesale price (AWP)   the published suggested wholesale price of a drug. It is often used by pharmacies as a cost basis for pricing prescriptions. While a reliable pricing reference for brand-name drugs, it can be misleading in the case of generic drugs since each manufacturer establishes its own AWP for the same generic drug. This can result in a broad range of prices for the identical product.

authorization   as it applies to managed care, authorization is the approval of care, such as hospitalization.

balance billing   1. a provider's billing of a covered person for charges above the amount reimbursed by the health plan (i.e., the difference between billed charges and the amount paid). This may or may not be appropriate, depending upon the contractual arrangements between the parties. 2. the fee amount remaining after patient co-payments.

base capitation   a stipulated dollar amount to cover the cost of health care per covered person, less mental health/substance abuse services, pharmacy and administrative charges.

basic benefits package   a core set of health benefits that everyone in the country should have—either through their employer, a government program, or a risk pool.

bed days/1000   the number of inpatient days per 1000 health plan members. The formula is: (# of days/member months) × 1000 members × # of months.

behavior modification   attempts to change patients' habits which bear on health status, such as diet, exercise, smoking, etc., especially through organized health education programs. This is also called lifestyle change or health promotion.

behavioral health care   assessment and treatment of mental and/or psychoactive substance abuse disorders.

beneficiary   a person designated by an insuring organization as eligible to receive insurance benefits.

benefit   a service provided under an insurance policy or prepayment plan.

benefit bank   a flexible spending arrangement under which a reimbursement account is established, reimbursements are made from the account, and the employee is entitled to any remaining amounts at the end of the year.

benefit level   the limit or degree of services a person is entitled to receive based on his/her contract with a health plan or insurer.

benefit maximum   a clause in the certificate of coverage or pharmacy rider description which specifies a dollar limit for the total reimbursement of drug costs during a benefit period.

benefit package   services an insurer, government agency, or health plan offers to a group or individual under the terms of a contract.

benefit payment schedule   list of amounts an insurance plan will pay for covered health care services.

best price   lowest price paid by any purchased.

bill review   third party review of medical bills for excessive or inappropriate charges. Some workers compensation state statutes mandate payers to examine bills.

billed claims   the fees or costs for health care services provided to a covered person, submitted by a health care provider.

biological equivalents   those chemical equivalents which, when administered in the same amounts, will provide the same biological or physiological availability, as measured by blood levels, urine levels, etc.

blue book (MDBT)   the generic name for a widely used pricing guide, entitled the *American Druggist Databank Directory of Pharmaceuticals.* Brand name and generic drugs are listed by product, manufacturer, National Drug or Universal price Codes, direct price, and average wholesale price (AWP). Other pricing guides are the *Red Book* and *Medispan's Pricing Guide.*

board certified   a physician who has passed an examination given by a medical specialty board and who has been certified as a specialist in that medical area.

board eligible   a physician who is eligible to take the specialty board examination by virtue of having graduated from an approved medical school, completed a specific type and length of training, and practiced for a specified amount of time.

brand-brand interchange   the dispensing of one name brand prescription product in place of another on the basis of chemical equivalency. See also *chemical equivalents.*

brand name   name identifying a drug as the product of a specific pharmaceutical company. Also known as proprietary trademark name.

brand-name drug   a drug protected by a patent issued to the original innovator or marketer. The patent prohibits the manufacture of the drug by other companies without consent of the innovator, as long as the patient remains in effect.

broker   the go-between for individuals or companies and health insurers. A broker may help locate, negotiate and finalize health insurance contracts. A broker may also be an agent for a specific insurance company.

buying group an organization representing multiple independent buying sources. A buying group obtains price concessions from manufacturers and wholesalers through the combined purchasing power of its members, and in turn, redistributes that benefit to its members, such as HMOs, PPOs, hospitals, and/or employees.

cafeteria plan an employee benefit plan under which all participants are permitted to choose among two or more benefit options according to their needs and/or ability to pay. Also called a *flexible benefit plan* or *flex plan.*

calendar year the period of time from Jan. 1 of any year through Dec. 31 of the same year, inclusive. Most often used in connection with deductible amount provisions of major medical plans providing benefits for expense incurred within the calendar year. Also found in provisions outlining benefits in basic hospital, surgical, medical plans.

call schedule the schedule for physician availability for afterhours care. Physicians usually rotate on-call responsibilities in order to ensure 24 hour a day access to medical advice or care.

capacity an organized system's ability to meet the demands of both routine, scheduled care, and afterhours care.

capitation in the strictest sense, a stipulated dollar amount established to cover the cost of health care delivered for a person. The term usually refers to a negotiated per capita rate to be paid periodically, usually monthly, to a health care provider. The provider is responsible for delivering or arranging for the delivery of all health services required by the covered person under the conditions of the provider contract.

capitation fund a fund based on the number of members multiplied by the budgeted or capitated amount each member pays. Some HMOs, in lieu of reimbursing physicians on a direct capitation basis, may establish such a fund. Physicians are then reimbursed on a fee-for-service basis from the capitation fund. The HMO monitors patient visits for over-utilization; patients exceeding the norm are notified.

card programs the use of a drug benefit identification card which, when presented to a participating pharmacy by employees or their dependents, usually entitles them to receive the medication for a minimal copay.

care coordinator see *gatekeeper.*

carrier an entity which may underwrite or administer a range of health benefit programs. May refer to an insurer or a managed health plan.

carve out a decision to purchase separately a service which is typically a part of an indemnity or HMO plan. Example: an HMO may "carve out" the behavioral health benefit and select a specialized vendor to supply these services on a stand-alone basis.

case management 1. a process whereby covered persons with specific health care needs are identified and a plan designed to efficiently utilize health care resources is formulated and implemented to achieve the optimum patient outcome in the most cost-effective manner. 2. A utilization management program that assists the patient in determining the most appropriate and cost-effective treatment plan. It is used for patients who have prolonged, expensive or chronic conditions, helps determine the treatment location (hospital, or other institution or home), and authorizes payment for such care if it is not covered under the patient's benefit agreement.

case manager an experienced professional (e.g., nurse, doctor or social worker) who works with patients, providers and insurers to coordinate all services deemed necessary to provide the patient with a plan of medically necessary and appropriate health care.

case mix the relative frequency and intensity of hospital admissions or services reflecting different needs and uses of hospital resources. Case mix can be measured based on patients' diagnoses or the severity of their illnesses, the utilization of services, and the characteristics of a hospital.

catastrophic health insurance insurance beyond basics and major medical insurance for severe and prolonged illness which poses a severe financial threat.

categorically needy under Medicaid, categorically needy causes are aged, blind, or disabled individuals or families and children who meet financial eligibility requirements for Aid to Families with Dependent Children, Supplemental Security Income, or an optional state supplement.

ceiling the highest amount of money that an insurance company will pay to cover a patient's care. Many HMOs have no ceiling on their coverage.

center-based HMO same as a staff model HMO

centers of excellence a network of health care facilities selected for specific services based on criteria such as experience outcomes, efficiency and effectiveness. For example, an organ transplant managed care program wherein employees/dependents access selected types of benefits through a specific network of medical centers.

certificate of authority (COA) a certificate issued by state government, licensing the operation of a health maintenance organization.

certificate of coverage (COC) a description of the benefits included in a carrier's plan. The certificate of coverage is required by state laws and represents the coverage provided under the contract issued to the employer. The certificate is provided to the employee.

certificate of need (CON) a certificate issued by a government body, where required, to an individual or organization proposing to construct or modify a health facility, acquire major new medical equipment, or offer a new or different health service. Such issuance recognizes that a facility or service, when available, will meet the needs of those for whom it is intended.

chain pharmacy one of a group of pharmacies, usually three or more, under the same management or ownership.

channeling use of incentives and plan design to encourage members to use network providers.

charged based payment system a system of paying for a health care service (usually a hospital or other facility) on the basis of what the provider furnishing the service usually charges all patients.

chemical dependency see *substance abuse*.

chemical equivalents those multiple-source drug products containing essentially identical amounts of the same active ingredients, in equivalent dosage forms, and meeting existing physical/chemical standards.

chronic care care for an individual with a long-term illness.

claim information, submitted by a provider or a covered person to establish that medical services were provided to a covered person, from which processing for payment to the provider or covered person is made. The term generally refers to the liability for health care services received by covered persons.

claims administration a carrier function involving the review of health insurance claims submitted for payment, by individual claim or in the aggregate. Claims administration, as it relates to professional review programs is an identification procedure, screening treatment or charge pattern, for subsequent peer review and adjudication.

claims clearinghouse system system which allows electronic claims submission through a single source.

claims review the method by which an enrollee's health care service claims are reviewed before reimbursement is made. The purpose of this monitoring system is to validate the medical appropriateness of the provided services and to be sure the cost of the service is not excessive.

clearinghouse capability company capable of submitting electronic and/or paper claims to several third-party payers.

clinical indicator a tool or marker used to monitor and evaluate care to assure desirable outcomes and to explain or prevent undesirable outcomes.

clinical outcome the status of the patient's health, especially after receipt of medical care services. Assessment of outcomes may be dependent upon targeted goals, clinical markers, and the ability to provide objective measurements.

clinical privileging process of reviewing a practitioners' credentials for the purpose of granting and delineating the scope of clinical privileges.

clinician a staff member providing technical medical services, especially a physician. Physicians, nurses in patient care, etc., are clinicians. Managers, marketing and finance staff, etc., are not clinicians.

closed access   a type of health plan in which covered persons are required to select a primary care physician from the plan's participating providers. The patient is required to see the selected primary care physician for care and referrals to other health care providers within the plan. Typically found in a staff, group or network model HMO. Also called *closed panel* or *gatekeeper model.*

closed panel HMO   a closed panel HMO generally offers the service of a relatively limited number of health care providers, e.g., physicians employed by the HMO. Staff- and group-model HMOs are usually referred to as being in this category.

coding systems   *ICD-9 System*—a diagnoses and procedure coding system for hospital care; *CPT-4 System*—used to identify physician services like injections and surgeries; *NDC Coding System*—a system used by insurers to pay outpatient pharmaceutical claims; *HCPCS System*—a Medicare system for identifying a wide variety of services including injectable drugs used in physicians' offices.

cognitive impairment   impairment in memory, reasoning or orientation to person., place or time; or an impairment requiring a person to be supervised to protect him/herself or others from harm.

coinsurance   the portion of covered health care costs for which the covered person has a financial responsibility, usually according to a fixed percentage. Often coinsurance applies after first meeting a deductible requirement.

combined audit   patient/medical care evaluation studies in which physicians, nurses and/or other health care disciplines jointly choose and utilize the same topic and the same sample of records, and utilize the same data retrieval process. Criteria development and variation analysis may or may not be conducted separately for the respective care provided.

commission   the portion of premiums or equivalent premium for self-funded groups to an insurance agent, sales representative, or broker as compensation for services provided. Commission are considered part of the selling administrative expenses.

community rating   a method of determining a premium structure that is influenced not by the expected level of benefit utilization by specific groups, but by expected utilization by the population as a whole. Most often based on the entire population of a metropolitan statistical area (MSA).

community rating by class (CRC)   the practice of community rating impacted by the group's specific demographics. Also known as *factored rating.*

competitive medical plan (CMP)   a status granted by the federal government to an organization meeting specified criteria, enabling that organization to obtain a Medicare risk contract.

completed audit written display of patient/medical care evaluation study data for which variation records have been analyzed and corrective actions formulated for problems identified. The audit procedure is not considered complete until follow-up of the problem has been planned and final reports forwarded to pertinent medical and professional staff and to the hospital governing body.

compliance the degree to which patients follow treatment recommendations.

complication 1. an unanticipated change in the patient's clinical status for which special clinical management is required to achieve desired patient outcomes; 2. complication rate; 3. the percent of records in a patient/medical care evaluation study that indicate that a particular complication developed during treatment

composite rate a group billing rate which applied to all subscribers within a specified group, regardless of whether they are enrolled for single or family coverage.

comprehensive benefits plan a variation of the major medical plan which carries copayment requirements, usually 10–20 percent of all health expenses and deductibles ranging from $100 to $1000.

concurrent certification see *admission certification.*

concurrent drug evaluation an electronic assessment of claims at the point of service to detect potential problems that should be addressed prior to dispensing drugs to patients.

concurrent monitors procedures for regular surveillance of patient care conducted while the care is being provided.

concurrent review 1. an assessment which determines medical necessity or appropriateness of services as they are being rendered; 2. an assessment of hospital admissions, conducted by trained managed care staff via telephone or on-site visits during a covered person's hospital stay, to ensure appropriate care, treatment, length of stay, and discharge planning.

conditionally renewable policy a policy that can be renewed up to a certain age limit, such as 65.

confinement an uninterrupted stay for a defined period of time (as reflected in a benefit contract) in a hospital, skilled nursing facility or other approved health care facility or program, followed by discharge from that same facility or program.

Consolidated Omnibus Budget Reconciliation Act (COBRA) a federal law that, among other things, requires employers to offer continued health insurance coverage to certain employees and their beneficiaries whose group health insurance coverage has been terminated.

consultant   an outside specialist not on regular staff. E.g., an independent specialty medical provider such as a cardiologist, gastroenterologist, or endocrinologist, who is called upon by an HMO to render services on a fee-for-service basis.

consumer price index (CPI)   formerly Cost of Living Index. A price index constructed monthly from Bureau of Labor statistics of the retail prices of 400 goods and services sold in large cities across the country. Weighs products in terms of importance (in terms of total expenditures) and compares prices to those of a selected base year. Expresses current expenditures as a percentage of the base.

continuation   a situation whereby a covered person who would otherwise lose coverage under a health plan due to certain occurrences such as termination of employment or divorce is allowed to "continue" his/her coverage under specified conditions.

continuity of care   the coordination of diagnoses and treatment among practitioners and health care settings to maximize treatment benefits for the patient.

continuous quality improvement (CQI)   a formal process of constantly seeking better ways to achieve stated goals.

continuum of care   a range of clinical services provided to an individual or group, which may reflect treatment rendered during a single inpatient hospitalization, or care for multiple conditions over a lifetime. The continuum provides a basis for analyzing quality, cost and utilization over the long term.

contract pharmacy system   pharmaceutical benefit delivery arrangement in which an HMO contracts with community pharmacies (chain or selected independents) to provide medications to members. Reimbursement may be by fee-for-service, capitation, or some other arrangement.

contract year   the period of time from the effective date to the expiration date of the contract.

contributory program   a method of payment for group coverage in which part of the premium is paid by the employee and part is paid by the employer or union.

conversion   the privilege given to a covered person to change his/her group medical care coverage to a form of individual coverage without evidence of insurability. The conditions under which conversion can be made are defined in the master group contract. Conversion is usually made when a covered person leaves the group.

coordination of benefits (COB)   a provision in a contract that applies when a person is covered under more than one group medical program. It requires that payment of benefits will be coordinated by all programs to eliminate overinsurance or duplication of benefits.

copay/copayment   a cost-sharing arrangement in which a covered person pays a specified charge for a specified service, such as $10 for an office visit. The covered person is usually responsible for payment at the time the health care is rendered. Typical copayments are fixed or variable flat amounts for physician office visits, prescriptions or hospital services. Some copayments are referred to as coinsurance, with the distinguishing characteristics that copayments are flat or variable dollar amounts with coinsurance is a defined percentage of the charges for services rendered.

cosmetic procedures   those procedures which involve physical appearance, but which do not correct or materially improve a physiological function and are not deemed medically necessary.

cost-based reimbursement   payment by third party insurers in which the amount is based on the cost to the provider of delivering services.

cost containment   control or reduction of inefficiencies in the consumption, allocation or production of health care services in order to lower health care costs.

cost contract   a formal agreement with HCFA to arrange for the provision of health services to plan members based on reasonable cost or prudent buyer concepts. The plan receives an interim capitated amount, derived from an estimated annual budget, which may be periodically adjusted during the course of the contract to reflect actual cost experience. The plan's expenses are audited at the end of the contract to determine the final rate the plan should have been paid. The AAPCC may be a factor in establishing the final payment rate.

cost-effectiveness   the degree to which a service meets a specified goal at an acceptable cost.

cost-effectiveness analysis   a study to determine the overall ratio of cost to benefit. The underlying premise of cost-effectiveness analysis in health-related decisions is that, for any given level of resources available, the decision maker wishes to maximize the aggregate health benefits conferred to the population of concern. Alternatively, a given health benefit goal may be set, the objective being to minimize the cost of achieving it. The cost-effectiveness ratio is the ratio of costs to health benefits and is expressed, for example, as the cost per year per life saved or the cost per quality-adjusted year per life saved.

cost sharing   a general set of financing arrangements via deductibles, copays and/or coinsurance in which a person covered by the health plan must pay some of the costs to receive care. See also *copayment*, *coinsurance* and *deductible*.

cost shifting   the redistribution of payment sources. Typically, cost-shifting occurs when a discount on provider services is obtained by one payer, and the providers increase costs to another payer to make up the difference.

counter detailing   a process of re-educating or influencing prescribers in a closed or controlled HMO plan. Usually done in order to gain more compliance with a formulary. In a counter-detailing program, techniques used by pharmaceutical sales representatives are adapted to a "counter" objective, i.e., to provide doctors with basic pharmacological information designed to influence their prescribing habits.

coverage   entire range of protection provided under an insurance contract.

covered expenses   medical and related costs, experienced by those covered under the policy, that qualify for reimbursement under terms of the insurance contract.

covered person   an individual who meets eligibility requirements and for whom premium payments are paid for specified benefits of the contractual agreement.

covered services/expenses   the specific services and supplies for which Medicaid will provide reimbursement. Covered services under Medicaid consist of a combination of mandatory and optional services within each state.

CPT   see *Physician's Current Procedural Terminology*.

credentialing   a process of review to approve a provider who applies to participate in a health plan. Specific criteria and prerequisites are applied in determining initial and ongoing participation in the health plan.

criteria set   a group of similar or related indicators of quality health care, usually for a given study topic.

custodial care   medical or non-medical services which do not seek to cure, are provided during periods when the medical condition of the patients is not changing, or do not require continued administration by medical personnel. For example, assistance in the activities of daily living.

customary, prevailing, and reasonable charges   method of reimbursement used under Medicare, which limits payment to the lowest of the following: physician's actual charge, physician's median charge in a recent prior period (customary), or the 75th percentile of charges in the same time period (prevailing).

customary charge   the charge a physician or supplier usually bills his patients for furnishing a particular service or supply is called the customary charge.

data retrieval and analysis form   written display of the audit committee assistant's medical record review, showing the details of each record's compliance/noncompliance with criteria and a committee decision after review of record for instances of noncompliance with criteria.

date of service   the date on which health care services were provided to the covered person.

days   the unit of measure of the length of a hospital confinement.

days/1000   see *bed days/1000.*

day supply maximum   the maximum amount of medication an employee may receive at one time, usually the amount needed for 30 (acute) or 90 (maintenance) days of therapy, as defined by the drug benefit.

decision tree   the decision tree, the fundamental analytic tool for decision analysis, is a way of displaying the temporal and logical sequence of a clinical decision problem. Its form highlights three structural components: the alternative actions that are available to the decision maker, the probabilistic events that follow from and affect these actions, such as clinical information obtained or the clinical consequences revealed; and the outcomes for the patient that are associated with each possible scenario of actions and consequences.

deductible   the amount of eligible expense a covered person must pay each year from his/her own pocket before the plan will make payment for eligible benefits.

deductible carry over credit   charges applied to the deductible for services during the last 3 months of a calendar year which may be used to satisfy the following year's deductible under some insurance plans. The deductible for the prior calendar year may or may not have been met.

defensive medicine   the medical practice of performing laboratory tests or other procedures to protect against potential malpractice lawsuits, although such services may not be necessary to diagnose or treat an illness.

deferred compensation administrator (DCA)   a company that provides services through retirement planning administration, third-party administration, self-insured plans, compensation planning, salary survey administration and workers compensation claims administration.

demand   the amount of care a population seeks to obtain through the health delivery system.

dependent   an individual who relies on an employee for support or obtains health coverage through a spouse, parent, or grandparent who is the covered person. See also *eligible dependent* and *member.*

depot price   means the price(s) available to any depot of the federal government, for purchase of drugs from the manufacturer through the depot system of procurement.

designated mental health provider   the organization or entity with which the health plan contracts to evaluate, diagnose, refer and/or provide mental health and substance abuse services.

detoxification   medical management while an individual goes through withdrawal from alcohol or other addictive substances.

diagnosis   the identification of a disease or condition through analysis and examination.

diagnosis related groups (DRGs)   a system of classification for inpatient hospital services based on principal diagnosis, secondary diagnosis, surgical procedures, age, sex and presence of complications. This system of classification is used as a financing mechanism to reimburse hospital and selected other providers for services rendered.

diagnostic related group (DRG)   a program in which hospital procedures are rated in terms of cost and taking into account the intensity of services delivered. A standard flat rate per procedure is derived from this scale, which is paid by Medicare for their beneficiaries, regardless of the cost to the hospital to provide that service.

Diagnostic and Statistical Manual—3rd Edition, Revised (DSMIII-R)   American Psychiatric Association's manual of diagnostic criteria and terminology, widely accepted as the common language of mental health clinicians and researchers.

diagnostic center   free-standing or hospital-based facility that specializes in diagnosing illness and injuries.

direct costs   direct costs are those that are wholly attributable to the service in question, for example, the services of professional and paraprofessional personnel, equipment, and materials.

disability   1. any condition which results in functional limitations that interfere with an individual's ability to perform his/her customary work and which results in substantial limitation in one or more major life activities. 2. condition(s) that prevent or limit an individual's ability to engage in normal activities. These may be temporary.

disability income insurance   type of health insurance that periodically pays a disabled subscriber to replace income lost during the period of disability.

disability management   a prevention and remediation strategy that seeks to prevent disability from occurring, and to promote a safe and appropriate return to work and achievement of optimal functional capabilities following a disabling illness or injury.

disallowance   a denial by the payer for portions of the claimed amount. Examples of possible disallows include coordination of benefits, non-covered benefits, or amounts over the maximum fee.

discharges   the number of patients who leave an overnight health care facility per time period. Usually refers to hospitals.

discharge planning   the evaluation of patients' medical needs in order to arrange for appropriate care after discharge from an inpatient setting.

disclosure   information released by a managed care organization or health care insurer on 1. policies and practices affecting access to covered care, 2. the scientific and clinical basis for those policies, 3. any relevant criteria used in such decision-making and 4. the decision-making process itself, including how public input is solicited and considered and the timing of revisions, Proposals for disclosure typically apply to all entities with policies and practices impacting patient care (e.g., insurers, plans, networks, HMOs and government health boards).

discounted charges   usually used with respect to hospital charges. For an HMO buying significant and/or predictable amount of hospital care, a hospital may reduce billed charges by some percent.

disease   a disorder with specific cause and recognizable signs and symptoms; any bodily abnormality leading to interruption, cessation, or disorder of proper physical or mental functions, systems, or organs, except those resulting directly from physical injury.

disease classification   a systematic arrangement of related diagnoses into a limited number of clinically homogenous categories, usually to support the analysis of the quality, access, utilization and cost of health care services.

disease episode   the entire time period in which a person has a specific disease

disease management   see STIIPCH

disease specific insurance   insurance that provides benefits should the insuree develop a specific illness such as cancer or heart disease. Disease-specific insurance is usually purchased as a supplement to conventional insurance policies that may have ceilings or limitations for such care.

disenrollment   the process of terminating individuals or groups from their enrollment with a carrier. See *delete*.

dismemberment   loss of body parts usually stemming from accidental physical injury.

dispense as written (DAW)   a prescribing directive issued by physicians to indicate that the pharmacy should not in any way alter a prescription. Such alterations are usually done in order to substitute a generic drug for the brand-name drug ordered.

dispensing, fill or professional fee   the amount paid to a pharmacy for each prescription, in addition to the negotiated formula for reimbursing ingredient cost.

disproportionate share payment   an amount added to government payment rates for providers, usually hospitals, which treat large numbers of patients unable to pay their bills.

drug detailing presenting information about a brand-name drug product to prescribers to educate them about its activity, uses, side effects, proper dosage and administration, etc.

drug formulary a listing of prescription medications which are preferred for use by a health plan and which will be dispensed through participating pharmacies to covered persons. This list is subject to periodic review and modification by the health plan. A plan that has adopted an "open or voluntary" formulary allows coverage for both formulary and non-formulary medications. A plan that has adopted a "closed, select or mandatory" formulary limits coverage to those drugs in the formulary.

drug use evaluation (DUE) an evaluation of prescribing patterns of prescribers to specifically determine the appropriateness of drug therapy. There are three forms of DUE: prospective (before or at the time of prescription dispensing), concurrent (during the course of drug therapy), and retrospective (after the therapy has been completed). Same as *drug utilization review*.

drug selection when the pharmacist is legally authorized to decide whether to dispense brand name drugs or generic equivalent.

drug utilization the prescribing, dispensing, administering and ingestion or use of pharmaceutical products.

drug utilization review (DUR) a quantitative evaluation of prescription drug use, physician prescribing patterns or patient drug utilization to determine the appropriateness of drug therapy.

dual choice (DC) a term used to describe a situation in which only two carriers are contracted by a specific group. For example, an employer offers its employees one HMO and one indemnity plan, or two HMOs and no indemnity plan.

dual diagnosis co-existence of more than one disorder in an individual patient. Commonly refers to a patient who is diagnosed with mental illness in conjunction with substance abuse.

duplicate coverage inquiry (DCI) a request to an insurance company or group medical plan by another insurance company or medical plan to find out whether coverage exists for the purpose of coordination of benefits.

duplication of benefits overlapping or identical coverage of an insured person under two or more health plans, usually the result of contracts with different service organizations, insurance companies or prepayment plans.

durable medical equipment (DME) equipment which can stand repeated use, is primarily and customarily used to serve a medical purpose, generally is not useful to a person in the absence of illness or injury, and is appropriate for use at home. Examples of durable medical equipment include hospital beds, wheelchairs and oxygen equipment.

Early and Periodic Screening, Diagnosis, and Treatment (EPSDT) a program which covers screening and diagnostic services to determine physical or mental defects in recipients under age 21, as well as health care and other measures to correct or ameliorate any defects and chronic conditions discovered.

effective date the date a contract becomes in force.

electronic data interchange (EDI) the computer-to-computer exchange of business or other information. The data may be in either a standardized or priority format.

eligibility date the defined date a covered person becomes eligible for benefits under an existing contract.

eligible dependent a dependent of a covered employee who meets the requirements specified in the group contract to qualify for coverage and for whom premium payment is made. See also *family dependent*.

eligible employee/person one who meets the requirements specified in the contract to qualify for coverage. Qualifications might include permanent, full time, 35 or more hours per week employment, or permanent, part time, 40 hours or more per 2-week pay period employment.

eligible expenses reasonable and customary charges or the agreed upon health services fee for health services and supplies covered under a health plan

emergency a serious medical condition resulting from injury, sickness or mental illness which arises suddenly and requires immediate care and treatment, generally within 24 hours of onset, to avoid jeopardy to the life or health of a person.

emergi-care center see *free-standing emergency medical service center*.

employee assistance program (EAP) services designed to assist employees, their family members, and employers in finding solutions for workplace and personal problems. Services may include assistance for family/marital concerns, legal or financial problems, elder care, child care, substance abuse, emotional/stress issues, and daily living concerns. EAPs may address violence in the workplace, sexual harassment, dealing with troubled employees, transition in the workplace, and other events that increase the rate of absenteeism or employee turnover, lower, productivity and other issues that impact an employer's financial success or employee relations management. EAPs also can provide the voluntary or mandatory access to behavioral health benefits through an integrated behavioral health program.

employee benefits program   health insurance and other benefits, beyond salaries, offered to employees at their place of work. The employer typically picks up all or part of the cost of the benefits.

employee contribution   the amount an employee must contribute toward the premium costs of the contract.

Employee Retirement Income Security Act of 1974, Public Law 93-406 (ERISA)   this law mandates reporting and disclosure requirements for group life and health plans. It also exempts many self-insured employers from many state health insurance regulatory requirements.

employer contribution   the amount an employer contributes toward the premium costs of the contract. This amount carries widely among employers and is a critical variable in any risk analysis. Employer contributions can be based on dollar amounts, percentages, employment status, length of service, single or family status, or other variables or combinations of the above.

employer coverage mandate   a government requirement that employers provide health care benefits for employees. A mandate may address a single service or a range/package of services, e.g., preventative care coverage.

employer mandate   under the federal HMO act, federally qualified HMOs can mandate or require an employer to offer at least one federally qualified HMO plan of each type (IPA/network or group/staff). Some state laws have similar provisions.

encounter   a face-to-face meeting between a covered person and a health care provider where services are provided.

encounters per member per year   the number of encounters related to each member on a yearly basis. The measurement is calculated as follows: total # of encounters per year/total # of members per year.

enrollee   an individual who is enrolled for coverage under a health plan contract and who is eligible on his/her own behalf (not by virtue of being an eligible dependent) to receive the health services provided under the contract.

enrolling unit   an employer or other entity with which a contract for participation is made.

enrollment   the total number of covered persons in a health plan. Also refers to the process by which a health plan signs up groups and individuals for membership, or the number of enrollees who sign up in any one group.

episode of care   treatment rendered in a defined time frame for a specified disease. Episodes provide a useful basis for analyzing quality, cost and utilization patterns.

ERISA   see *Employee Retirement Income Security Act.*

Estimated Acquisition Cost (EAC) estimated acquisition cost based on price information supplied at regular intervals by the DHHS. This information will show estimated costs to groups of providers classified by dollar volume of drug sales.

evidence of coverage see *certificate of coverage.*

evidence of insurability (EOI) proof presented through written statements (e.g., an application form) and/or a medical examination that an individual is eligible for a certain type of insurance coverage. This form is required for eligibles who do not enroll during the open enrollment period (generally a 31-day period), or who apply for excess amounts of group life insurance. Also known as *evidence of good health.*

exclusions specific conditions or circumstances listed in the contract or employee benefit plan for which the policy or plan will not provide benefit payments.

exclusive provider organization (EPO) a term derived from the phrase preferred provider organization (PPO). However, where a PPO generally extends coverage for non-preferred provider services as well as preferred provider services, an EPO provides coverage only for contracted providers. Technically, many HMOs also can be described as EPOs.

expected claims the projected claim level of a covered person or group for a defined contract period. This level also becomes known as a desired loss ratio or break even point in relationship to projected premium. See also *experience rating.*

expenditure limits a limit set by a public body on the total amount to be spent on various health services. Used to help determine provider payment levels and utilization of services.

expenditures under Medicaid, "expenditures" refers to an amount paid out by a state agency for the covered medical expenses of eligible participants.

experience rating the process of setting rates based partially or in whole on previous claims experience and projected required revenues for a future policy year for a specific group or pool of groups. See also *expected claims.*

experimental, investigational or unproven procedures medical, surgical, psychiatric, substance abuse or other health care services, supplies, treatments, procedures, drug therapies or devices that are determined by the health plan (at the time it makes a determination regarding coverage in a particular case) to be either: not generally accepted by informed health care professionals in the U.S. as effective in treating the condition, illness or diagnosis for which their use is proposed; or not proven by scientific evidence to be effective in treating the condition, illness or diagnosis for which their use is proposed.

explanation of benefits (EOB) the statement sent to covered persons by their health plan listing services provided, amount billed, and payment made.

extended care facility   a nursing home or nursing center licensed to operate in accordance with all applicable state and local laws to provide 24-hour nursing care. Such a facility may offer skilled, intermediate or custodial care, or any combination of these levels of care.

extension of benefits   a provision of many insurers' policies which allows medical coverage to continue past the termination date of the policy for employees not actively at work and for dependents hospitalized on that date. Such extended coverage usually applies only to the specific medical condition which has caused the disability only until the employee returns to work or the dependent leaves the hospital. Not as common since the implementation of COBRA regulations.

factored rating   see *community rating by class*.

family dependent   a person enrolled for coverage under a health plan contract who is: the enrollee's spouse; or an unmarried dependent child (including stepchildren or legally adopted children) of either the enrollee or the enrollee's spouse, and whose principal place of residence is with the enrollee unless other arrangements have been made with the health plan. the definition also may be subject to certain conditions and limitations spelled out in the contract.

favored nations discount   see *most favored nations*.

family planning services   any medically approved means, including diagnosis, treatment, drugs, supplies and devices, and related counseling which are furnished or prescribed by or under the supervision of a physician for individuals of childbearing age for purposes of enabling such individuals freely to determine the number of spacing of their children.

federal qualification   a designation made by HCFA after conducting an extensive evaluation process of an HMO's entire method of doing business: documents, contracts, systems, facilities, etc. An organization must be federally qualified or a designated competitive medical plan to be eligible to participate in certain Medicare cost and risk contracts.

fee-for-service equivalency   a quantitative measure of the difference between the amount a physician and/or other provider receives from an alternative reimbursement system, e.g., capitation, compared to fee-for-service reimbursement.

fee-for-service reimbursement   the traditional health care payment system, under which physicians and other providers receive a payment that does not exceed their billed charge for each unit of service provided. Fees are paid as care is rendered.

fee maximum   the maximum amount a participating provider may be paid for a specific health care service provided to a covered person under a specific contract. Sometimes called *fee max.*

fee schedule a listing of codes and related services with pre-established payment amounts which could be percentages of billed charges, flat rates or maximum allowable amounts.

field underwriting the process whereby health plan sales personnel screen prospective buyers of the plan's products in order to ensure profitable contracting. Field underwriting also may include authority to quote premium rates of specific products for defined types and sizes of groups.

first-dollar coverage health policies that pay all medical expenses up to a predetermined limit, without a deductible charge.

fiscal agent a fiscal agent is a contractor that processes or pays vendor claims on behalf of the Medicaid agency.

fiscal intermediary the agent that has contracted with providers of service to process claims for reimbursement under health care coverage. In addition to handling financial matters, it may perform other functions such as providing consultative services or serving as a center for communication with providers and making audits of providers' records.

fixed fee an established "fee"schedule for pharmacy services allowed by certain government and private third-party programs in lieu of cost-of-doing business mark-ups.

flexible benefit plan a type of benefit program offered by some employers in which employees are presented annually with a number of benefit options, allowing employees to tailor benefits to their specific needs.

formulary see *drug formulary.*

free-standing emergency medical service center a health care facility that is physically, organizationally and financially separate from a hospital and whose primary purpose is the provision of immediate, short-term medical care for minor but urgent medical conditions. Also called *emergi-center* or *urgi-center.*

free-standing outpatient surgical center a health care facility, physically separate from a hospital, that provides pre-scheduled, outpatient surgical services. Also called *surgi-center.*

frequency the number of times a service was provided.

funding level the amount of revenue to finance a medical care program. Under an insured program, this is usually premium rate. Under a self-funded program, this amount is usually assessed per expected claim costs, plus stop loss premium, plus all related fees.

funding method the means by which an employer pays for the employee health benefit plan. Several funding methods shift risk from the employer to a carrier, or an employer may self-fund the employee health benefit plan. The most common methods are: prospective and/or retrospective premium payments, refunding products, self-funding, and shared risk arrangements.

gatekeeper   a primary health care practitioner, (1) who provides primary care services to an enrollee, (2) who is generally responsible for coordinating the enrollee's health care, and (3) with whom, other than in an emergency, a patient must consult to obtain a referral to a specialist provider in order to obtain the highest level of benefits under a health plan. Gatekeepers are sometimes called *care coordinators*.

gatekeeper model   a situation in which primary care physician, serves as the patient's "gatekeeper" or the initial contact for medical care and referrals. Also called *closed access*.

generic drug   a chemically equivalent copy designed from a brand-name drug whose patent has expired. A generic is typically less expensive and sold under a common or "generic" name for that drug. Also called *generic equivalent*.

generic equivalent   see *generic drug*.

generic substitution   dispensing a generic drug in place of a brand-name medication.

global budget   a budget that would determine the total amount of money that a geographic area could spend each year for health care. Under a global budget, providers and hospitals receive predetermined payments. As an enforcement mechanism for staying within budget, providers and hospitals would supposedly not receive additional funding if their costs exceeded their budgeted payments.

global target   a financing method identical to a global budget except that no strict enforcement mechanism is used to keep providers and hospitals within budget (i.e., providers and hospitals would receive additional funding if their costs exceeded their budgeted payments).

grace period   a set number of days past the due date of a premium payment during which medical coverage may not cancelled and the premium payment may be made. This period varies by health plan contract, generally 30, 60, 90 or 120 days.

group   a collection of individuals treated as a single entity; usually, an employer purchasing medical coverage on behalf of its full-time employees.

group contract   the application and addenda, signed by both the health plan and the enrolling unit, which constitutes the agreement regarding the benefits, exclusions and other conditions between the health plan and the enrolling unit. Also, the agreement with persons who obtain coverage for themselves and their children, whether under a group or individual program.

group model HMO a health care model involving contracts with physicians organized as a partnership, professional corporation, or other association. The health plan compensates the medical group for contracted services at a negotiated rate, and that group is responsible for compensating its physicians and contracting with hospitals for care of their patients.

Group Health Association of America (GHAA) merged with AMCRA to form the American Association of Health Plans (AAHP).

group insurance any insurance policy or health services contract by which groups of employees (and often their dependents) are covered under a single policy or contract, issued by their employer or other group entity.

group practice without walls typically a network of physicians who have formed a single entity but maintain their individual practices. The assets of individual practices may be acquired by the larger entity, but some autonomy is retained at each site. The central management provides administrative support. See *integrated delivery system.*

guaranteed renewability the assurance that an insurance company will continue to offer a policy to an individual or group that has made premium payments on a timely basis. An insurance company could not drop coverage due to specific circumstances, including high medical claims or illness.

HCFA 1500 a universal form, developed by the government agency known as Health Care Financing Administration (HCFA), for providers of services to bill professional fees to health carriers.

HCFA Common Procedural Coding System (HCPCS) a listing of services, procedures and supplies offered by physicians and other providers. HCPCS includes Current Procedural Terminology (CPT) codes, national alpha-numeric codes and local alpha-numeric codes. The national codes are developed by HCFA in order to supplement CPT codes. They include physician services not included in CPT as well as non-physician services such as ambulance, physical therapy and durable medical equipment. The local codes are developed by local Medicare carriers in order to supplement the national codes. HCPCS codes are 5-digit codes, the first digit a letter followed by four numbers. HCPCS codes beginning with A through V are national, those beginning with W through Z are local.

health alliances or regional alliances purchasing pools which would be responsible under some forms of proposed health care reform, for negotiating health insurance arrangements for employers and/or employees. Alliances would use their leverage to negotiate contracts that would ensure care is delivered in economic and equitable ways. (Also referred to as *health insurance purchasing cooperatives* or *health plan purchasing cooperatives.*)

health benefits package   the services and products (coverage) a health plan offers a group or individual.

Health Care Financing Administration (HCFA)   the federal agency responsible for administering Medicare and overseeing states' administration of Medicaid.

health care prepayment plan (HCPP)   a cost contract with the HCFA that prepays a health plan a flat amount per month to provide Medicare-eligible Part B medical services to enrolled members. Members pay premiums to cover the Medicare coinsurance, deductibles and copayments, plus any additional non-Medicare covered services that the plan provides. The HCPP does not arrange for Part A services.

health coverage   protection that provides payment of benefits for covered sickness or injury. This may include short and long term disability, dental, medical and vision care, and sometimes accidental death coverage as well as other benefits.

health history   a form used by underwriting personnel for evaluating the medical history of individuals to determine acceptable risk. See also *evidence of insurability*.

health insurance purchasing cooperatives (HIPC)   the purchasing entity under a managed competition health care reform proposal that would permit individuals and employer groups to band together to achieve greater purchasing power in negotiating insurance contracts than they otherwise would achieve alone. HIPCs would usually collect and distribute premiums, as well as distribute health plan information on prices, patient satisfaction and health outcomes to consumers. HIPCs might or might not compete with other HIPCs. See *health alliances*.

health IRAs   proposed tax-preferred plans to encourage saving for future medical expense. Funds in health IRAs could be later cashed out for medical expenses.

health maintenance organization (HMO)   1. an entity that provides, offers or arranges for coverage of designated health services needed by plan members for a fixed, prepaid premium. There are four basic models of HMOs: staff model, group model, network model and individual practice association; 2. Under the federal HMO Act, an entity must have three characteristics to call itself an HMO: a. an organization system for providing health care or otherwise assuring health care delivery in a geographic area. b. an agreed upon set of basic and supplemental health maintenance and treatment services, and c. a voluntary enrolled group of people.

health plan   health maintenance organization, preferred provider organization, insured plan, self-funded plan or other entity that covers health care services, may also refer to an employer's arrangements to cover health care needs of its employees which could include a combination of any of the above.

Health Plan Employer Data and Information Set (HEDIS) a core set of performance measures to assist employers and other health purchasers in understanding the value of health care purchases and evaluating health plan performance. HEDIS 2.0 is currently used and distributed by NCQA (National Committee for Quality Assurance). HEDIS 3.0 is under development.

health service agreement (HSA) the detailed procedure and benefit description given to each enrolled employer. This agreement is the basis for discussion and/or explanation between the employer and the health plan on enrollment, eligibility limitations, benefit descriptions, etc.

home health agency (HHA) a facility or program licensed, certified or otherwise authorized pursuant to state and federal laws to provide health care services in the home.

hospice a facility or program engaged in providing palliative and supportive care of the terminally ill, and licensed, certified or otherwise pursuant to the law of jurisdiction in which services are received.

hospital affiliation a contractual relationship between a health plan and one or more hospitals whereby the hospital provides the inpatient benefits offered by the health plan.

hospital alliance a group of voluntary hospitals that have joined together to reduce costs by sharing common services and developing group purchasing programs. Hospital alliances are formed to improve competitive positions over other voluntary institutions and chains.

human risk management a service designed to reduce the demand for treatment by identifying, assessing, and managing individuals' medical or behavioral health risks before treatment becomes imperative. Human risk management is designed to respond proactively to employee risk areas and to address problem/issues before they become psychological, medical, or financial crises.

hybrid model HMO an HMO that combines attributes of more than one of the four principal HMO models and hence is not classifiable in any one of the four categories.

impairment any loss or abnormality of psychological, physiological or anatomical structure of function (e.g., hearing loss).

in-area services health care received within the authorized service area from a participating provider of the health plan.

incurred but not reported (IBNR) costs associated with a medical service that has been provided, but for which a claim has not yet been received by the carrier. IBNR reserves are recorded by the carrier to account for estimated liability based on studies of prior lags in claim submissions.

incurred claims   the actual carrier liability for a specified period, including all claims with dates of service within a specified period (usually called the experience period). Due to the time lag between dates of service and the dates of claims payments are actually processed, adjustments must be made to any paid claims data to determine incurred claims.

incurred claims loss ratio   the result of incurred claims divided by premiums. A defined time period is usually specified.

indemnity   an insurance program in which the insured person is reimbursed or the provider is paid for covered expenses after services are rendered.

independent medical evaluation (IME)   an examination carried out by an impartial health care provider, generally board certified, for the purpose of resolving a dispute related to the nature and extent of an illness or injury.

independent practice association   see *individual practice assoc.*

independent practice organization (IPO)/independent practice network (IPN)   a group of medical providers which contract services to managed care plans. Currently, some IPOs/IPNs seek to contract directly with employers.

individual practice association (IPA) model HMO   a health care model which contracts with physicians and other community health care providers, to provide services in return for a negotiated fee. Physicians continue in their existing individual or group practices and are compensated on a per capita, fee schedule, or fee-for-service basis.

initial eligibility period   the period of time specified in the contract during which eligible persons may enroll themselves and dependents under the health plan, usually without providing evidence of good health.

injury   physiological damage other than sickness, including all related conditions and recurrent symptoms.

inpatient   an individual who has been admitted to a hospital as a registered bed patient and is receiving services under the direction of a physician (customarily for at least 24 hours).

integrated behavioral health   a carve-out benefit plan that combines independent managed care services into what is designed as a seamless delivery system for behavioral health concerns. Components could include employee assistance services, a telephone counseling triage, utilization management, behavioral health treatment networks, claims payment, and data management.

integrated delivery system   a generic term referring to a joint effort of physician/hospital integration for a variety of purposes. Some models of integration include physician-hospital organization, group practice without walls, integrated provider organization and medical foundation.

integrated provider organization a corporate umbrella for the management of a diversified health care delivery system. The system may include one or more of the following: hospitals, physician group practices, and other health care operations. Physicians practice as employees of the organization or in closely affiliated physician group. See *integrated delivery system*.

integrated service network (ISN) see *organized delivery systems*.

intensive care skilled nursing services, usually in a hospital, prescribed by a physician for individuals with serious medical conditions and delivered with the guidance of a registered nurse.

intermediate care facility (ICF) a facility providing a level of care that is less than the degree of care and treatment that a hospital or skilled nursing facility (SNF) is designed to provide, but greater than the level of room and board.

International Classification of Diseases, 9th Edition (Clinical Modification)(ICD-9-CM) a listing of diagnoses and identifying codes used by physicians for reporting diagnoses of health plan enrollees. The coding and terminology provide a uniform language that can accurately designate primary and secondary diagnoses and provide for reliable, consistent communications on claim forms.

investigational treatments medical treatments, including drugs waiting for FDA approval, that are considered experimental and, therefore, may not be covered by insurance plans. The definition of experimental currently varies from plan to plan.

Jackson Hole Group an ad hoc group of health executives, business leaders and policy experts that authored the health reform initiative known as "managed competition." The group is named after its meeting place in Jackson Hole, Wyoming. See *managed competition*.

job-lock the inability of an individual to change employers for fear of losing health coverage, particularly if the employee or a dependent has a pre-existing condition which might not be covered, at least for an initial period of new employment.

Joint Commission on Accreditation of health care Organizations (JCAHO) a private, not-for-profit organization that evaluated and accredits hospitals and other health care organizations providing home care, mental health care, ambulatory care, and long term care services.

large claim pooling a practice in experience rating which isolates claim amounts per individuals over a defined level (e.g., $30,000). These isolated amounts are charged to a pool funded by a contribution charged to all groups who share this same pooling level. (Handling large claim amounts in this manner helps stabilize significant premium fluctuations more prominent with smaller group sizes. Smaller groups generally will have lower pooling points and larger groups will have larger ones.)

legend drug   a drug that, by law, can be obtained only by prescription and bears the label, "Caution: federal law prohibits dispensing without a prescription." See *prescription drug.*

length of stay (LOS)   the number of days that a covered person stays in an inpatient facility.

lifetime maximum benefit   a limitation on financial coverage for health care for an individual stated by an insurer. This amount serves as a cap on contractual liability and can be exceeded only in rare and unusual circumstances.

long term care   assistance and care for persons with chronic disabilities who require help with the activities of daily living or who suffer from cognitive impairment. Long term care's goal is to help people with disabilities be as independent as possible; thus it is focused more on caring than on curing.

long term care insurance   insurance coverage designed to help pay some or all of any necessary long term care costs.

loss ratio   the result of paid claims and incurred claims plus expenses divided by the paid premiums. See also *incurred claims loss ratio, net loss ratio, paid claims loss ratio* and *medical loss ratio.*

maintenance list   see *additional drug benefit list.*

major diagnostic category (MDC)   a clinically coherent grouping of ICD-9-CM diagnoses by major organ system or etiology that is used as the first step in assignment of most diagnosis related groups (DRGs). MDCs are commonly used for aggregated DRG reporting.

malpractice reform   changing the laws that apply to lawsuits against physicians and other health care providers alleging improper care.

managed care   1. a system of health care delivery that influences utilization and cost of services and measures performance. The goal is a system that delivers value by giving people access to high quality, cost-effective health care; 2. a systemized approach which seeks to ensure the provision of the right health care at the right time, place and cost.

managed competition   a proposed policy approach whereby health plans would compete on the basis of cost and other factors. Purchasers would join cooperatives and be given the ability to compare plans across several dimensions of performance. The principle behind this approach is improvement of the health economy through increased health plan competition.

managed health care plan   a health care organization that provides managed care (see definition). Such organizations generally share the following hallmarks: integration of financing and management with the delivery of health care services to an enrolled population; employment or contracting with an organized provider network which delivers services and which (as a network or individual provider) either shares financial risk or has some incentive to deliver quality, cost-effective services; use of an information system capable of monitoring and evaluating patterns of covered persons' use of medical services and the cost of those services.

management service organization (MSO)   a legal entity that provides practice management, administrative and support services to individual physicians or group practices. An MSO may be a direct subsidiary of a hospital or may be owned by investors. See *integrated delivery system.*

managing general underwriter   a firm that specializes in guaranteeing risks on behalf of an insurance company. Usually a formal management agreement delineates duties, allowable risk type and limits of authority (e.g., $1 million per person). Its services usually are used for a specific niche market, such as HMO reinsurers.

mandated benefits   those benefits that health plans are required by state or federal law to provide to policy holders and eligible dependents.

mandated providers   providers of medical care, such as psychologists, optometrists, podiatrists and chiropractors, whose licensed services must, under state or federal law, be included in coverage offered by a health plan.

manual rates   rates developed based upon the health plan's average claims data and adjusted for group specific demographic, industry factor or benefit variations.

master group contract   a legal document between the enrolling unit and the carrier, setting forth in detail the rights and obligations of the enrolling unit, covered person and carrier, and terms and conditions of the coverage provided by the contract.

maximum allowable cost (MAC) list   specified multi-source prescription medications that will be covered at a generic product cost level established by the plan. This list, distributed to participating pharmacies, is subject to periodic review and modification by the plan. The MAC list may require covered persons to pay a cost differential for a brand name product.

maximum allowable fee schedule   a health care payment system which reimburses up to a specified dollar amount for services rendered.

maximum out-of-pocket costs   the limit on total member copayments, deductibles and coinsurance under a benefit contract.

Medicaid   a federal program administered and operated individually by participating state and territorial governments which provides medical benefits to eligible low income persons needing health care. The program's costs are shared by the federal and state governments. (Established under Title XIX of the Social Security Act).

Medicaid buy-in   a provision in certain health reform proposals whereby the uninsured would be allowed to purchase Medicaid coverage by paying premiums on a sliding scale based on income.

medical expense trend   the rate at which medical costs are increasing or decreasing, influenced by, for example, utilization, new technology and billed charges.

medical foundation   a not-for-profit entity associated with a physician group that provides medical services under a professional services contract. The foundation acquires the business and clinical assets of the group practice, holds the provider number, and manages the business for both parties. See *integrated delivery system*.

medical loss ratio   the cost ratio of health benefits used, compared to revenue received. Calculated as follows: total medical expenses/premium revenue.

medical necessity   the evaluation of health care services to determine if they are: medically appropriate and required to meet basic health needs; consistent with the diagnosis or condition and rendered in a cost-effective manner; and consistent with national medical guidelines regarding type, frequency and duration of treatment.

medical savings account (MSAs)   a non-taxable savings account used to cover medical expenses. Based loosely on the idea of individual retirement accounts.

Medicare   a nationwide, federally-administered health insurance program which covers the costs of hospitalization, medical care, and some related services for eligible persons. Medicare has two parts: Part A covers inpatient costs. Medicare pays for pharmaceuticals provided in hospitals, but not for those provided in outpatient settings. Also called *Supplementary Medical Insurance Program*. Part B covers outpatient costs for Medicare patients.

Medicare beneficiary   a person designated by the Social Security Administration as entitled to receive Medicare benefits.

Medicare supplement policy   a policy guaranteeing that a health plan will pay a policyholder's coinsurance, deductible and copayments and will provide additional health plan or non-Medicare coverage for services up to a predefined benefit limit. In essence, the product pays for the portion of the cost of services not covered by Medicare. Also called *Medigap* or *Medicare wrap*.

medigap   see *Medicare supplement policy.*

member assistance program (MAP)   a human risk management program that focuses on lowering behavioral and medical health costs by proactively reducing demand on the treatment system. This employee assistance type program is targeted to covered persons of health plans and insurers.

members   participants in a health plan (subscribers/enrollees and eligible dependents), who make up the plan's enrollment. "Member" also is used to describe an individual specified within a subscriber contract who may or may not receive health care services according to the terms of the subscriber policy.

members per year   the number of members effective in the health plan on a yearly basis. Calculation is: member months/12.

mental health provider   a psychiatrist, licensed consulting psychologist, social worker, or hospital or other facility duly licensed and qualified to provide mental health services under the law or jurisdiction in which treatment is received.

minimum premium   medical benefit financing mechanism in which an employer remits only a portion of the conventional premium to an insurer to cover the cost of administering the benefits program and of providing specific and aggregate stop-loss insurance. The employer, usually referred to in this case as self-insured, funds a "bank account" which the insurance company draws upon for the payment of claims.

modified community rating (MCR)   a separate rating of medical service usage in a given geographic area (community) using age-sex data, etc.

modified fee-for-service   a system in which providers are paid on a fee-for-service basis, with certain fee maximums for each procedure.

morbidity (morbidity rate)   1. an actuarial determination of the incidence and severity of sicknesses and accidents in a well-defined class or classes of people; 2. the actual state of being diseased.

mortality (mortality rate)   an actuarial determination of the death rate in a given population in a given period.

most favored nations discount or clause   a contractual agreement that stipulates that a vendor must provide to a particular payor the lowest prices that would be available to any purchaser. The federal government often invokes most favored nations clauses for health care contracts.

multidisciplinary   determination of treatment plans and delivery of care through professionals with a wide range of specialties.

multiple option plan   a health care plan design which offers employees the option of electing to enroll under one of several types of coverages and usually from among an HMO, a PPO and a major indemnity plan.

national drug code (NDC)   a national classification system for identification of drugs. Similar to the Universal Product Code (UPC).

national health board   a federally established entity that, under various managed competition health care proposals, would have been charged with overall implementation and oversight of the reforms to the health care system. Duties would have likely included designing a standard benefit plan, specifying cost-sharing requirements, developing a formula for premium risk-adjustments and constructing and overseeing a national cost-containment strategy.

net loss ratio   the result of total claims liability and all expenses divided by premiums. This is the carrier's loss ratio after accounting for all expenses.

network model HMO   an HMO type in which the HMO contracts with more than one physician group, and may contract with single- and multi-specialty groups. The physician works out of his/her own office. The physician may share in utilization savings, but does not necessarily provide care exclusively for HMO members.

non-contributory   a term describing a situation in which the plan sponsor pays the entire cost of premium for coverage. Employees do not contribute towards the cost of the coverage.

non-participating provider (non-par)   a term used to describe a provider that has not contracted with the carrier or health plan to be a participating provider of health care.

non-participating provider indemnity benefits   a type of health care coverage for services rendered by providers who are not under contract with the health plan. The benefits are covered on an indemnity basis, typically carrying high copayment requirements and deductibles. See *Point of Service*.

office visit   provision of health care services in an office setting, usually that of a physician.

open access (OA)   a self-referral arrangement allowing members to see participating providers for specialty care without a referral from another doctor. Typically found in an IPA HMO. Also called *open panel*.

open enrollment period   a time which subscribers in a health benefit program have an opportunity to re-enroll or select an alternate health plan being offered to them, usually without evidence of insurability or waiting periods.

open panel HMO   open panel HMOs contract with private office physicians and other health care providers to assure care of their members. This usually allows enrollees a wider choice of health care providers and freer movement among participating providers than is seen in closed panel models. The IPA model HMOs fall into this category.

organized delivery systems proposed networks of providers and payers which would provide care and compete with other systems for enrollees in their region. Systems could include hospitals, primary care physicians, specialty care physicians, and other providers and sites that could offer a full range of preventative and treatment services. Also referred to as accountable health plans (AHP), coordinated care networks (CCN), community care networks (CCN), integrated health systems (IHS), and integrated service networks (ISN).

outcome measures assessments which gauge the effect or results of treatment for a particular disease or condition. Outcome measures include such parameters as: the patient's perception of restoration of function, quality of life and functional status, as well as objective measures of mortality, morbidity and health status.

outcomes results achieved through a given health care service, prescription drug use or medical procedure.

outcomes management systematically improving health care results, typically by modifying practices in response to data gleaned through outcomes measurement, then remeasuring and remodifying—often in a formal program of continuous quality improvement.

outcomes research studies aimed at measuring the effect of a given product, procedure, or medical technology on health or costs.

outlier an observation in a distribution that is outside a certain range, often defined as two or three standard deviations from the mean or exceeding a specific percentile. Frequently refers to a case or hospital stay that is unusually long or expensive for its type, or to a physician practice that uses an abnormally high or low volume of resources.

out-of area (OOA) coverage for treatment obtained by a covered person outside the network service area.

out-of-pocket costs/expenses (OOPs) the portion of payments for health services required to be paid by the enrollee, including copayments, coinsurance and deductibles.

out-of-pocket limit the total payments toward eligible expenses that a covered person funds for him/herself and/or dependents: i.e., deductibles, copays and coinsurance–as defined per the contract. Once this limit is reached, benefits will increase to 100% for health services received during the rest of that calendar year. Some out-of-pocket costs (e.g., mental health, penalties for non-precertification, etc.) are not eligible for out-of-pocket limits.

outpatient a person who receives health care services without being admitted into a hospital.

over-the-counter (OTC) a drug product that does not require a prescription under federal or state law.

paid claims   the amounts paid to providers to satisfy the contractual liability of the carrier or plan sponsor. These amounts do not include any covered person liability for ineligible charges or for deductibles or copayments. If the carrier has preferred payment contracts with providers (e.g., fee schedules or capitation arrangements), lower paid claims liability will usually result.

paid claims loss ratio   the result of paid claims divided by premiums.

partial hospitalization services   a mental health or substance abuse program operated by a hospital that provides clinical services as an alternative or follow-up to inpatient hospital care.

participating provider   a provider who has contracted with the health plan to deliver medical services to covered persons. The provider may be a hospital, pharmacy or other facility or a physician who has contractually accepted the terms and conditions as set forth by the health plan.

participation   the number of employees enrolled for medical coverage, usually identified as a percentage relative to the total eligible population. A 75% participation requirement means that at least 75% of eligible employees must enroll for coverage. Participation requirements also apply to eligible dependent units.

payer   a public or private organization that pays for or underwrites coverage for health care expenses.

peer review   the evaluation of quality of total health care provided, by medical staff with equivalent training.

peer review organization (PRO)   an entity established by the Tax Equity and Fiscal Responsibility Act of 1982 (TERFA) to review quality of care and appropriateness of admissions, readmissions and discharges for Medicare and Medicaid. These organizations are held responsible for maintaining and lowering admissions rates, and reducing lengths of stay while insuring against inadequate treatment. Also known as *professional standards review organization*.

per contract per month (PC/PM)   the dollar amount related to each effective contract holder, subscriber or member for each month (PS/PM–per subscriber per month and PM/PM–per member per month).

per member per month (PM/PM)   the unit of measure related to each effective member for each month the member was effective. The calculation is: # of units/member months (MM).

pharmacy and therapeutics (P & T) committee   an organized panel of physicians from varying practice specialties, who function as an advisory panel to the plan regarding the safe and effective use of prescription medications. Often compromises the official organizational line of communication between the medical and pharmacy components of the health plan. A major function of such a committee is to develop, manage and administer a drug formulary.

physician   any doctor of medicine (M.D.) or doctor of osteopathy (D.O.) who is duly licensed and qualified under the law of jurisdiction in which treatment is received.

physician contingency reserve (PCR)   "at-risk" portion of a claim deducted and withheld by the health plan before payment is made to a participating physician as an incentive for appropriate utilization and quality of care. This amount—for example, 20% of the claim—remains within the plan and is credited to the doctor's account. Can be used where the plan needs additional funds to pay for claims. The withhold may be returned to the physician in varying levels which are determined based on analysis of his/her performance or productivity compared against his/her peers. Also called *withhold*.

physician-hospital organization (PHO)   a legal entity formed and owned by one or more hospitals and physician groups in order to obtain payer contracts and to further mutual interests. Physicians usually maintain ownership of their practices while agreeing to accept managed care patients under the terms of the PHO agreement. The PHO serves as a negotiating, contracting and marketing unit. See *integrated delivery system*.

Physician Payment Review Commission (PPRC)   a bipartisan congressional advisory group established in 1986 to advise Congress on setting Medicare and Medicaid reimbursement. In 1990, PPRC's responsibilities were expanded to include other payment policy issues.

Physician's Current Procedural Terminology (CPT)   list of medical services and procedures performed by physicians and other providers. Each service and/or procedure is identified by its own unique 5-digit code. CPT has become the health care industry's standard for reporting of physician procedures and services, thereby providing an effective method of nationwide communication.

place of service   the location where health services are rendered (e.g., office, home, hospital, etc.).

play-or-pay   in any health care reform scheme, a system that would require employers to provide health insurance benefits or pay a tax that government would use to provide coverage.

point-of-service (POS) plan   a health plan allowing the covered person to choose to receive a service from a participating or non-participating provider, with different benefit levels associated with the use of participating providers. POS can be provided in several ways: an HMO may allow members to obtain limited services from non-participating providers; an HMO may provide non-participating benefits through a supplemental major medical policy; a PPO may be used to provide both participating and non-participating levels of coverage and access; or various combinations of the above may be used.

pool (risk pool)   a defined account (e.g., defined by size, geographic location, age health states, etc.) to which revenue and expenses are posted. A risk pool attempts to define expected claim liabilities of a given defined account as well as required funding to support the claim liability.

pooling   the process of combining risk for all groups or a number of groups.

portability   an individual changing jobs would be guaranteed coverage with the new employer without a waiting period or having to meet additional deductible requirements.

practice guidelines   systematically developed statements on medical practice that assist a practitioner and a patient in making decisions about appropriate health care for specific medical conditions. Managed care organizations frequently use these guidelines to evaluate appropriateness and medical necessity of care. Terms used synonymously include practice parameters, standard treatment protocols and clinical practice guidelines.

pre-admission certification (PAC)   a review of the need for inpatient hospital care, done prior to the actual admission. Established review criteria are used to determine the appropriateness of inpatient care.

pre-certification review   see *utilization review*.

pre-existing condition (PEC)   any medical condition that has been diagnosed or treated within a specified period immediately preceding the covered person's effective date of coverage under the master group contract.

preferred provider organization (PPO)   a program in which contracts are established with providers of medical care. Providers under such contracts are referred to as preferred providers. Usually, the benefit contract provides significantly better benefits (fewer copayments) for services received from preferred providers, thus encouraging covered persons to use these providers. Covered persons are generally allowed benefits for non-participating providers' services, usually on an indemnity basis with significantly higher copayments. A PPO arrangement can be insured or self-funded. Providers may be, but are not necessarily, paid on a discounted fee-for-service basis.

preferred providers   physicians, hospitals, and other health care providers who contract to provide health services to persons covered by a particular health plan. See also *preferred provider organization*.

premium   the amount paid to a carrier for providing coverage under a contract. Premiums are typically set in coverage classifications such as: individual, two-party and family; employee and dependent unit; employee only, employee and spouse, employee and child, and employee, spouse and child.

prepaid group practice plans   organized medical groups of essentially full-time physicians in appropriate specialties, as well as other professional and subprofessional personnel, who, for regular compensation, undertake to provide comprehensive care to an enrolled population for premium payments that are made in advance by the consumer and/or their employers.

prescription medication   a drug which has been approved by the Food and Drug Administration and which can, under federal and state law, be dispensed only pursuant to a prescription order from a duly licensed prescriber, usually a physician.

preventive care   comprehensive care emphasizing priorities for prevention, early detection and early treatment of conditions, generally including routine physical examinations, immunization and well person care.

primary care   basic or general health care, traditionally provided by family practice, pediatrics and internal medicine. See also *secondary care* and *tertiary care*.

primary care network (PCN)   a group of primary care physicians who have joined together to share the risk of providing care to their patients who are covered by a given health plan.

primary care physician (PCP)   a physician the majority of whose practice is devoted to internal medicine, family/general practice and pediatrics. An obstetrician/gynecologist may be considered a primary care physician.

primary coverage   under coordination of benefit rules, the coverage plan which considers and pays its eligible expenses without consideration of any other coverage.

principal diagnosis   the condition established after study to be mainly responsible for the patient's seeking health care services from a provider. Commonly refers to the condition most responsible for a patient's admission to the hospital.

prior authorization   the process of obtaining prior approval as to the appropriateness of a service or medication. Prior authorization does not guarantee coverage.

professional review organization (PRO)   a physician-sponsored organization charged with reviewing the services provided patients. The purpose of the review is to determine if the services rendered are medically necessary; provided in accordance with professional criteria, norms and standards; and provided in the appropriate setting.

Prospective Payment Assessment Commission (ProPAC)   a federal commission established under the Social Security Act amendments of 1983 to advise and assist Congress and the Department of Health and Human Services in maintaining and updating the Medicare prospective payment system.

prospective rating   see *adjusted community rating.*

prospective reimbursement   any method of paying health care providers for a defined period (usually one year) according to amounts of rates of payment established in advance.

provider   a physician, hospital, group practice, nurse, nursing home, pharmacy or any individual or group of individuals that provides a health care service.

qualified Medicare beneficiary (QMB)   a person whose income falls below a set percentage of federal poverty guidelines, often 100% but sometimes higher, for whom the state must pay the Medicare Part B premiums, deductibles and copayments.

quality reassurance   a formal set of activities to review and affect the quality of services provided. Quality assurance includes quality assessment and corrective actions to remedy any deficiencies identified in the quality of direct patient, administrative and support services.

quality improvement   a continuous process that identifies problems in health care delivery, tests solutions to those problems and constantly monitors the solutions for improvement.

rate   the amount of money per enrollment classification paid to a carrier for medical coverage. Rates are usually charged on a monthly basis.

rating process   the process of evaluating a group or individual to determine a premium rate in regard to the type of risk it presents. Key components of the rating formula are the age/sex factor, location, type of industry, base capitation factor, plan design, average family size and the administration allowance.

rational drug therapy   prescribing the right drug for the right patient, at the right time, in the right amounts, and with due consideration of relative costs.

RBRVS   see *Resource Based Relative Value Scale.*

reasonable and customary (R&C)   a term used to refer to the commonly charged or prevailing fees for health services within a geographic area. A fee is considered to be reasonable if it falls within the parameters of the average or commonly charged fee for the particular service within that specific community.

rebate   a monetary amount that is returned to a payer from a prescription drug manufacturer based upon utilization by a covered person or purchases by a provider.

recidivism   the frequency of the same patient returning to the hospital for the same presenting problems. Refers to the inpatient hospitalization.

referral   the recommendation by a physician and/or health plan for a covered person to receive care from a different physician or facility.

referral provider   a provider that renders a service to a patient who has been sent to him/her by a participating provider in the health plan.

reinsurance   insurance purchased by an HMO, insurance company, or self-funded employer from another insurance company to protect itself against all or part of the losses that may be incurred in the process of honoring the claims of its participating providers, policy holders, or employees and covered dependents. Also called *risk control insurance* or *stop-loss insurance*.

renewal   continuance of coverage under a policy beyond its original term by the acceptance of a premium for a new policy term.

report card on health care   an emerging tool that can be used by policy makers and health care purchasers, such as employers, government bodies, employer coalitions and consumers, to compare and understand the actual performance of health plans. The tool provides health plan performance data in major areas of accountability, such as health care quality and utilization; consumer satisfaction, administrative efficiencies and financial stability; and cost control.

reserve   see *physician contingency reserve*.

reserves   funds for incurred but not reported health services or other financial liabilities. Also refers to deposits and/or other financial requirements that must be met by an entity as defined by various state or federal regulatory authorities.

Resource Based Relative Value Scale (RBRVS)   a fee schedule introduced by HCFA to reimburse physicians' Medicare fees based on the amount of time and resources expended in treating patients, with adjustments for overhead costs and geographical differences.

retention   that portion of the cost of a medical benefit program which is kept by the insurance company or health plans to cover internal costs or to return a profit. Can also be referred to as *administrative costs*.

retrospective rate derivation (retro)   an addendum to insurance coverage that provides for risk sharing, with the employer being responsible for all or part of that risk. The employer can be at risk for a pre-negotiated percentage of the group's health care cost in excess of total premium dollars paid by the employer during the contract year. The carrier may also be required to refund to the employer a pre-negotiated percentage of premium dollars paid if actual health care costs of the group are less than the premium dollars paid during the contract year.

retrospective review   determination of medical necessity and/or appropriate billing practice for services already rendered.

risk analysis   the process of evaluating expected medical care costs for a prospective group and determining what product, benefit level and price to offer in order to best meet the needs of the group and the carrier.

risk contract 1. an agreement between HCFA and an HMO or competitive medical plan requiring the HMO to furnish at a minimum all Medicare covered services to Medicare eligible enrollees for an annually determined, fixed monthly payment rate from the government and a monthly premium paid by the enrollee. The HMO is then liable for services regardless of their extent, expense or degree; 2. an agreement between a provider and payer, or intermediary, on behalf of a payer, that requires the provider to furnish all specified services for specified enrollee for a set fee, usually prepaid, and for a set period of time (usually one year). The provider is then liable for services regardless of their extent, expense or degree. Such stated limitations for such liability are stated in advance and may be subject to reinsurance.

risk control insurance see *reinsurance*.

risk pool see *pool*.

sanction a reprimand, for any number of reasons, of a participating provider.

second opinion an opinion obtained from an additional health care professional prior to the performance of a medical service or a surgical procedure. May relate to a formalized process, either voluntary or mandatory, which is used to help educate a patient regarding treatment alternatives and/or to determine medical necessity.

secondary care services provided by medical specialists, such as cardiologists, urologists and dermatologists, who generally do not have first contact with patients. See also *primary care* and *tertiary care*.

secondary coverage the plan that has the responsibility for payment of any eligible charges not covered by the primary coverage. See also *coordination of benefits*.

Section 125 plan a term used to refer to flexible benefit plans. The reference derives from the section of the IRS code which defines such plans and stipulates that employee contributions to such plans may be made with pre-tax dollars.

self-funding, self-insurance a health care program in which employers fund benefit plans from their own resources without purchasing insurance. Self-funded plans may be self-administered, or the employer may contract with an outside administrator for an administrative services only (ASO) arrangement. Employers who self-fund can limit their liability via stop-loss insurance on an aggregate and/or individual basis.

service area the geographic area serviced by the health plan as approved by state regulatory agencies and/or as detailed in the certification of authority.

single carrier replacement   the process by which a purchaser of group health care coverage covers all eligibles through one carrier and drops all other carriers.

single-payer system   a health care financing arrangement in which money, usually from a variety of taxes, is funneled to a single entity (usually the government) which then is responsible for the financing and administration of the health system. Single payer systems can be regional, statewide or nationwide.

skilled nursing facility (SNF)   a facility either freestanding or part of a hospital, that accepts patients in need of rehabilitation and medical care that is of a lesser intensity than that received in a hospital.

small group pooling   combining all or segments of small group businesses into a pool or pools. Expected claims, and therefore premium rates, are determined by pool and not on a group-specific basis. See also *pool* and *pooling*.

staff model HMO   a health care model that employs physicians to provide health care to its members. All premium and other revenues accrue to the HMO, which compensates physicians by salary and incentive programs.

standard benefit package   a set of specific health care benefits that would be offered by delivery systems. Benefit packages could include all or some of the following: preventive care; hospital and physician services; prescription drugs; limited mental health and chemical dependency services; and long-term care.

standard class rate (SCR)   a base revenue requirement on a per member or per employee basis, multiplied by group demographic information to calculate monthly premium rates.

standard prescriber identification number (SPIN)   under development by the National Council of Prescription Drug Programs in conjunction with other professional organizations, this standard number could be used to identify prescribers.

stop-loss insurance   insurance coverage taken out by a health plan or self-funded employer to provide protection from losses resulting from claims greater than a specific dollar amount per covered person per year (calendar year or illness-to-illness). Types of stop-loss insurance: 1. Specific or individual—reimbursement is given for claims on any covered individual which exceeded a predetermined deductible, such as $25,000 or $50,000; 2. Aggregate—reimbursement is given for claims which in total exceed a predetermined level, such as 125% of the amount expected in an average year. See also *reinsurance*.

subrogation   a procedure under which an insurance company can recover from third parties all or some proportionate part of benefits paid to an insured.

subscriber   the person responsible for payment of premiums or whose employment is the basis for eligibility for membership in an HMO or other health plan.

subscriber contract   a written agreement, which also may be called a subscriber certificate or member certificate, describing the individual's health care policy.

substance abuse   the taking of alcohol or other drugs at dosages that place a person's social, economic, psychological and physical welfare in potential hazard, or endanger public health, morals, safety or welfare, or a combination thereof. Also called *chemical dependency*.

summary plan description   a description of the entire benefits package available to an employee as required to be given to persons covered by self-funded plans.

superbill   a modified claim form that lists specific and/or specialty medical services provided by a physician. A superbill is not acceptable in place of the standard AMA form. See also *claim*.

supplemental services   optional services that a health plan may cover to provide in addition to its basis health services.

surgi-center   see *free-standing outpatient surgical center*.

systems management of medicine   synonym for STIIPCH.

systematic, totally integrated, individualized, patient-centered health care (STIIPCH)   a term referring to medical care provided based on needs of individual patients. Under STIIPCH, all care would be coordinated with each provider having access to integrated health data management records.

systematic, totally integrated, individualized, *person*-centered health care (STIIPCH 2.0)   a term referring to total health care provided based on needs of individual consumers. Under STIIPCH 2.0, all health care (including preventative care) would be coordinated with every provider having access to complete electronic records that would list not only medical data, but sociologic information.

table rates   see *age/sex rates*.

Tax Equity and Fiscal Responsibility Act of 1982 (TEFRA)   the federal law which created the current risk and cost contract provisions under which health plans contract with HCFA and which defined the primary and secondary coverage responsibilities of the Medicare program.

termination date   the date that a group contract expires; or, the date that a subscriber and/or covered person ceases to be eligible.

tertiary care   those health care services provided by highly specialized providers such as neurosurgeons, thoracic surgeons and intensive care units. These services often require highly sophisticated technologies and facilities.

therapeutic alternatives drug products containing different chemical entities but which should provide similar treatment effects, the same pharmacological action or chemical effect when administered to patients in therapeutically equivalent doses.

therapeutic substitution the practice of dispensing one therapeutic alternative for another. Requires the physician's authorization before the substitution may occur.

third party administrator (TPA) an independent person or corporate entity (third party) that administers group benefits, claims and administration for a self-insured company/group. A TPA does not underwrite the risk.

third party payer a public or private organization that pays for or underwrites coverage for health care expenses or another entity, usually an employer (examples: Blue Cross, Blue Shield; Medicare; Medicaid; commercial insurers).

tort reform an umbrella term used to encompass proposed changes in malpractice liability laws.

treatment facility a residential or non-residential facility or program licensed, certified or otherwise authorized to provide treatment of substance abuse or mental illness pursuant to the law or jurisdiction in which treatment is received.

trending a calculation used to predict future utilization of a group based upon past utilization.

triage the classification of sick or injured persons according to severity in order to direct care and ensure the efficient use of medical and nursing staff facilities.

triple option a type of health plan in which employees may choose from an HMO, PPO, or indemnity plan, depending on how much they are willing to contribute to cost. See also *multiple option plan.*

trust fund an organization established to control, invest and otherwise administer moneys, securities or other property for the benefit of others. The fund is operated under the guidance of a trust agreement by trustees whose fiduciary responsibility requires a prudent, successful administration of the fund's purpose. Most common to the group health field are those created by unions for the benefit of their members and by trade associations for the benefit of the employees of association members.

turnaround time (TAT) the measure of a process cycle from the date a transaction is received to the date completed. (For claims processing, the number of calendar days from the date a claim is received to the date paid.)

unbundling   separately packaging units that might otherwise be packaged together. For claims processing, this includes providers billing separately for health care services that should be combined according to industry standards or commonly accepted coding practices. Also refers to the practice of providing separate prices and administrative support for services such as prescription drug benefit management, mental health/substance abuse services and utilization review.

Uniform Billing Code of 1992 (UB-92)   a revised version of the UB-82, a federal directive requiring a hospital to follow specific billing procedures, itemizing all services included and billed for on each invoice, which was implemented October 1, 1993.

upcoding   in claims submission, using a higher level procedure code than the level of service actually provided.

URAC accreditation   verification that a utilization review organization meets national utilization review standards for prospective and concurrent review services.

URAC Standards   national utilization review guidelines developed by URAC's member organizations and used to evaluate utilization review organizations for accreditation. See *URAC Accreditation*.

urgi-center   see *free-standing emergency medical service center*.

usual, customary and reasonable (UCR)   see *reasonable and customary*.

utilization   the extent to which the members of a covered group use a program or obtain a particular service, or category of procedures, over a given period of time. Usually expressed as the number of services used per year or per 100 or 1,000 persons eligible for the service.

utilization management (UM)   a process of integrating review and case management of services in a cooperative effort with other parties, including patients, employers, providers, and payers.

utilization review (UR)   a formal assessment of the medical necessity, efficiency, and/or appropriateness of health care services and treatment plans on a prospective, concurrent or retrospective basis.

Utilization Review Accreditation Commission (URAC)   a Washington-based, not-for-profit corporation formed in 1990 and dedicated to improving the quality of utilization review in the health care industry by providing a method of evaluation and accreditation of utilization review programs.

vendor   a medical vendor is an institution, agency, organization, or individual practitioner that provides health or medical products and/or services either to a medical provider, who in turn interfaces with patients, or directly to the public.

voluntary formulary   see *drug formulary*.

waiver   a rider or clause in a health insurance contract excluding an insurer's liability for some sort of pre-existing illness or injury. Also refers to a plan amendment, such as a HCFA waiver or plan modification.

withhold   see *physician contingency reserve*.

workers compensation   a state-governed system designed to address work-related injuries. Under the system, employers assume the cost of medical treatment and wage losses arising from a worker's job-related injury or disease, regardless of who is at fault.

Workgroup for Electronic Data Interchange (WEDI)   a task force formed in 1991 by the Secretary of Health and Human Services to develop recommendations for government and industry relating to the advancement of electronic data in health care. WEDI's steering committee consists of senior executives from more than 25 insurance and health care organizations.

wrap-around coverage or plan   insurance to cover copays or deductible not covered by a basic insurance plan.

Procter & Gamble: The Health Care Company

Many do not realize the breadth and depth of Procter & Gamble's heritage and commitment to health care—to the patients who benefit from our products and technologies, the professionals who recommend them, and to the retail and wholesale partners who distribute them.

BUSINESS OPERATIONS

P&G brings to the Health Care sector the same capacity for technical innovation, understanding of consumers and marketing expertise that has made possible the success of the Company's consumer products, such as Oil of Olay®, Tide®, Pampers®, and Bounty®. Health Care brands include nonprescription medicines such as Vicks®, Metamucil®, and ThermaCare®; prescription products such as Actonel® (risedronate) and Asacol® (mesalamine); and oral care products such as Crest® and Fixodent®.

CUSTOMER AND CONSUMER UNDERSTANDING

One of Procter & Gamble's hallmarks is the depth of understanding of customers and consumers. Through market research and consumer relations operations, P&G talks to over one million consumers about health care every year. Hundreds of quantitative and qualitative studies are done with thousands of pharmacists, physicians and other health professionals annually. Insights from these efforts lead to new and improved products and packaging.

INNOVATION

Innovation is another hallmark of Procter & Gamble. Advanced science and technology are focused to discover, develop and deliver products to improve the lives of consumers. That is P&G's corporate mission, and nowhere is this more evident than in the Health Care business. Procter & Gamble has deep roots in health care research beginning with the first dentifrice clinically proven effective in the prevention of tooth decay, Crest®, through the discovery of entirely new classes of medicines such as the bisphosphonates (Didronel® and Actonel®). Discovery—seeing and understanding things in new ways—is at the heart of our work in health care.

FUTURE FOR HEALTH CARE

In 1995, Procter & Gamble opened a new research campus that is dedicated to the discovery and development of prescription and nonprescription medicines and health care products. Sited on 253 acres, the complex covers 1.3 million square feet of laboratory and office space and houses nearly 2,500 personnel. This center serves as the hub linking facilities in North America, Europe, Asia and Latin America.

Research and development focus areas in prescription medicines include anti-infective, bone, cardiac, gastrointestinal and hormone replacement. In the nonprescription medicines areas the focus is on respiratory, gastrointestinal and oral care.

PROCTER & GAMBLE'S STRENGTHS IN HEALTH CARE

Procter & Gamble's health care business has grown tenfold in the last 12 years. It will continue to grow because we're using our proven strengths in this business.

Employees   We understand consumers the world over, in part because we operate from multiple facilities with a highly diverse, expertly skilled and multi-cultural group of professionals. Our people are our greatest asset.

Discovery and Innovation   A commitment to always be an innovative company, with strong links to the scientific community and leading-edge technologies in the company's other product sectors, helps us make breakthrough discoveries and develop products faster.

Consumer Understanding   We lead the industry in consumer loyalty because we understand consumers thoroughly and anticipate and satisfy their needs with better products.

Company Culture   Cross-functional teams manage projects, with emphasis on the total needs of the business, as opposed to single function considerations.

Customer Satisfaction   We build on strong relationships with our customers, pharmacists and other health care professionals, managed care organizations, regulatory agencies, scientists and retailers.

Global Growth   We maximize Procter & Gamble's worldwide resources to create a truly integrated global health care company, in both prescription and nonprescription medicines.

Licensing and Acquisition   We pursue acquisitions and alliances with the right partners, then add value with product development, clinical, sales and marketing capabilities.

THE PROCTER & GAMBLE STATEMENT OF PURPOSE

We will provide products of superior quality and value that improve the lives of the world's consumers. As a result, consumers will reward us with leadership sales and profit growth, allowing our people, our shareholders and the communities in which we live and work to prosper.

PRINCIPLES

We show respect for all individuals.
The interests of the Company and the individual are inseparable.
We are strategically focused in our work.
Innovation is the cornerstone of our success.
We are externally focused.
We value personal mastery.
We seek to be the best.
Mutual interdependency is a way of life.

Notes

Notes

Notes

Notes